I0054650

Sport Injury Psychology

Written by a team of international experts and emerging talents from around the world, *Sport Injury Psychology: Cultural, Relational, Methodological, and Applied Considerations* challenges the status quo of the field of sport injury psychology and opens new and exciting future research trajectories by critically considering:

- How to evolve from an individual-focused and single, scientific discipline into a cultural and relational-focused and interdisciplinary discourse.
- How to shift from the dominant positivist foundation toward a more inclusive scholarship with divergent epistemologies, theories, and methodologies.
- How to replace the attempt to establish "best practice" and desire for "clean" findings with the need for continuous innovation and multifaceted applied experiences.

Each chapter stimulates debate and encourages theoretical, methodological, and/or applied diversification, and closes with future research directions that provide novel and rigorous programs of research that have the potential to advance the field of sport injury psychology into an interdisciplinary discourse that strives for and embraces collaboration between academic disciplines and with practitioners working in the field. Cutting edge, timely, and comprehensive, *Sport Injury Psychology: Cultural, Relational, Methodological, and Applied Considerations* is essential reading for undergraduate students, postgraduate students, and more established scholars in the fields of sport communication, sports medicine, sport psychology, sports sociology, and other related sport science disciplines.

Ross Wadey, PhD, is an Associate Professor at St Mary's University, UK.

Routledge Psychology of Sport, Exercise and Physical Activity

This series offers a forum for original and cutting edge research exploring the latest ideas and issues in the psychology of sport, exercise and physical activity. Books within the series showcase the work of well-established and emerging scholars from around the world, offering an international perspective on topical and emerging areas of interest in the field. This series aims to drive forward academic debate and bridge the gap between theory and practice, encouraging critical thinking and reflection among students, academics and practitioners. The series is aimed at upper-level undergraduates, research students and academics, and contains both authored and edited collections.

Series Editor: Andrew M. Lane, University of Wolverhampton, UK

Available in this series:

For more information about this series, please visit: www.routledge.com/sport/series/RRSP

Sport Injury Psychology

Cultural, Relational, Methodological, and Applied Considerations

Edited by Ross Wadey

Routledge
Taylor & Francis Group

NEW YORK AND LONDON

First published 2020
by Routledge
605 Third Avenue, New York, NY 10017

and by Routledge
2 Park Square, Milton Park, Abingdon, Oxon, OX14 4RN

Routledge is an imprint of the Taylor & Francis Group, an informa business

© 2020 Taylor & Francis

The right of Ross Wadey to be identified as the author of the editorial
material, and of the authors for their individual chapters, has been asserted
in accordance with sections 77 and 78 of the Copyright, Designs and
Patents Act 1988.

All rights reserved. No part of this book may be reprinted or reproduced
or utilised in any form or by any electronic, mechanical, or other means,
now known or hereafter invented, including photocopying and recording,
or in any information storage or retrieval system, without permission in
writing from the publishers.

Trademark notice: Product or corporate names may be trademarks or
registered trademarks, and are used only for identification and explanation
without intent to infringe.

Library of Congress Cataloging-in-Publication Data
A catalog record for this title has been requested

ISBN: 978-0-367-22382-3 (hbk)
ISBN: 978-0-367-56914-3 (pbk)
ISBN: 978-0-367-85499-7 (ebk)

Typeset in Baskerville
by Deanta Global Publishing Services, Chennai, India

To Becky, Phoebe, and George, for everything and forever

Contents

Figures

Tables

Contributors

Renee Newcomer Appaneal
Australian Institute of Sport, Canberra, Australia

Monna Arvinen-Barrow
University of Wisconsin-Milwaukee, USA

Michael Atkinson
University of Toronto, Canada

Britton W. Brewer
Springfield College, USA

Tanya Bunsell
University of Bath, UK

Francesca Cavallerio
Anglia Ruskin University, UK

Sarah Cecil
English Institute of Sport

Damien Clement
West Virginia University, USA

Melissa Day
University of Chichester, UK

Nikolaus A. Dean
The University of British Columbia, Canada

Mark Doidge
University of Brighton, UK

Rachel Dunn
University of Toronto, Canada

Lynne Evans
Cardiff Metropolitan University, UK

Ciara Everard
St Mary's University, UK

Sarah Gairdner
University of Toronto, Canada

Brian Hemmings
Private Practice, UK

Karen Howells
Cardiff Metropolitan University, UK

Kimberley Humphrey
University of Chichester, UK

Sunita Kerai
St Mary's University, UK

Nicole Kimpton
Swansea University, UK

Camilla J. Knight
Swansea University, UK

Kirsty Ledingham
Cardiff Metropolitan University, UK

Fiona J. Leggat
St Mary's University, UK

Laura Martinelli
Peter Symonds College, UK

Kerry R. McGannon
Laurentian University, Canada

Jenny McMahon
University of Tasmania, Australia

Robert Morris
University of Stirling, UK

Katherine A. Tamminen
University of Toronto, Canada

Ross Wadey
St Mary's University, UK

Tom Williams
University of South Wales, UK

Toni L. Williams
Leeds Beckett University, UK

Foreword

I never really thought about getting injured when I was an athlete. In fact, from an early age I thrived across most sports, excelling into elite teams whereby I found things relatively easy, and as far back as I can remember, I don't think I had to cope with much adversity along the way. At a young age, my sporting success inflated my popularity both in and outside of school and I found myself embedded in numerous social networks developing strong relationships with others of varying ages and levels of sporting ability. I played professional football, captained my country, and also represented Great Britain at the World Student Games. I was fortunate in that I grew up in an extremely supportive environment, both from an educational and a sporting point of view. Both of my parents were teachers and valued highly the development of knowledge and academic career pathways.

Experiencing a major injury is not something that I would wish on any athlete as it can have a significant impact not just on the individual but on others around you. I ruptured my anterior cruciate ligament (ACL), tore my medial collateral ligament and meniscus, together with a Tibial plateau fracture. Throughout my rehabilitation I was reflective, particularly around my emotional and behavioral responses; driven by the normal challenging goals that I was used to, I stayed connected to my teammates, which resulted in feeling a sense of belonging with others, and, importantly, I kept perspective on everything. I tapped into every coping resource that I had and that others could offer me to manage the ever-increasing demand that I was experiencing; I was most definitely displaying resilience behaviors. I fully recovered from my injury and although advised not to continue for much longer by specialists, played for a number of years after, constantly looking back on my injury experience. It was during that period of time that I recognized the need for a more in-depth understanding of my own injury experience and perhaps how that may help me support others as a sport psychologist. Under the supervision of Professor Lynne Evans, it was during this period of time that I signed up to pursue a PhD.

There is a 400-year-old Japanese technique known as the "golden repair" or Kintsugi which is the art of putting broken pottery pieces back together through the combination of lacquer and gold; the piece through its flaws and imperfections is more beautiful (and stronger) than the original. Indeed, this is a befitting metaphor for the injured athlete journey. The pain and fears that athletes feel and the struggles that they experience have the ability to change them. My own injury experience was just that. The adversity afforded opportunities for me to grow, to further develop my skillset as a practitioner, and to develop as a person; my character matured through a deeper understanding of both humility and wisdom.

It's been 20 years since my injury experience, and I have been very fortunate to work at the highest level of sport where I have supported athletes in performance and injury-related areas. Athletes who I spend time with after becoming injured sometimes struggle with understanding how they are thinking and feeling, and with the respective responses. As a practitioner, my support has been influenced by my own journey but also through an understanding of the sport injury research. My early work was largely directed by Kübler-Ross' (1969) grief response model, Brewer's (1994) cognitive appraisal model, and Wiese-Bjornstal, Smith, Shaffer, and Morrey's (1998) integrated model of response to injury. All of these initially helped me to understand psychological responses to a sport injury and how they can shape behavioral responses and recovery outcomes. Additionally, I was introduced to the fascinating area of social support by Professor Tim Rees. I started to understand the importance of the interconnectedness of people and how that may have a protective influence and aid in the regulation of behavior and the functions that are provided by social relationships, particularly their ability to influence outcomes in times of stress but also their beneficial effect upon outcomes irrespective of stress. There is no doubt that research plays a key role in the development of evidence-based practice and must be able to affect the performance and preparation of the athletes that we work with. I have been fortunate to collaborate with key stakeholders when athletes get injured and through relevant research knowledge I have been able to develop intervention strategies to implement the best available evidence into applied practice.

There is a real opportunity to create competitive advantage through our culture. We must strive to create a sense of belonging and identity that is aligned to the athlete and performance context; a rehabilitation culture (both pre- and post-injury) is demonstrated by the behaviors that we display, role model, and tolerate. We can display a sense of identity through an enabling culture that outlines the higher purpose of the work – work that is over and above self-interest, work that encourages highly collaborative behaviors, and work that demands a high-learning and high-accountability rehabilitation environment. Relational aspects afford the opportunity to reflect on the identity of the athlete and what it represents. The rehabilitation context will be much stronger if it reflects the athlete's own story and journey; valued aspects such as resilience, character, and humility will emerge that authentically underpin what is expected of someone as they progress through the process. Creating opportunities for injured athletes to develop deep levels of trust through sharing personal journeys will provide further athlete insights and the use of consistent language with an honest and compassionate narrative will encourage and develop a curious and healthy feedback culture. As practitioners, we can reinforce that culture through our own leadership: shared leadership that observes and listens carefully to the athlete and respective social context, that is seen to represent the values of the athlete and the context and provides opportunities to realize goals and athlete potential. A strong and healthy culture will undoubtedly maintain belief and focus on the athlete's North Star throughout rehabilitation – the vision beyond recovery.

This text, *Sport Injury Psychology: Cultural, Relational, Methodological, and Applied Considerations*, offers a fresh perspective on an ever-growing area of Sport Psychology. The selection of content could not be more relevant to strengthen the need for current and critical thinking around applied practice. The content has been presented by a diverse group of exciting authors that will challenge the more conventional understanding of sport injury psychology and enable discussion and action around supportive cultures and facilitative rehabilitation teams. I am sure that you will enjoy the book and confident that it will be a resource that is used both in and out of academic environments. Challenging the way that we look at familiar aspects in unfamiliar ways is certainly something that will enable shifts in culture and this book will most certainly do that in a number of ways.

Dr Ian Mitchell C. Psychol. HCPC

Head of Performance Psychology, The Football Association (The FA)

References

Brewer, B. (1994). Review and critique of models of psychological adjustment to athletic injury. *Journal of Applied Sport Psychology*, *6*, 87–100. doi: 10.1080/10413209408406467

Kübler-Ross, E. (1969). *On death and dying*. London: Tavistock.

Wiese-Bjornstal, D. M., Smith, A. M., Shaffer, S. M., & Morrey, M. A. (1998). An integrated model of response to sport injury: Psychological and sociological dynamics. *Journal of Applied Sport Psychology*, *10*, 46–69. doi:10.1080/10413209808406377

Preface

Welcome to *Sport Injury Psychology: Cultural, Relational, Methodological, and Applied Considerations*, a book that challenges the status quo and opens new and exciting trajectories for this field of research. From the outset, the book sets out to evolve sport injury psychology from an individual-focused and single, scientific discipline into a cultural and relational-focused and interdisciplinary discourse. Up until now, research interest in cultural and relational thought and practice has been marginal, if not completely eschewed, in sport injury psychology. Therefore, the opening chapters in this text consider how future researchers in this field can connect their work with the larger social-cultural environment in and outside of sport, and forge links and reciprocity with related disciplines (e.g., sport communication, sport sociology, social psychology, organizational psychology, cultural psychology). A barrier to this interdisciplinary scholarship, however, is the positivist foundation of the field of sport injury psychology, which inhibits inclusive scholarship and practice with divergent epistemologies, theories, and methodologies. While some authors in this book provide several helpful recommendations on how to improve the methodological rigor of studies informed by positivism, it is anticipated by others that future researchers might consider embracing alternative research paradigms guided by other philosophical assumptions that incorporate diverse qualitative methodologies and methods, which might involve working "with" rather than "on" our participants to increase the uptake of research in practice.

Congruent with this more collaborative agenda, the final consideration discussed in this book is the tension that exists between academic researchers and applied practitioners. In an effort to bridge the research-to-practice "gap" and encourage greater diversification in applied practice rather than relying on the same old "usual suspects" (i.e., psychological skills), the authors in the closing chapters draw upon their craft knowledge to "lift the veil" on applied practice, which challenges the dominant positivistic discourse and desire for "clean" findings and provides more multifaceted and nuanced illustrations of the challenges of working with injured athletes in the field. It is also recommended that future researchers replace the attempt to establish "best practice" or *the* "single best practice" with the need for continuous innovation and diversification of applied practices at micro (i.e., intrapersonal), meso (i.e., interpersonal), and macro levels (e.g., institutional, cultural) that ultimately seek to prevent injury occurrence or nurture recovery.

Written by a team of international experts and emerging talents from around the world, this book is cutting-edge, timely, and comprehensive. The narrative in each chapter encourages theoretical, methodological, and/or applied diversification, and closes with future research directions that provide exciting, novel, and rigorous programs of research that have the potential to advance the field of sport injury psychology into an interdisciplinary discourse that strives for and embraces collaboration between academic disciplines and with practitioners working in the field. This book is essential reading for undergraduate students, postgraduate students, and more established scholars in the fields of sport psychology, sport communication, sports sociology, sports medicine, and other related sport science disciplines.

Ross Wadey is an Associate Professor in the Faculty of Sport, Health, and Applied Sciences at St Mary's University, Programme Director of the MSc Applied Sport Psychology course, Chair of Injury and Rehabilitation Research Group, and a Chartered Psychologist with the British Psychological Society. His current research projects involve working with external stakeholders to co-construct tailored programs of research to inform practice and policy. His own research interests integrate psychological and sociological approaches to advancing knowledge in the prevention of and rehabilitation from sport injury. Ross has published widely in sport and health psychology journals and has won national and international awards for the rigor and scope of his research. Ross sits on the editorial board for *The Sport Psychologist* and *Journal of Applied Sport Psychology*. In addition to his research activities, Ross is a trustee to the charity LimbPower that aims to engage amputees and individuals with limb impairments in physical activity to improve quality of life and aid lifelong rehabilitation. Ross is married to Becky and has two children, Phoebe and George.

Introduction

Challenging the Status Quo of Sport Injury Psychology

Ross Wadey

Introduction

I've never experienced a meaningful sport injury. Yet, I find myself sat at my desk at home writing this introduction, for a book on "sport injury" psychology. As I sit here trying to make sense of how I came to edit this book, I recall various key turning points during my academic career that led me to this field of research and ultimately the aim and scope of this book. At the start of my academic career (2001–2005), my research interests were on the acritical notion of helping athletes to improve their sporting performance via examining concepts such as mental toughness. Unbeknown to me at the time, I was naively seduced by the sport ethic (Hughes & Coakley, 1991) and culture of risk (Nixon, 1992) that continues to permeate high-performance sport. Falling into an individualistic and neoliberal trap, the purpose of my early research was to understand how to help athletes become more "mentally tough" by identifying self-help strategies to enable them to become more dedicated and committed to sport and to push through pain and injury in their ultimate pursuit of athletic success; all "personal" qualities I didn't possess myself (and still don't) in my amateur athletic career!

At this time in academia, mental toughness was a "hot topic"; the workshops and presentations at academic conferences were well attended and at prime times-lots, and my early research in this area was well received by the academic community. I received praise from scholars I admired, which validated to me that I was focusing on the "right" research topic and "doing good". However, as my postgraduate studies in applied sport psychology were ending and I looked for funded PhD opportunities, none on mental toughness became available. It was at this time in my career that I experienced my first turning point; I was approached by Professor Lynne Evans and Professor Sheldon Hanton about doing a funded PhD in sport injury psychology. Given my limited experience of injury, I wasn't overly keen, but I was drawn in by Lynne's enthusiasm for this field of research. I applied, went for the interview, got offered the PhD, and my career as a sport injury researcher had begun.

As my PhD and other offshoot programs of research unfolded, the seductive charms of the dominant sport ethic and culture of risk remained with me and led me to identify, and subsequently explore, the concepts of personal resilience and post-traumatic growth in injury and rehabilitation contexts to identify how injured athletes can return to sport quicker and stronger (two concepts I am now far more critical of due to their individualistic and neoliberal underpinning; Wadey, Day, & Howells, 2020). Yet, Despite researching these topics and finishing the first study of my PhD, I remained disinterested in sport injury psychology and kept my eye on the emerging field of research of mental toughness in sport. For my second research study, however, I shifted from a quantitative (nomothetic) to qualitative (ideographic) methodological design; a shift that would represent the second turning point in my academic career.

Having the opportunity and privilege to hear injured athletes' stories, my interest and curiosity grew. I heard stories of loss, suffering, despair, and woe. I can remember one injured athlete I was interviewing who was completely distraught; tears were streaming down her face as she described to me in vivid detail how her injury had had a devastating impact on her and her life as she'd known it. She told me how she didn't know who she was anymore, how her coach and teammates didn't care, and how she didn't know where to turn for help; this was a story that lingered with me for several weeks and months afterward (it still does) and went on to impact my research interests. Over time, I became less interested in sporting performance and related concepts such as mental toughness, and far more concerned about the health and well-being of athletes; a shift that continues to sit well with me. Although I hadn't experienced a meaningful injury myself before, it was at this time that I started to adopt the role of being an advocate for injured athletes. I wanted to understand how to prevent injury and nurture recovery back to or away from sport. I wanted to help.

From continuing to listen to countless stories from injured athletes, as well as reading numerous autobiographies and trying to talk with as many support staff as possible (e.g., physiotherapists) to better understand injury and rehabilitation, I soon found myself becoming critical of the sport injury literature published in sport psychology journals. I realized the individualistic nature of the discipline in terms of the concepts examined (e.g., *self*-efficacy, *self*-determination) and the "self-help" applied skills and recommendations (e.g., self-talk, imagery, relaxation), as well as how it was largely underpinned by cognitivism. For example, the two most well-cited models that continue to lead this field of research focus on, and center around, injured athletes' cognitive appraisals, which are suggested to affect athletes' emotions and behaviors (Williams & Andersen, 1998; Wiese-Bjornstal, Smith, Shaffer, & Morrey, 1998). However, this dominant intrapersonal perspective could be criticized for being reductionist (e.g., emotions arise solely from within the individual). It does not account for how sport injury might also be a cultural, intersubjective, situated, and embodied experience (cf. Gergen, 2011; Laurendeau, 2014; Sparkes, 1996; Spencer, 2012). These early musings were further developed by speaking with and learning from Dr Ian Mitchell about social psychology and Dr Chris Wagstaff about organizational psychology, both of whom were doing their PhDs at the same time as me. However, my musings didn't materialize much further than this – "life got in the way" so to speak; I was finishing my PhD, starting a new job, and I had just met my future wife, leaving me with little time to develop and refine these ideas by engaging with and learning from these other fields of research. As time went by over the next five or so years, I continued to research what I knew and what I was comfortable with.

The next turning point in my career, which I would argue has been the most significant, was when I met Dr Melissa Day at the British Association of Sport and Exercise Sciences annual conference in Glasgow. Aside from sharing a passion for tea, Melissa shared an interest in sport injury psychology and was also critical of the research landscape. From discussing and debating this field of research with her, we were able to develop and refine our arguments further.[1] Melissa also had a wealth of knowledge about qualitative research and she challenged me to reflect on my research philosophy and encouraged me to consider new bodies of research and revisit ones I had already read but not yet fully considered. To illustrate, she drew upon the groundbreaking research by Professor Brett Smith and Professor Andrew Sparkes on athletes who had experienced spinal cord injuries (Smith & Sparkes, 2002, 2004, 2005) and the use of narrative inquiry as a way of theorizing about and doing research (Smith & Sparkes, 2009). Reading and rereading this program of research helped me to think more critically about the broader social-cultural narratives that circulate in sporting and non-sporting cultures and within rehabilitation settings, and how these narratives do things on, in, and for those who operate within them – a discourse seldom considered in sport injury psychology.

The next turning point in my career was when I moved to a new academic institution. On day one, I was told I was convening and teaching two postgraduate modules I hadn't previously taught: "social psychology of sport" and "qualitative research methods". For several months, I became immersed in new bodies of research ranging from cultural sport psychology (e.g., Schinke & Hanrahan, 2008), organizational psychology (e.g., Wagstaff, 2016), team dynamics (e.g., Beauchamp & Eys, 2014), to interpersonal relations (e.g., Jowett & Lavallee, 2006) – all vibrant areas of research that I hadn't fully engaged with before, which not only reignited my curiosity to explore other fields of research, but also fueled my frustration with the dominant individualistic underpinning of sport injury psychology. From teaching qualitative research methods, I also became better-versed in research philosophy and qualitative traditions, methods, analyses, and forms of representation (e.g., Sparkes, 1992, 2002; Richardson & St Pierre, 2005; Sth & Sparkes, 2016). This scholarly work, alongside attending and talking with researchers at the international conference for *Qualitative Research in Sport, Exercise and Health*, opened my eyes to new ways of doing research and taught me, among other things, about subjectivity and the multiple meanings that people attach to their experiences and the social structures and processes that shape these meanings. Familiarizing myself with this literature also made me increasingly aware of the positivist foundation of sport injury psychology research and practice and the critical need for more inclusive scholarship and practice with divergent epistemologies, theories, and methodologies.

At my new academic institution, I was also fortunate enough to meet, and learn a great deal from, Dr Tanya Bunsell, who taught sport sociology and soon became a regular coffee-buddy. She introduced me to the work of researchers I had never been taught in my academic studies (e.g., Michel Foucault, Pierre Bourdieu, Erving Goffman) and fields of research that I had limited awareness of (e.g., physical cultural studies, gender studies, feminism). When not putting the world to rights, we also shared a common interest in the injury literature. However, conversations on injury between us weren't easy (for me, at least). I was drawing from the sport injury psychology literature and Tanya was drawing from the sport sociology literature. These ongoing conversations led us to debate whether the disciplines could ever work together in an interdisciplinary manner and to discuss the barriers that deter them from doing so (e.g., journal outlets, epistemologies). A cursory glance at the sport injury research landscape soon reveals that these two disciplines have traditionally always worked in isolation, which can be evidenced, for example, from the early books published in both fields: *Sporting Bodies, Damaged Selves: Sociological Studies of Sports-Related Injury* by Kevin Young (2004) and *Psychology of Sport Injury* by John Heil (1993). While I was able to find a few books and papers that have operated at the intersection of psychology and sociology in my search for interdisciplinary research (see Curry, 1993; Collinson, 2005; Howe, 2004), I would argue these have been the exception rather than the rule. However, in my search I did come across a special issue of *Sociology of Sport Journal* on the subject of new conversations between sociology and psychology (Thorpe, Ryba, & Denison, 2014). The aim of this special issue was to open conversations about the potential and politics of working at the intersection between these two disciplines. This special issue gave me hope for interdisciplinary discourse that sought to provide a more cultural and relational understanding of injured athletes' psychological experiences and offered several ideas for collaborative projects on how to do just that (see e.g., Butryn, LaVoi, Kauer, Semerjian, & Waldron, 2014; Markula, 2014); however, from examining the literature and conference abstracts since this special issue I have seen little evidence of interdisciplinary research between these two professions (or between them and others). Mainstream research in sport injury psychology remains an individual-focused and single, scientific discipline, which I find to be a shortcoming of the literature. As Diane Wiese-Bjornstal (2019) has written: "Most aspects of sport, and therefore, sport injuries, are fundamentally as much a social and cultural in nature as they are personal" (p. 18).

The final turning point in my career stemmed from reaching out and having ongoing conversations with practitioners working in the field with injured athletes. Like the divide between sport psychology and sport sociology, I have noticed, over the years, similar tensions between applied practitioners and researchers. On the one hand, academic researchers convey their desire to me to reduce complex behavior to simplistic isolated components that can be controlled, manipulated, and tested. They also complain to me that practitioners don't read their work and take up their applied recommendations. Yet, academics do little to translate their findings beyond academic journals and conferences. On the other hand, practitioners tell me they are more concerned with experiential or craft knowledge. They critique the inadequacy of research (e.g., it's inaccessible, it doesn't address "real-world" issues) and as a result they engage little, if at all, with academic research. Yet, practitioners converse little with academic researchers about their frustrations with the research landscape and appear reluctant to share their craft knowledge. If practitioners *do* publish their experiences of working with injured athletes at all, they are often highly polished, sanitized accounts of successful interventions that met the injured athletes' needs. The more multifaceted, uneven, and somewhat fragmented picture of sport injury experiences that they describe to me, gets pushed aside to align with the positivistic desires for "clean" findings. While I am not the first to share these frustrations in the applied sport psychology literature (see e.g., Martens, 1987), I would argue that these tensions between practitioners and academics have not been grappled with in the sport injury psychology literature. To embrace the complexity of injury and provide more nuanced insights into the working alliance between practitioners and injured athletes, I would argue we need to "lift the veil" on applied practice to, among other things, inform theoretical knowledge, improve the training of applied practitioners, and enhance the effectiveness of professional practice.)

Academics also need to recognize that sometimes practitioners cannot wait for established theory and practice, and perhaps there is a need to report findings retrospectively (see e.g., Henschen & Heil, 1992). It might also be wise for future applied intervention research in sport injury psychology to replace the attempt to establish "best practices" or *the* "single-best practice" with continuous innovation and future-making practices (Gergen, 2016). From my perspective and in agreement with Gergen, the broader the array of available practices that aim to prevent injury or nurture recovery, the greater the number of athletes who can find help. As Gergen reported, "… the very attempt to use evidence-based evaluation to winnow out ineffective practices in misconceived … In effect, depending on time and place, evidential support may be garnered for virtually any form of therapy" (p. 12). Moving forward, rather than continuing to streamline our practices, I believe it is important that we encourage greater diversification of interventions to prevent injury or nurture recovery back to or away from sport. To expand, psychological skills don't always work with injured populations (Wadey, 2019) and therefore we need to consider other strategies beyond the "usual suspects" (e.g., goal setting, imagery, and self-talk) that operate at micro (i.e., individual), meso (e.g., dyadic, multidisciplinary team), and macro (e.g., organizational policies and practices) levels (e.g., Bolling, van Mechelen, Pasman, & Verhegen, 2018; Bianco & Eklund, 2001; Hess, Gnacinski, & Meyer, 2019; Wadey, Day, Cavallerio, & Martinelli, 2018; Wiese-Bjornstal, 2019). Importantly, "we do not just need to make athletes more 'mentally tough' and 'resilient', we also need to ensure that policies and practices are put in place the support their safety, well-being and welfare" (Wadey et al., 2019, p. 338).

Taken together, all these turning points have led me to this area of research and have shaped the aim and scope of this book, which is to challenge the status quo of sport injury psychology and open new and exciting trajectories for established researchers in this field and to encourage a new generation of scholars. From the outset, the book sets out to evolve sport injury psychology from an individual-focused and single, scientific discipline into a cultural and relational-focused and interdisciplinary discourse. Up until now, I argue, research interest on cultural and relational thought and practice has been marginal, if not completely eschewed, in sport injury psychology. Therefore, the opening chapters in this text consider how future researchers in this field can connect their work with the larger social-cultural environment in and outside of sport, and forge links and reciprocity with related disciplines (e.g., sport communication, sport sociology, social psychology, organizational psychology, cultural psychology). In Chapter 1, Toni Williams considers social-cultural narratives and how they can help injured athletes make sense of their experiences. The chapter provides a description and overview of narrative theory, with illustrative examples of how different social-cultural narrative types can shape how athletes story their injury experiences. The chapter concludes with considerations of how a narrative approach can inform future research and practice in sport injury psychology. Chapter 2, written by Kerry McGannon and Jenny McMahon, reviews the benefits of studying the media as a cultural site to expand sport injury psychology research by bringing together sport sociology, sport communication, and sport psychology. The meaning of "sport media research" is outlined, with research examples focusing on sport injury. Future research directions are offered that consider mainstream media forms (e.g., news media, television) and new media forms (e.g., Instagram, Twitter, Facebook), and how social agents (e.g., athletes, coaches, parents) engage with and/or react to these media stories about injury.

Tanya Bunsell and Mark Doidge, in Chapter 3, draw from research in sport sociology to consider how gender structures attitudes toward, expectations about, and experiences of pain and injury within sporting milieus, which may threaten the presentation of the gendered self. While the authors recommend that sport injury psychology can ill afford to ignore gender and should move beyond the traditional gender binary in their future research endeavors, it is also recommended that it should also take into account the various intersections of athlete identity (e.g., sexuality, ethnicity, age (dis)ability, and religion). In Chapter 4, Nikolaus Dean critically explores the various ways in which sport-related concussion has been studied within academic literature and, importantly, considers how it could be explored in the future. For example, instead of limiting the scope of research to more analyses of hockey, rugby, and football sporting cultures, Nikolaus contends examining sport-related concussion in alternative, individualized, and non-contact sporting environments. He also draws attention to the advantages of expanding one's methodological tool kit and how researchers studying concussion could (better) disseminate their research. Chapter 5, written by Michael Atkinson, reviews a broad range of substantive and theoretical approaches to the study of pain (and injury) in sport and considers some of the virtues of studying sport from a "cell to society" perspective. Emphasis is given to viewing sports and exercise worlds as "pain communities", and future researchers are encouraged to stretch research boundaries to reveal new ground in pain research yet to be traversed.

Jenny McMahon and Kerry McGannon, in Chapter 6, critically consider how culturally accepted bodies within elite sporting cultures point to entrenched "slim-to-win" ideologies, whereby the "slim" and "fatless" body shape is perceived to enhance competitive performance. Providing rich illustrative examples from athletes' stories, the chapter considers how the sport context of swimming has led athletes and other cultural insiders (e.g., coaches, managers, other athletes) to compromise their health through forms of self-injury (e.g., taking medications), which puts their bodies at risk of physical injury and creates mental health issues. Future research suggestions are offered, which include implementing education interventions using, for example, narrative pedagogy, with the possibility of social action being initiated. Chapter 7, written by Karen Howells and Ciara Everard, critically considers the often-celebrated storyline championed in sport of *growth following adversity* and associated research in sport injury psychology that has considered athletes' accounts of overcoming injury and returning physically and mentally stronger. In the chapter, Karen and Ciara question whether injured athletes' experiences of growth are genuine or whether, for example, they are adhering to a broader cultural script to demonstrate they are coping. While there is no shortage of evidence documenting the importance of emotions and emotional responses in athletes' injury experiences, in Chapter 8, Katherine Tamminen, Rachel Dunn, and Sarah Gairdner, critically review the way the emotions have been conceptualized and studied in the sport injury literature until now. For example, they highlight the limited work examining the interpersonal processes at play surrounding emotions among injured athletes and encourage future researchers to advance research by investigating how athletes' emotions are socialized or constrained through interactions with teammates, coaches, and athletic therapists.

Sunita Kerai, in Chapter 9, calls for a cultural and relational understanding of the physiotherapist–injured-athlete relationship. Critiquing the dominant individualistic literature in sport injury psychology, she encourages future researchers in sport injury psychology to think more dyadically and to consider how the wider sporting culture influences interpersonal processes between physiotherapists and injured athletes. As the chapter closes, a broader representation of the physiotherapist–injured-athlete relationship is also encouraged in future research endeavors, such as the gender structure (e.g., female physiotherapist–male athlete, male physiotherapist–female athlete). In Chapter 10, Laura Martinelli and Melissa Day consider the guilt experienced by coaches following athlete injury. This chapter recognizes the interpersonal nature of injury and that members of injured athletes' networks may be impacted by injury. Drawing from their groundbreaking research in this area, Laura and Melissa consider guilt as an interpersonal emotion and why it may be a commonplace experience for coaches after witnessing an athlete's injury. Chapter 11, by Francesca Cavallerio, Nicole Kimpton, and Camilla Knight, considers the role of parents in relation to their children's sport injuries and how they can impact and be impacted by injury. Drawing from autoethnographic extracts from Nicole, the authors encourage readers to think with the illustrative examples provided and to consider the quandary parents of elite child athletes may face. The chapter closes with considerations of how we can better support parents and disseminate knowledge in ways that are creative and accessible (e.g., creative nonfiction, poetry).

However, a barrier to the cultural and relational discourse outlined in Chapters 1–11 is the positivist foundation of the field of sport injury psychology, which inhibits inclusive scholarship and practice with divergent epistemologies, theories, and methodologies. Aligned with this more inclusive agenda, in Chapter 12, Melissa Day and Kimberley Humphrey consider the future of qualitative injury research. In this chapter, the authors call for methodological diversification and challenge sport injury researchers to "go beyond" their usual practice to consider other ways of doing qualitative research to enable participants to tell or show their injury stories in a variety of different ways. Specifically, Melissa and Kimberley encourage future researchers to consider alternative sampling strategies (e.g., extreme or deviant cases), new forms of data collection (e.g., visual methods), and how research can be disseminated in more creative, user-friendly ways (e.g., ethnodrama). However, this is not to say that all future research should be qualitative in nature and that we should abandon the dominant positivism paradigm in sport injury psychology; quite the contrary: this book encourages a shift toward more *inclusive* scholarship. Given the dominant positivism foundation in sport injury psychology, however, it is perhaps surprising there are so few rigorous methodological experimental sport injury studies. For those adopting a positivist paradigm, in Chapter 12, Kirsty Ledingham, Tom Williams, and Lynne Evans, consider why the increased proliferation of injury research has not yet extended to injury interventions and, importantly, how this can be addressed in future research. Following a systematic review of the sport injury psychology literature, the authors pool together a body of research to help inform the design of future methodologically rigorous intervention studies. Considerations include recruiting large and homogenous samples, ensuring baseline equivalence, blinding, standardized treatment protocols, and validity and reliability of measures. In Chapter 14, Fiona Leggat, introduces a new methodological approach, knowledge translation, into the field of sport injury psychology to enhance research uptake in practice. Not only does Fiona introduce knowledge translation, with a specific focus on *integrated* knowledge translation, she also explains to readers how it can be utilized from drawing from her own experiences of using the methodology and from drawing from other fields of research (e.g., implementation science). This chapter represents an exciting and timely methodology for future researchers who are keen to make an impact in their research endeavors.

The final consideration discussed in the closing chapters of this book addresses the tension that exists between academic researchers and applied practitioners. To close the research–practice "gap" and encourage greater diversification in applied practice rather than relying on the same old "usual suspects" (i.e., psychological skills), the authors in the closing chapters draw upon their craft knowledge to "lift the veil" on applied practice, which challenges the dominant positivistic discourse and desire for "clean" findings and provides more multifaceted and nuanced illustrations of the challenges of working with injured athletes in the field. In Chapter 15, Robert Morris draws from his experiential knowledge of working with an injured athlete (Joanne) and the challenges of using rational emotive behavior therapy. He goes on to illustrate the importance of understanding the context in which practitioners find themselves working and the need to be flexible when working with injured athletes. The chapter closes with future research recommendations, which include, among other things, the need for practice-based evidence of "unsuccessful" consultancy. Chapter 16, by Sarah Cecil, draws upon her experiences of using acceptance and commitment therapy (ACT) with injured athletes, which has received limited research attention in sport injury psychology. Drawing from five years of practice in an intensive rehabilitation unit, she outlines her reflections of using the ACT "Hexaflex" in a multidisciplinary setting to enabled injured athletes to move forward in their rehabilitation in a valued direction. She encourages future researchers to get into the consultancy space to explore the interplay between therapeutic approach, practitioner, and injured athlete. Monna Arvinen-Barrow, Damien Clement, and Brian Hemmings, in Chapter 17, consider storytelling within the context of sport injury rehabilitation. While storytelling has become a well-versed strategy in different healthcare domains, it has been marginal in sport injury psychology. Drawing from and weaving in their own applied experiences, the authors describe different types of stories, elaborate on the potential outcomes of storytelling, and critically consider its intricacies. In the final applied chapter, Chapter 18, Renee Newcomer Appaneal further challenges the dominant discourse in applied research. She argues that "textbooks don't tell it like it is", and rather than drawing from her own "success" stories from working with injured athletes, she provides three vignettes that reflect some of her more uncomfortable applied experiences. The chapter closes with Renee describing her "survival pack" to navigate the diverse and challenging terrain of professional practice, and the need for practitioners working with injured athletes to develop their cultural competence.

Rather than writing the concluding chapter myself, I wanted to invite Britton Brewer, who is the leading scholar in sport injury psychology. The field of research owes him a great deal for his theoretical advancements (i.e., biopsychosocial model of sport injury rehabilitation; Brewer, Andersen, & Van Raalte, 2002), periodic and timely reviews of the literature (e.g., Brewer, 1994, 2001, 2007, 2010), and for the methodological rigor and quality of his research to create a sound evidence base to support professional practice. Drawing from three decades' worth of research the chapter starts by providing a review of the historical developments and advancements in sport injury psychology from a theoretical, research, and applied perspective. Interwoven within this narrative, projections of future developments in sport injury psychology are made, among the formidable theoretical and methodological challenges and considerable applied obstacles that need to be overcome for sport injury psychology to fulfill its potential. Given the absence of professional organizations, journals, or conferences devoted exclusively to sport injury psychology, he outlines that the success of this field of research relies on parties from disparate backgrounds coming together to best serve the athlete they study and with whom they work. One question the chapter closes with is: "What are the most vital research questions facing sport injury psychology? What would a 'focused and united' agenda for the field look like?" I do hope this chapter, like all the chapters in this book, sparks conversations that ultimately lead to research and collegiate action to fulfill the potential of sport injury psychology in helping to prevent injury occurrence or nurture recovery.

Note

1   I did ask Melissa to co-author this book with me, but she declined (much to my frustration) because she had several other ongoing programs of research at the time. That said, I would like to acknowledge that many of my musings in this chapter have come from ongoing conversations with her, and I would like to thank her for being such a supportive colleague and friend to work with over the years. I hope there are many more to come.

References

Beauchamp, R. R., & Eys, M. A. (2014). *Group dynamics in exercise and sport psychology*. London, UK: Routledge.

Bianco, T., & Eklund, R. C. (2001). Conceptual considerations for social support research in sport and exercise settings: The case of sport injury. *Journal of Sport and Exercise Psychology*, *23*(2), 85–107. doi: 10.1123/jsep.23.2.85

Bolling, C., van Mechelen, W., Pasman, H. R., & Verhagen, E. (2018). Context matters: Revisiting the first step of the 'Sequence of Prevention' of sports injuries. *Sports Medicine*, *48*(10), 2227–2234. doi: 10.1007/s40279-018-0953-x

Brewer, B. W. (1994). Review and critique of models of psychological adjustment to athletic injury. *Journal of Applied Sport Psychology*, *6*(1), 87–100. doi: 10.1080/10413209408406467

Brewer, B. W. (2001). Psychology of sport injury rehabilitation. In R. N. Singer, H. A. Hausenblas, & C. M. Janelle (Eds.), *Handbook of sport psychology* (2nd ed.) (pp. 787–809). Hoboken, NJ: Wiley.

Brewer, B. W. (2007). Psychology of sport injury rehabilitation. In G. Tenenbaum & R. C. Eklund (Eds.), *Handbook of sport psychology* (3rd ed.) (pp. 404–424). Hoboken, NJ: Wiley.

Brewer, B. W. (2010). The role of psychological factors in sport injury rehabilitation outcomes. *International Review of Sport and Exercise Psychology*, *3*(1), 40–61. doi: 10.1080/17509840903301207

Brewer, B. W., Andersen, M. B., & Van Raalte, J. L. (2002). Psychological aspects of sport injury rehabilitation: Toward a biopsychosocial approach. In D. L. Mostofsky & L. D. Zaichkowsky (Eds.), *Medical and psychological aspects of sport and exercise* (pp. 41–54). Morgantown, WV: Fitness Information Technology.

Butryn, T. M., LaVoi, N. M., Kauer, K. J., Semerjian, T. Z., & Waldron, J. J. (2014). We walk the line: An analysis of the problems and possibilities at the sport psychology-sport sociology nexus. *Sociology of Sport Journal*, *31*(2), 162–184. doi: 10.1123/ssj.2012-0169

Cavallerio, F., Wadey, R., & Wagstaff, C. R. D. (2016). Understanding overuse injuries in rhythmic gymnastics: A 12-month ethnography. *Psychology of Sport and Exercise*, *25*, 100–109. doi: 10.1016/j.psychsport.2016.05.002

Curry, T. J. (1993). A little pain never hurt anymore: Athletic career socialization and the normalization of sports injury. *Symbolic Interactionism*, *16*(3), 273–290. doi: 10.1525/si.1993.16.3.273

Gergen, K. J. (2011). Relational being: beyond self and community. New York, NY: Oxford University Press.

Gergen, K. J. (2016). Toward a visionary psychology. *The Humanistic Psychologist*, *44*(1), 3–17. doi: 10.1037/hum0000013

Heil, J. (1993). *Psychology of sport injury*. Champaign, IL: Human Kinetics.

Henschen, K. R., & Heil, J. (1992). A retrospective study of the effect of an athlete's sudden death on teammates. *Journal of Death and Dying, 25*(3), 217–223. doi: 10.2190%2FTUU3-Y7J9-QLRG-C08G

Hess, C. W., Gnacinski, S. L., & Mayer, B. B. (2019). A review of the sport injury and rehabilitation literature: From abstraction to application. *The Sport Psychologist, 33*(3), 232–243. doi: 10.1123/tsp.2018-0043

Howe, D. P. (2004). *Sport, professionalism, and pain: Ethnographies of injury and risk*. London, UK: Routledge.

Hughes, R., & Coakley, J. (1991). Positive deviance among athletes: The implications of overcomformity to the Sport Ethic. *Sociology of Sport Journal, 8*(4), 307–325. doi: 10.1123/ssj.8.4.307

Jowett, S., & Lavallee, D. (2006). *Social psychology in sport*. Champaign, IL: Human Kinetics.

Laurendeau, J. (2014). "Just tape it up for me, ok?" Masculinities, injury and embodied emotion. Emotion, Space and Society, 12, 11–17

Markula, P. (2014). Embodied subjectivities: Intersections of discursive and critical psychology with social-cultural exercise research. *Sociology of Sport Journal, 31*(2), 139–161. doi: 10.1123/ssj.2013-0049

Martens, R. (1987). Science, knowledge, and sport psychology. *The Sport Psychologist, 1*(1), 29–55.

Nixon, H. (1992). A social network analysis of influences on athletes to play with pain and injuries. *Journal of Sport and Social Issues, 16*(2), 127–135. doi: 10.1177%2F019372359201600208

Richardson, L., & St. Pierre, E. A. (2005). Writing: A method of inquiry. In N. K. Denzin & Y. S. Lincoln (Eds.), *The Sage handbook of qualitative research* (pp. 959–978). Los Angeles: Sage.

Sparkes, A., (1996). The fatal flaw: a narrative of the fragile body-self. Qualitative Inquiry, 2, 463–494

Sparkes, A. C. (2002). Telling tales in sport and physical activity: A qualitative journal. Human Kinetic Publishers.

Spencer, D.C. (2012). Narratives of despair and loss: pain, injury and masculinity in the sport of mixed martial arts. Qualitative Research in Sport, Exercise and Health, 4, 117–137

Schinke, R. J., & Hanrahan, S. J. (2008). *Cultural sport psychology*. Champaign, IL: Human Kinetics.

Smith, B., & Sparkes, A. C., (2016). *Routledge handbook of qualitative research in sport and exercise*. London: Routledge.

Smith, B., & Sparkes, A. (2002). Men, sport, spinal cord injury, and the construction of coherence: Narrative practice in action. *Qualitative Research, 2*(2), 143–171. doi: 10.1177%2F146879410200200202

Smith, B., & Sparkes, A. (2004). Men, sport, and spinal cord injury: An analysis of metaphors and narrative types. *Disability and Society, 19*(6), 509–612. doi: 10.1080/0968759042000252533

Smith, B., & Sparkes, A. (2005). Men, sport, and spinal cord injury and narratives of hope. *Social Science and Medicine, 61*(5), 1095–1105. doi: 10.1016/j.socscimed.2005.01.011

Smith, B., & Sparkes, A. (2009). Narrative inquiry in sport and exercise psychology: What can it mean, and why might we do it? *Psychology of Sport and Exercise, 10*(1), 1–11. doi: 10.1016/j.psychsport.2008.01.004

Sparkes, A. (1992). *Research in physical education and sport: Exploring alternative visions*. London: The Falmer Press.

Thorpe, H., Ryba, T., & Denison, J. (2014). Toward new conversations between sociology and psychology. *Sociology of Sport Journal, 31*(2), 131–138. doi: 10.1123/ssj.2013-0109

Wadey, R. (2019). Reaction to returning to the decks: Melissa Scruton, professional disc jockey. In M. Arvinen-Barrow & D. Clement (Eds.), *The psychology of sport and performance injury: An interprofessional case-based approach* (pp. 100–112). London, UK: Routledge.

Wadey, R., Day, M., Cavallerio, F., & Martinelli, L. (2018). The Multi-Level Model of Sport Injury: Can coaches impact and be impacted by injury? In R. Thelwell & M. Dicks (Eds.), *Professional advances in sports coaching: Research and Practice* (pp. 408–440) London: Routledge.

Wadey, R., Day, M., & Howells, K. (2020). Taking stock and making hay: Growth following adversity research in applied sport psychology. In R. Wadey, M. Day & K. Howells (Eds.), *Growth following adversity in sport: A mechanism to positive change* (pp. 257–274). London, UK: Routledge.

Wadey, R., Roy-Davis, K., Evans, L., Howells, K., Salim, J., & Diss, C. (2019). Sport psychology consultants' perspectives on facilitating sport injury-related growth. *The Sport Psychologist, 33*(3), 244–255. doi: 10.1123/tsp.2018-0110

Wagstaff, C. R. D. (2016). *The organizational psychology of sport: Key issues and practical applications.* London: Routledge.

Wiese-Bjornstal, D. M. (2019). Sociocultural aspects of sport injury and recovery. In E. O. Acevedo (Ed.), *Oxford encyclopedia of sport, exercise, and performance psychology* (pp. 841–863). New York: Oxford University Press.

Wiese-Bjornstal, D. M., Smith, A. M., Shaffer, S. M., & Morrey, M. A. (1998). An integrated model of response to sport injury: Psychological and sociological dimensions. *Journal of Applied Sport Psychology, 10*(1), 46–69. doi: 10.1080/10413209808406377

Williams, J. M., & Andersen, M. B. (1998). Psychosocial antecedents of sport injury: Review and critique of the stress and injury model. *Journal of Applied Sport Psychology, 10*(1), 5–25. doi: 10.1080/10413209808406375

Young, K. (2004). *Sporting bodies, damaged selves: Sociological studies of sports-related injury.* Bingley, UK: Emerald Publishing.

1 Narratives Matter!

Storying Sport Injury Experiences

Toni L. Williams

Introduction

Stories are everywhere: in the books we read, in the songs we listen to, in the movies we watch, in the media we engage with, and in our conversations with others. Importantly, formulating and sharing stories helps people create an identity and sense of self, while also bringing meaning and coherence to our lives (Charmaz, 1999; Crossley, 2000). Through a narrative lens, it is understood that although we tell unique stories of our own personal experiences, we draw upon dominant sociocultural narratives to structure our tales (Frank, 2013). Thus, the stories out there – in the locker room, on the sports field, embedded within social and cultural settings – act as narrative resources to make sense of experiences such as sport injury. Yet limited research attention has been afforded to the social-cultural context in sport injury psychology. Answering calls for future research in this area (Wadey, Day, Cavallerio, & Martinelli, 2019; Wiese-Bjornstal, 2010), this chapter will provide a brief description and overview of narrative before turning to the possibilities narrative inquiry can offer in understanding the impact of injury through sport. Here, two examples are drawn upon to illustrate how different sociocultural narrative types can shape interpretations of sport injury. Finally, the importance of taking a narrative approach in the professional practice of sport injury psychology (and beyond) is critically discussed with suggestions for further research within this field.

Why do Narratives Matter?

Narrative is a form of inquiry that has been extensively used to interpret the embodied experience of illness and injury. This is because narratives are essential means by which people make sense of their lives and experiences. As Frank (2013) explains, serious illness and injury represent a loss in the *destination* and *map* that have previously guided an individual's life. For example, for athletes, sporting injuries may result in losing a medal, not qualifying for a major event, the premature end of an athletic career, or even permanent disability. These experiences bring disruption and confusion into people's lives as an imagined future is no longer possible. Accordingly, telling stories is a way that people make sense of experience, produce and maintain a sense of identity, and reconstruct a sense of order in their lives disrupted by illness and injury (Charmaz, 1999; Crossley, 2000; Frank, 2010, 2013).

Before exploring the role of narrative in shaping interpretations of sport injury, it is important to expand upon what narrative is. First, humans have been widely accepted as storytellers, and therefore this forms an underlying assumption that people lead *storied lives* (Crossley, 2000; Phoenix & Sparkes, 2006). In other words, people express themselves through stories and make sense of their lives and experiences by telling stories. Second, people transmit meaning by telling stories, and understanding meaningful experience is a central component of narrative inquiry. As Garro and Mattingly (2000) explain, "Narrative is a fundamental human way of giving meaning to experience. In both telling and interpreting experiences; narrative mediates between an inner world of thought–feeling and an outer world of observable actions and states of affairs" (p. 1). Similarly, Mayer (2014) suggests "Stories imbue our experience with 'meaning'. Events become meaningful to the extent that they can be fit into or evoke some larger narrative about ourselves or our world... It is impossible to say who we are without telling a story" (p. 7).

Third, narratives are conceptualized as both personal and sociocultural. The stories people tell about their lives convey, express, and formulate *personal* thoughts and feelings in relation to particular experiences. Yet while these experiences are personal to the individual, the stories people tell are *socially* and *culturally* constructed (Frank, 2013). As Phoenix and Sparkes (2006) illuminate:

> People resort to a mode of telling with which they feel familiar. In this sense, narrative is a form of social practice in which individuals draw from a cultural repertoire of stories that they then assemble into personal stories ... . It is through this social aspect of narrative that the dominant narratives available in culture may act to shape not only who we think we are, but also who we think we can become in the future.
>
> (p. 109)

Therefore, the dominant narratives available in society and culture – the stories that are widely retold in this context – act as a resource, or template, which people can draw upon to tell their own stories (Frank, 2010). Here, a useful distinction between narrative and story can be made. Broadly speaking, a narrative can be understood as "a complex genre that routinely contains a *point* and *characters* along with a *plot* connecting *events* that unfold *sequentially* over *time* and in *space* to provide an overarching *explanation* or *consequence*" (Smith & Sparkes, 2009a, p. 2). Stories on the other hand, are individual tales, or specific acts of telling, constructed from narratives that social relations, culture, and society make available to us. This is not to suggest that people do not have agency in telling their own stories. Rather, people adapt established and recognizable narrative resources to tell individual tales (Frank, 2013). The distinction between narrative and story can be hard to sustain as "narratives only exist in particular stories, and all stories are narratives" (Frank, 2013, p. 224). Yet, this distinction between narrative and story is valuable to "recognise the uniqueness of each individual story, while at the same time understanding how individuals do not make up stories by themselves" (Frank, 2010, p. 119).

Fourth, narratives are not only resources for telling personal stories; they are also actors, in that they *do* things on, in, for, and with us (Frank, 2010). In other words, narratives are crucial actors in helping create and shape experiences through the ordering of events. Stories have a capacity to *act* in a way that guides and informs our actions and future possibilities. For example, stories work *for* people by providing a map or destination to follow, and act *on* people by teaching what to pay attention to and how to respond to certain actions. As Frank (2010) describes:

> People do not simply listen to stories. They become *caught up*, a phrase that can only be explained by another metaphor: stories get under people's skin. Once stories are under people's skin, they affect the terms in which people think, know and perceive.
>
> (p. 48)

Furthermore, as Mayer (2014) illustrates, "stories motivate our actions. When we act we are often to a great extent *enacting*, we are acting out the story as the script demands, acting in ways that are meaningful in the context of some story" (p. 7).

A Narrative Approach to Sport Injury

The dominant narratives that circulate within society and culture influence our understanding of health and performance. These stories circulating "out there" are extremely powerful resources for framing experiences of sport injury. For example, within sporting contexts, Douglas and Carless (2006, 2009) identified the *performance narrative* as a dominant cultural script which shapes and constrains elite sport experience (i.e., sport is life, life is sport). The performance narrative storyline reflects a single-minded dedication to winning where sacrifice, discipline, and pain are accepted in the quest for success, and feelings of shame accompany failure. Athletes have been shown to go to extreme lengths to align their lives to the performance narrative, including identity foreclosure, compromising education, reduced family time and social relationships (Carless & Douglas, 2013; Douglas & Carless, 2009). Thus, when an athlete becomes ill or injured, and personal embodied experiences fail to align with the culturally dominant performance narrative, sense of self, athletic identity, and mental well-being can be threatened.

The narrative resources available in society and culture are therefore important in helping people regain a sense of coherence following the disruption to their lives through life-threatening events or unexpected crisis (Crossley, 2000). For example, Bury (1982) conceptualized chronic illness as a form of *biographical disruption* as illness ruptures the structure of everyday life. Similarly, when sport injury breaks our anticipated life path – such as losing out on being selected for the Olympic Games or sustaining catastrophic injury through sport – our narratives lose coherence. As a result, meaning and identity as a sport person are also lost (Douglas & Carless, 2006, 2009). Thus, people need to create new stories, and reconstruct their narrative and identity, to regain coherence in their life stories following illness or injury.

One of the most comprehensive narrative studies on experiences of illness comes from Arthur Frank and his influential work *The Wounded Storyteller* ([1995], 2013). Through an in-depth and prolonged exploration of experiences of cancer, Frank identified three broad narrative typologies that underpin stories of illness. These were restitution, chaos, and quest. In brief, Frank proposed that the restitution narrative is the *metanarrative* of modern Western culture with a basic storyline of "Yesterday I was healthy, today I'm sick, but tomorrow I'll be healthy again" (p. 77). In stories of restitution, the ill or injured individual is seeking to regain their former healthy self. As Frank contends: "For the individual teller, the ending is to return to just before the beginning: 'good as new' or status quo ante. For the culture that prefers restitution stories, this narrative affirms that breakdowns can be fixed" (p. 90). Chaos on the other hand, is the opposite of restitution. Following injury or illness, chaos narratives envisage life never getting better:

> Stories are chaotic in their absence of narrative order. Events are told as the storyteller experiences life: without sequence or discernible causality. The lack of coherent sequence is an initial reason why chaos stories are harder to hear; the teller is not understood as telling a "proper" story. But more significantly, the teller of the chaos story is not heard to be living a "proper" life, since life as in story, one event is expected to lead to another.
>
> (Frank, 2013, p. 97)

Finally, the quest narrative differs from both restitution and chaos in that the individual seeks to gain something positive from their illness or injury experience. Accordingly,

> quest stories meet suffering head on; they accept illness and seek to use it … What is quested for may never be wholly clear, but the quest is defined by the ill person's belief that something is to be gained from the experience.
>
> (Frank, 2013, p. 115)

Many authors have drawn upon Frank's theoretical framework to interpret unexpected events such as sport injury. Two examples are illustrated below. The first features the story of acquiring a spinal cord injury and becoming disabled through playing sport. The second draws upon the story of an elite athlete whose injuries prevent him from qualifying for the Olympic Games.

Becoming Disabled Through Sport: The Case of Spinal Cord Injury

Smith and Sparkes (2005) conducted a life history study of a small group of men who suffered a spinal cord injury (SCI) and became disabled through playing the sport of rugby union. They identified that the restitution narrative framed the majority of the men's stories. In relation to SCI, the restitution narrative followed the plot "yesterday I was able-bodied, today I'm disabled, but tomorrow I'll be able-bodied again" (Smith & Sparkes, 2005, p. 1096). Within these stories, the restitution narrative was acting to shape experiences of injury as the people following this plot had *concrete hope* of recovery from SCI. In restitution stories, concrete hopes are linked to technological or medical breakthroughs, to restore the individual to their pre-injured self and pre-disabled identity.

Similarly, Williams, Hunt, Papathomas, and Smith (2018) identified restitution as a dominant narrative structure in stories of exercise following SCI. In this instance, a form of exercise called activity-based rehabilitation (ABR) – rather than medical interventions or technology – was the means by which people were seeking to return to their former able-bodied self. This new narrative read: "yesterday I was able-bodied, today I'm disabled, but tomorrow through exercise, I'll be able-bodied again" (Papathomas, Williams, & Smith, 2015, p. 4). Here, exercise was perceived to be a route to cure (Williams et al., 2018, p. 445):

Interviewer: Do you have any specific goals that you have in mind from exercise?

Daniel: Get back to how I was. Yeah, get walking … I know I'm progressing, getting fitter and everything just as a whole … I haven't seen no massive improvement, no like all of sudden my foot started moving, like being able to control my foot and stuff. I don't know, I've just heard a lot of stories of people in the chair and stuff and I think like 18 months or whatever, and getting stuff back. And funny enough there is one guy in the gym and he like took his first step after 3 years … I'll just keep going, trying you know.

The above quote from Daniel – a young man injured in the sport of motocross – highlights the power of the restitution narrative to *interpellate* (i.e., hail; Frank, 2010) people to participate in ABR. The anticipation of restored function and cure from exercise *acted on* Daniel to motivate initial engagement and facilitate continued participation in ABR even when functional restoration was not forthcoming (Williams et al., 2018). As Frank (2013) explains, restitution is the most culturally preferred narrative; anyone who is ill or injured wants to be healthy again. Thus, friends and family are crucial in relationally sustaining this preferred narrative (Smith & Sparkes, 2005; Williams et al., 2018). Yet, there is a danger of living by restitution. That is, what happens when recovery is not forthcoming? As Frank (2013) warns, "Restitution stories no longer work when the person is dying or when impairment remains chronic. When restitution does not happen, other stories have to be prepared or the narrative wreckage will be real" (p. 94). Without another story to live by, individuals can be plunged into chaos. For individuals living in chaos, life is expressed as meaningless, devoid of purpose, and effectively over, as all hopes of a future worth living are lost (Frank, 2013). This is illustrated in the following words from Jamie following his SCI (Smith & Sparkes, 2005, p. 1101):

I have no future, no. Then, I won't walk again … It's just. You have an accident in life. I don't know, but, but it's, it's, a jumble. I've been given a chance of life, but it's not a life, not living. It's, then, then, see, the accident happened and I can't do anything now. That's the way it is. What can I do? My life, it's, it's, not here. It's over … I have nothing left to live. I have no hope of a life. I have nothing. There is no hope for me.

One way to move out of chaos is to tell stories. Storytelling can play an important role in repairing narrative wreckage as the self is gradually reclaimed in the act of telling (Frank, 2013). Thus, wounded storytellers need the opportunity and support to recover and reclaim the voices that injury has taken away from them (Smith & Sparkes, 2005). In other words, chaos stories need to be tolerated and honored, otherwise the world in all its possibilities is denied: "people can only be helped out when those who care are willing to become witnesses to the story. Chaos is never transcended but must be accepted before new lives can be built and new stories told" (Frank, 2013, p. 110). An important counter-narrative to restitution and chaos is quest. For Smith and Sparkes (2005), people who framed their stories by the quest narrative, resisted concrete hope, as they were not actively seeking a cure. Rather, the quest narrative offered *transcendent hope* which embraces the unknown and provides a narrative scaffold that allows the teller to flexibly adapt to an uncertain future (Frank, 2013; Smith & Sparkes, 2005). Here, an uncertain future was embraced as being full of challenging and exciting possibilities and tied to developing their identity as disabled men.

Elite Sport Disruptions: Injury and Non-Qualification for an Olympic Games

Barker-Ruchti, Schubring, Post, and Pettersson (2019) examined the case of one elite athlete – Mark – who sustained several injuries and failed to qualify for the Rio 2016 Olympic Games. For the authors, Frank's conceptualization of narrative disruptions resonated with the precarious nature of elite sport due to common experiences of injury, illness, and de/non-selection. In this example, Mark's investment in the performance narrative (Douglas & Carless, 2006, 2009) led to the downgrading of serious injury and dangerous simplifying of recovery. With a lack of alternative elite sport narratives to draw upon, the athlete was compelled to adopt a number of restitution strategies (e.g., dismissing serious injury; alternative training/competition plans) to adhere to the performance narrative. Unfortunately, these restitution strategies resulted in further injury and devastatingly ended Mark's qualification attempt (Barker-Ruchti et al., 2019, p. 10):

Athlete: It's how we in … it was so much like … when the first rupture happened, it was so much that I was still so focused about qualifying because I still believed in it. So, every week, I kind of just pushed the thoughts of not qualifying away, so when it happened, it as SO many of weeks of just (long break)
Interviewer: Of still hoping …
Athlete: Yes.
Interviewer: And then it was like immediate.

Athlete: Yes, exactly. So it was … I just felt that there's nothing else to do than to give up the dreams.

As these comments demonstrate, when Mark's injuries were no longer following the path of restitution, and he could not conform to the performance narrative, he was temporarily drawn into chaos. Yet as his injury was not permanent, his narrative did not remain without hope. Barker-Ruchti et al. (2019) noted a process that resembled the quest narrative as Mark reconstructed the self in this time of crisis. During this reconstruction, Mark found an opportunity to make sense of non-qualifying as he reflected upon the training schedule developed by his coach and his own actions during this qualification phase. Although Mark's injury temporarily wrecked his performance narrative, by drawing upon other narrative resources, such as quest, Mark was able to approach training with more caution and control. However, this reconstruction of his career remained constrained by the performance narrative as Mark was even more determined to reach his career goal of qualifying for an Olympic Games.

Mark's story also demonstrates how elite athletes draw upon the dominant cultural script of the performance narrative, yet move in and out of alternative narratives when faced with unexpected events (Barker-Ruchti et al., 2019). This change reflected a *shift* in narrative as chaos and quest temporarily moved to the forefront of Mark's story while the performance narrative remained in the background (Williams, 2018). Furthermore, as this and other studies highlight (see Papathomas et al., 2015; Williams, 2018), no actual story conforms exclusively to one narrative type. As Frank (2010, p. 119) explains, "a typology of *narratives* recognizes that experience follows from the availability of narrative resources, and people's immense creativity is in using these resources to fabricate their stories. The types in a typology are of *narratives*, not people". In reality, people operate within these typologies which act as resources for telling stories and expectations when listening to stories.

Narrative Practice in Sport Injury Psychology (and Beyond)

Narrative practice has much to offer sport psychologists as they are in the profession of dealing with athletes' experience. As Sparkes and Partington (2003) explain:

> In both practice and for research purposes we often ask athletes to share with us their personal accounts of key moments or phases in their career. In so doing, we are inviting stories. Thus, for example, we have stories of winning against the odds, stories of heroic losses, injury stories and comeback stories … Indeed, both athletes and researchers swim in a sea of sporting stories and tales that we hear or read or listen or see.
>
> (p. 293)

Furthermore, as Smith and Sparkes (2009a, 2009b) illustrate, narrative may do things for sport psychologists. Given the potential of stories to engage, inspire, and persuade, narratives may help athletes and practitioners find inspiration to handle specific challenges in new and different ways. This narrative function may be particularly useful when we need the stories of others, or we need to tell stories with others, to help us make sense of events such as career-ending sport injury or becoming disabled through sport. In this instance, narrative inquiry may be beneficial when listening to stories of injured athletes as the underlying narrative of the story being told may be identified, and any possible problems associated with it anticipated (Smith & Sparkes, 2009b, p. 283):

> Thus, intervention strategies could be put in place *before* they occur rather than *after* they happen. In this sense, partly by turning one's analytic lens on the structure of stories, a psychologist working with an athlete could anticipate roadblocks to and avenues for their healing.

Accordingly, sport psychologists are in a valuable position to expand athletes' narrative repertoire by offering multiple and alternative narratives. The more stories an athlete has access to, the more opportunities and flexibility they have to live differently. For example, following a traumatic injury such as SCI, the restitution narrative can be crucial for keeping people engaged in rehabilitation, and a key motivator to start a physically active lifestyle (Papathomas et al., 2015; Perrier, Smith, & Latimer-Cheung, 2013). Yet restitution stories are often told on the edge of chaos. A continued hope for cure can be counterproductive as this may constrain a person's ability to narratively reconstruct their life following injury (Smith & Sparkes, 2005). Furthermore, people may experience psychological distress and reduced well-being if recovery is not forthcoming in the long term. Thus, sharing stories can expand people's narrative resources by providing different perspectives and alternative maps regarding sport injury. This is illustrated in the following passage with Doug as he took the narrative turn toward quest through the stories made available by others (Smith & Sparkes, 2005, p. 1100):

Interviewer: How did you feel after breaking your neck?
Doug: Depressed. Angry. A complete mess. I admit that after the accident I was pretty messed up. I never thought at that point that I would be here right now. But, while the journey to where I am right now hasn't been easy, I've managed to turn the road.
Interviewer: How did you do that?
Doug: How did I turn the road and change? ... One reason for this, and my whole change in who I am, I suppose, has to do with the help that other people have given me. Disabled and able-bodied, have taught me that being disabled isn't the end of the world. Quite the contrary. You can be happy and live a very good life ...

Similarly, Barker-Ruchti et al. (2019) demonstrated the need for alternative narratives within elite sport. In this example an investment in the dominant performance narrative left elite athlete Mark without an alternative script to story his struggles with injury. As such, Mark's narrative realignment restitution strategies resulted in risky behavior including dismissing the seriousness of injury, quick return to training from injury, and unrealistic expectations of qualification for the Olympic Games. Drawing upon Hydén's (1997) concept of narrative as illness, the danger here is that if people are unable to story unexpected events and experiences such as illness and injury, these negative events become normalized and part of an accepted narrative script. Therefore, as Barker-Ruchti et al. (2019) argue, the performance and restitution narratives not only normalize extreme training methods and associated health risk behaviors, but integrate injury as an expected outcome and ultimately endanger athlete welfare. In line with the recommendations proposed by Barker-Ruchti et al. (2019), sport psychologists are in a unique position to offer storytelling sessions in a safe environment in which athletes can voice their stories with a compassionate and understanding audience. Here, alternative narrative resources – such as relational and discovery narratives – can be provided to help athletes shape negative experiences and "re-story" their self and identity (see Carless & Douglas, 2013; Douglas & Carless, 2006). Such opportunities would support elite athletes in managing disruptions such as sport injury, reduce the adoption of risk-taking behavior, and ease personal trauma.

Future Research Implications

To further advance our understanding of sport injury psychology, and push the boundaries of narrative research, there are several future research avenues to be considered. First, adopting a longitudinal approach to data collection can highlight the temporal dynamics of storytelling and provide a more nuanced understanding of how narratives shift over time (Barker-Ruchti et al., 2019; Williams, 2018). Second, integrating multiple methods such as interviews, participant observation, and visual methods may allow participants to express their stories in a variety of complementary and congruent ways (Phoenix & Rich, 2016; Williams, 2018) (see Chapter 12). Third, researchers may wish to explore narrative as a knowledge translation tool as evidence-based stories could be used a resource to share alternative scripts with both injured athletes and sport psychologists (Smith, Tomasone, Latimer-Cheung, & Martin Ginis, 2015) (see Chapter 14). Finally, one innovative strategy is to take on the role of a storyteller, rather than story analyst, and delve into methods such as autoethnography (Allen-Collinson & Hockey, 2001), or creative non-fiction (Cavallerio, Wadey, & Wagstaff, 2016; Ivarsson et al., 2018) to deliver inspiring, emotive, multilayered accounts of culturally situated injury experiences (see Papathomas, 2016 for further examples).

Conclusion

This chapter highlights how dominant narrative types are powerful actors in shaping and constraining stories of sport injury. For example, culturally available resources such as the restitution and performance narrative no longer work for people when their injury is permanent or prematurely ends an athletic career.

When there are few narrative resources to draw upon to make sense of these experiences, narrative wreckage may occur as people are propelled into a meaningless chaotic existence. This chapter also demonstrates the important role sport psychologists can play in providing new stories and alterative narrative scripts which more closely align with personal experience during these disruptive events. It is hoped that this chapter has provided an introduction to the possibilities narrative inquiry has to offer to sport injury psychology and is a starting point for critical thinking and future conversations in the field.

Critical Discussion Questions

1) What dominant cultural narratives can you identify from your experience in sport contexts (e.g., personal stories vs. stories in the media)?
2) How might different qualitative methods be useful in illustrating a nuanced understanding of participants' stories of sport injury over time?
3) What practical and ethical challenges and/or limitations might need to be considered when researching disruptive events such as becoming injured through sport?

References

Allen-Collinson, J., & Hockey, J. (2001). Runners' tales: Autoethnography, injury and narrative. *Auto./Biography*, *9*(1), 95–106.

Barker-Ruchti, N., Schubring, A., Post, A., & Pettersson, S. (2019). An elite athlete's storying of injuries and non-qualification for an Olympic Games: A socio-narratological case study. *Qualitative Research in Sport, Exercise and Health*, *11*(5), 687–703. doi: 10.1080/2159676X.2019.1605405

Bury, M. (1982). Chronic illness as biographical disruption. *Sociology of Health and Illness*, *4*(2), 167–182. doi: 10.1111/1467-9566.ep11339939

Carless, D., & Douglas, K. (2013). Living, resisting, and playing the part of athlete: Narrative tensions in elite sport. *Psychology of Sport and Exercise*, *14*(5), 701–708. doi: 10.1016/j.psychsport.2013.05.003

Cavallerio, F., Wadey, R., & Wagstaff, C. R. D. (2016). Understanding overuse injuries in rhythmic gymnastics: A 12-month ethnographic study. *Psychology of Sport and Exercise*, *25*, 100–109. doi: 10.1080/1612197X.2018.1462227

Charmaz, K. (1999). Stories of suffering: Subjective tales and research narratives. *Qualitative Health Research*, *9*(3), 362–382. doi: 10.1177%2F104973239900900306

Crossley, M. L. (2000). *Introducing narrative psychology: Self, trauma and the construction of meaning*. Buckingham: Open University Press.

Douglas, K., & Carless, D. (2006). Performance, discovery, and relational narratives among women professional tournament golfers. *Women in Sport and Physical Activity Journal*, *15*(2), 14–27. doi: 10.1123/wspaj.15.2.14

Douglas, K., & Carless, D. (2009). Abandoning the performance narrative: Two women's stories of transition from professional sport. *Journal of Applied Sport Psychology*, *21*(2), 213–230. doi: 10.1080/10413200902795109

Frank, A. W. (2010). *Letting stories breathe: A socio-narratology*. London, UK: University of Chicago Press.

Frank, A. W. (2013). *The wounded storyteller* (2nd ed.). London, UK: University of Chicago Press.

Garro, L., & Mattingly, C. (2000). Narrative as construct and construction. In C. Mattingly & L. Garro (Eds.), *Narrative and the cultural construction of illness and healing* (pp. 1–49). Berkley, CA: University of California Press.

Hydén, L. C. (1997). Illness and narrative. *Sociology of Health and Illness*, *19*(1), 48–69. doi: 10.1111/j.1467-9566.1997.tb00015.x

Ivarsson, A., Johnson, U., Karlsson, J., Börjesson, M., Hägglund, M., Andersen, M. B., & Waldén, M. (2018). Elite female footballers' stories of sociocultural factors, emotions, and behaviours prior to anterior cruciate ligament injury. *International Journal of Sport and Exercise Psychology*, *17*(6), 630–646. doi: 10.1080/1612197X.2018.1462227

Mayer, F. W. (2014). *Narrative politics: Stories and collective action*. New York: Oxford University Press.

Papathomas, A. (2016). Narrative inquiry: From cardinal to marginal…and back? In B. Smith & A. C. Sparkes (Eds.), *International handbook of qualitative methods in sport and exercise* (pp. 37–48). London, UK: Routledge.

Papathomas, A., Williams, T. L., & Smith, B. (2015). Understanding physical activity participation in spinal cord injured populations: Three narrative types for consideration. *International Journal of Qualitative Studies on Health and Well-Being*, *14*, 272–295. doi: 10.3402/qhw.v10.27295

Perrier, M.-J., Smith, B., & Latimer-Cheung, A. E. (2013). Narrative environments and the capacity of disability narratives to motivate leisure-time physical activity among individuals with spinal cord injury. *Disability and Rehabilitation*, *35*(24), 2089–2096. doi: 10.3109/09638288.2013.821179

Phoenix, C., & Rich, E. (2016). Visual methods research. In B. Smith & A. C. Sparkes (Eds.), *International handbook of qualitative methods in sport and exercise* (pp. 139–151). London, UK: Routledge.

Phoenix, C., & Sparkes, A. C. (2006). Young athletic bodies and narrative maps of aging. *Journal of Aging Studies*, *20*(2), 107–121. doi: 10.1016/j.jaging.2005.06.002

Smith, B., & Sparkes, A. C. (2005). Men, sport, spinal cord injury and narratives of hope. *Social Science and Medicine*, *61*(5), 1095–1105. doi: 10.1016/j.socscimed.2005.01.011

Smith, B., & Sparkes, A. C. (2009a). Narrative inquiry in sport and exercise psychology: What can it mean, and why might we do it? *Psychology of Sport and Exercise*, *10*(1), 1–11. doi: 10.1016/j.psychsport.2008.01.004

Smith, B., & Sparkes, A. C. (2009b). Narrative analysis and sport and exercise psychology: Understanding lives in diverse ways. *Psychology of Sport and Exercise*, *10*(2), 279–288. doi: 10.1016/j.psychsport.2008.07.012

Smith, B., Tomasone, J. R., Latimer-Cheung, A. E., & Martin Ginis, K. A. (2015). Narrative as a knowledge translation tool for facilitating impact: Translating physical activity knowledge to disabled people and health professionals. *Health Psychology*, *34*(4), 303–313. doi: 10.1037/hea0000113

Sparkes, A., & Partington, S. (2003). Narrative practice and its potential contribution to sport psychology: The example of flow. *The Sport Psychologist*, *17*(3), 292–317. doi: 10.1123/tsp.17.3.292

Wadey, R., Day, M., Cavallerio, F., & Martinelli, L. (2019). Multilevel model of sport injuries (MMSI): Can coaches impact and be impacted by sport injury? In R. Thelwell & M. Dicks (Eds.), *Professional advances in sports coaching: Research and practice* (pp. 540–580). London: Routledge.

Wiese-Bjornstal, D. M. (2010). Psychology and socioculture affect injury risk, response, and recovery in high-intensity athletes: A consensus statement. *Scandinavian Journal of Medicine and Science in Sports, 20* Suppl. 2, 103–111. doi: 10.1111/j.1600-0838.2010.01195.x

Williams, T. L. (2018). Exploring narratives of physical activity and disability over time: A novel integrated qualitative methods approach. *Psychology of Sport and Exercise, 37*, 224–234. doi: 10.1016/j.psychsport.2017.09.004

Williams, T. L., Hunt, E. R., Papathomas, A., & Smith, B. (2018). Exercise is Medicine? Most of the time for most; but not always for all. *Qualitative Research in Sport, Exercise and Health, 10*(4), 441–456. doi: 10.1080/2159676X.2017.1405363

2 Sport Media Research

Examining the Benefits for Sport Injury Psychology and Beyond

Kerry R. McGannon and Jenny McMahon

Introduction

"Those of you posting and tagging me in the video of my injury, I am asking you to please stop," Cerio reportedly Tweeted Wednesday, before taking her account private on Thursday. "Going through the pain and seeing my knees bent unnaturally in real life was horrible enough, but to continue to see it from videos/pictures because some people feel entitled to repost it is not okay. My pain is not your entertainment", she added.

(Bieler, 2019)

The above quote comes from a news media story about US Collegiate gymnast Samantha Cerio, who suffered a horrific injury (i.e., broke both legs and dislocated both knees) while performing a difficult skill in her floor routine, on 5 April 2019. In the hours, days, weeks, and months that followed this "media incident", the impact of the injury on Cerio's life publicly unfolded in various media forms. The quote above refers to a video of the injury posted on YouTube and circulated across digital media platforms, in which Cerio was "tagged" through her account and hashtags. Each time this occurred, she relived the incident, all the while facing an uncertain future. An updated search for this video reveals circulation of the incident in other storied video forms in the past four months, totalling over 3.5 million views and comments. Several days following the initial posting of the video, Cerio took to her social media accounts (i.e., Twitter, Instagram) to "clap back", noting the trauma that re-viewing the injury caused her. She has continued to post her experiences on Instagram in conjunction with mainstream media stories. To date, over 10,000 news stories have been produced on Cerio's injury, recovery, and experiences. A google search of Cerio's injury garners over 89,000 matches, showing continued public interest in the story.

Stories about athletic injury – recreational, youth, collegiate, elite – are ubiquitous in the media landscape, generating personal, public, and commercial interest (Young, 2019). Cerio's story alludes to different forms of "intertextual significance" (i.e., multiple and different meanings are generated in relation to surrounding media texts; Millington & Wilson, 2016) concerning media-generated injury meanings, sport values, and the lifeworld of an athlete. Related to the point of intertextuality, Cerio's story also shows the blurring of boundaries of media production, consumption, and representation, as athletes and social agents (e.g., coaches, teammates, spectators) interacted with mainstream media stories, to (re)produce, reconfigure, or resist them in digital spaces. What value and benefit does studying media representations about athletes and sport injury hold for sport injury psychology and beyond in this regard?

Within the present chapter, this complex question is explored by bringing together research in the sociology of sport, sport communication, and sport psychology, to outline some benefits of studying the media for sport injury psychology. The goal is to answer calls within the sport injury psychology literature to explore the sociocultural context to further understand injury meanings, response, and recovery of injured athletes more holistically (Wadey, Day, Cavallerio, & Martinelli, 2019; Wiese-Bjornstal, 2010; Wiese-Bjornstal, Smith, Shaffer, & Morrey, 1998). To accomplish this purpose, an overview of what constitutes sport media research and why it is of value is first outlined, followed by research in sport sociology concerning risk culture to contextualize sport media work on injury. Media research focusing on sport injury is then presented to show the value of studying the media as a sociocultural site of analysis. We conclude with future research avenues and critical discussion questions to pique conversations and interest on media work in sport injury psychology and beyond.

Critical Review of Literature

Sport Media Research: Clearing Some Ground

What is "sport media research"? Given the dynamic media landscape and way(s) in which media-related sources and technologies afford, and limit, sport-related values and identities (e.g., fans, athletes, coaches), answering this question is not straightforward (Millington & Wilson, 2016; Wenner, 2015). While some media sources were alluded to in our opening, within the present chapter "media research" refers to the systematic study of "media" focusing on at least one of three interconnected elements: production, representation, and consumption (Millingon & Wilson, 2016, p. 153). Sources of media data might include text and images found in news media (print, digital), television and film (documentary, narrative fiction), sport magazines, photographs, advertisements, drawings, and artwork. Sport media researchers may explore digital/social media such as blogs, websites, chat rooms, Facebook, Instagram, Twitter, and YouTube (Bundon, 2016). Sport media using verbal and auditory communication, such as podcasts and radio, are also sources of media production, representation, and consumption research topics. Although it is not possible to explore the advantages of studying all of these media sources, they are noted so that readers gain a sense of the vast, and as yet, untapped area of media research in sport injury psychology. Although sport media injury research examples will be shown, given that such research is limited some of these media data sources will be revisited when making future research suggestions.

Sport media research is extensive within sociology of sport and sport communication scholarship. This work can be found in handbooks (Billings & Hardin, 2014; Pederson, 2013), edited books (Bundon, 2017), and chapters in edited books (Bundon, 2016; Millington & Wilson, 2016; Wenner, 2015). While sport psychology researchers have engaged less with media data, McGannon and McMahon (2016) outlined the benefits of studying the media in relation to identity formation and representation issues in sport psychology. Drawing on cultural studies of sport research, they argued that exploring the media's role in the social construction of athlete identities was important to expand taken-for-granted understanding of identity meanings and implications in cultural sport psychology research (McGannon & Smith, 2015). Broadly grounded in social constructionist forms of theorizing, the media is viewed as a powerful source of cultural representation and circulation of ideologies (i.e., expected behaviors based on cultural values and norms) concerning sport and athletic identities (Andrews & Jackson, 2001), which influences how athletes are perceived by society and how they may perceive themselves (McMahon & Barker-Ruchti, 2016; McMahon, McGannon, & Zehntner, 2017). Examples of media research in sport psychology can be found in a growing body of work on a range of topics, including, but not limited to, career retirement (Cosh, Crabb, & Tully, 2015), career trajectory, and performance of professional athletes (Bonhomme, Seanor, Schinke, & Stabulova, 2020), elite athlete mother identities (McGannon, Gonsalves, Schinke, & Busanich, 2015), and leadership and elite athletic performance (Slater, Barker, Coffee, & Jones, 2015).

Contextualizing Sport Injury Media Research: Culture of Pain and Risk

Research from sport sociology provides compelling evidence that psychosocial issues concerning sport injury can be further understood within the context of sociocultural influences, which has been less examined within sport injury psychology (Wadey et al., 2019). In order to contextualize sport injury media research as a sociocultural influence, some additional discussion of sport sociology research on the culture of pain and risk is warranted. Unlike sport psychology, which formed an interest in sport injury research in the 1970s (Wadey et al., 2019), prior to the 1990s sport sociologists considered sport injury research the domain of sports medicine (Roderick, 2006). The early 1990s ushered in research on a culture of risk in sport to explore injury and pain-related issues, which continued into the early 2000s and beyond (Atkinson, 2019; Young, 2019). Such work is relevant toward expanding sport psychology injury research, as it has problematized taken-for-granted aspects of sport culture that may compromise athlete health, well-being, and performance. Risk culture has been shown to encourage and/or reward pain and injury so that athletes will gain respect and/or put athletic performance ahead of health and safety (Nixon, 1992, 1993; Safai, 2003; Young, 1993, 2004). Within a culture of risk, pain and/or injury tolerance have socially constructed meanings linked with desirable athlete attributes of toughness, strength, and commitment, which create the parameters of the "sport ethic" (Hughes & Coakley,

1991; Young, 2004). When athletes demonstrate hard work, mental toughness, and winning at all costs, through physical training and performance practices, they conform to the sport ethic (Hughes & Coakley; Sabo, 2009).

Risk culture and the tolerance of pain and injury in sport is further normalized through a network of social relationships – termed "sportsnets" by Nixon (1992) – that pressures athletes to play with, and through, pain, thus reinforcing conforming to the "sport ethic" (Hughes & Coakley, 1991). While both male and female athletes' identities, experiences, and behaviors are impacted by a culture of risk (Nixon, 1992; Safai, 2003) male athletes who give in to their pain and/ or resist playing injured have their masculinity and athleticism questioned, while those who do not give in to their pain are lauded and rewarded (Nixon, 1992, 1993; Young, 2004; Young, McTeer, & White, 1994). Athletes learn from a young age that if they want to succeed in sport, playing with, and accepting, injury and pain are "meritocratic acts" that afford access to sporting rewards and success (Sabo, 2009; Young, 2004). Pain and risk culture in sport is so ingrained that some athletes will over-conform to the sport ethic, even when social agents (e.g., family, coaches, medical staff, teammates) express concern, and suggest modification, rest, or treatment (Howe, 2004; Sabo, 2009; Safai, 2003). Chapter 9 (physiotherapists and injury), Chapter 10 (coaches and injury), and Chapter 11 (parents and injury) provide additional perspectives on social influences and sport injury.

Young et al.'s (1994) sociological study on male athletes' injury-related "body talk" further showed that athletes used strategies (e.g., ignoring pain, adopting an irreverent attitude), to supress emotions and rationalize pain and injury to themselves and others. Research on women's experiences shows that they also normalize playing with pain and injury, and hide pain and injury from others (e.g., coaches, medical staff) so that they do not appear too "feminine" or "weak" (Young et al., 1994). As a consequence of risk culture and the associated pain, injury meanings, and practices, athlete health and well-being may be compromised, and at times health and sport science professionals are complicit in the process (Howe, 2004; Roderick, 2006; Young, 2004; Safai, 2003).

Sport Media and Injury: Research Examples

When Young (2004) took stock of the research on pain, risk, and injury 15 years ago, he noted that while people may experience the tactile, lived, and emotional sides of sports-related pain and injury, "it is nevertheless the case that sports injury reaches most people indirectly as a set of images transmitted by the mass media" (p. 16). The media serves in this case not simply as a conveyer of risk-culture meanings in sport, but as another normalizing force that reinforces taken-for-granted cultural meanings about what an "athlete" is (e.g., tough, committed strong, can withstand pain and injury) and what it means to be "injured" (e.g., broken, needs to be fixed, less of an athlete, less strong or weak, less masculine) (Anderson & Kian, 2012; Nixon, 1993; Sabo & Jones, 1998). Conversely, as noted in our opening media incident example, cultural meanings concerning risk, pain, injury, and athletic identity can be contested or resisted in, and through, the media. Despite the potential for learning more by studying media texts and images concerning pain, injury, and risk culture, relatively few sport sociologists had systematically studied mediated pain and injury when Young (2004) called for more work in this regard. Our updated search yielded a surprisingly limited number of articles in the sociology of sport and sport psychology literature. Before outlining some of this work, it should be noted that there is related media research under the umbrella of "sport, violence, and society". Reviewing this work is outside our scope, but interested readers are referred to Young's (2019) overview on sport, violence, and the media in contact sports.

Sport sociologist Nixon (1993) provided one of the first media studies on sport injury and the media. Cultural meanings of risk, pain, injury, and coming back to play in American sport, were explored through a broad content analysis of *Sports Illustrated* magazine articles between 1969 and 1991. Nixon sought to connect the broader meanings produced within the texts to athlete's willingness to risk their bodies and health to play in professional sports. Media items and/or stories primarily came from journalists, coaches, retired athletes, doctors, and trainers, providing the opportunity to explore the social (re)production of meanings. The results of the content analysis identified six overarching themes, which showed that male athletes are exposed to a set of mediated beliefs that coalesce the message that they must accept risks of pain and injury in sport as normal and necessary. These themes related to structural influences (e.g., constraints about what it means to be an athlete), structural inducements (e.g., prospects, rewards, and encouragements for athletes), cultural values of sport (e.g., good character, pain tolerance), and athletic socialization (e.g., multiple others in the sport context reinforcing pain and injury tolerance), that collectively conveyed the message that athletes should accept the risks, pain, and injuries of sport. Of particular interest to sport injury psychology was that Nixon linked findings concerning risk culture and the sport ethic to athlete health and well-being, which was compromised due to athletes "suffering in silence". Issues identified included guilt, shame, job insecurity, and depression among those with disabling injuries. Although this study is over 25 years old, it shows the value of systematically studying the media to learn more about sport culture, pain, and injury meanings, and a prevalent issue still shown to compromise injured athletes' health: returning to play after injuries (McGannon, Cunningham, & Schinke, 2013).

Nixon's study is one in which media representation was the focus, rather than the interrelated aspects of production and/or consumption, although the consumption of the mediated messages and meanings were implied given Nixon's (1993) findings were connected to athletes' identities, performances, and lives. The majority of media research on sport injury has followed a similar track, exploring media representations and the health, injury, and safety implications for athletes and other social agents. A recent example of this work explored mainstream print news media's framing of two injury incidents involving two prominent National Football League (NFL) quarterbacks – Jay Cutler and Robert Griffin II – who became injured during games (Sanderson, Weathers, Grevious, Tehan, & Warren, 2016). Cutler incurred a serious knee injury during the second quarter and tried to return but ceased playing and remained on the sidelines to watch his team, while Griffin sustained an injury with only six minutes remaining and left the field. Analysis of 177 print news representations of these two incidents showed contradictory portrayals of the athletes and injury meanings. Cutler's masculinity and toughness was questioned in some portrayals by downplaying the severity of injury, while other portrayals supported him for taking care of his health. Griffin was given heroic status in portrayals for sacrificing his body for his team by incurring the injury due to its severity. This media analysis also showed that some news media portrayals of the injuries that both athletes incurred shifted blame to social agents (e.g., coaches, the organization) with some noting aspects of risk culture (e.g., inherent pressures to play injured to demonstrate masculinity). This study shows the advantages of centralizing a particular media incident and high-profile athletes to learn more about the narratives that reinforce the sport ethic, but also beginning to question it, shifting some blame and responsibility off the athlete to others' role in the sociocultural sport context.

Additional media work on sport injury has primarily focused on concussion and/or the progressive degenerative disease of the brain, chronic traumatic encephalopathy (CTE), in sport media forms. An example of this work comes from Anderson and Kian's (2012) exploration of the news media's characterization of NFL player Aaron Rodger's self-withdrawal after hitting his head. An analysis of ten news media outlets from print media and internet sources also showed that news media were beginning to draw attention to athlete health and CTE, questioning a pain and risk narrative, and noting a "softening of masculinity". This study is of value and interest to sport injury psychology because it highlights how media narratives surrounding the portrayal athlete's injuries can resist dominant narratives surrounding risk and the sport ethic, allowing for male athletes taking care of their bodies and health.

The media has undoubtedly played a role is raising awareness concerning concussion and CTE, pain, and risk culture in sport, as further shown in Furness' (2016) analysis of the television documentary "League of Denial" which exposed the NFL and pro-football's complicity in concussion and CTE injury. This analysis showed that concussion was framed as a "crisis" through resistance of the sport ethic and of risk culture that position injury and violence as necessary parts of the game. Importantly, this analysis also drew attention to the film's critiques of the media's role – and use as a cultural site – in constructing football, pain, and injury as a spectacle that has contributed to the cultural context in which the "concussion crisis" has emerged. Ventresca's (2019) recent analysis is a rare exploration of how multiple media sources (news stories, documentary films, popular books) and scientific studies further coalesce dominant understandings of CTE as an "urgent public health problem" but remains characterized by scientific uncertainty, and downplaying athletes' voices and experiences.

Finally, McGannon et al. (2013) explored news media portrayals of National Hockey League (NHL) star Sidney Crosby's incurrence of a concussion (see Chapter 4) from controversial hits in back-to-back games that sidelined him for ten months. This study was the only one positioned in sport psychology. Analysis of 150 articles showed that injury meanings were constructed within an over-arching narrative: a culture of risk and its impact on athletes. Multiple meanings of concussion within the risk narrative were linked to three sub-narratives: (a) Crosby's concussion as a cautionary tale, (b) Crosby's concussion as a political platform, and (c) concussion as an ambiguous injury. These findings drew attention to previous media portrayals of concussion being based solely on physical risks and symptomology, with little, if any, discussion of psychosocial issues and concussion. This is problematic given that sport psychology research on athlete concussion has repeatedly identified psychological and social consequences, which can result in anxiety, depression, and isolation for athletes.

Future Research Implications

The foregoing media research examples provide a glimpse of what sport injury and media investigations might focus on. These studies show that the media is a valuable data resource to explore narratives and representations of sport injury and some of the implications (e.g., social, psychological, health, awareness of injury issues in sport). While this work is of benefit for researchers interested in socio-cultural and psychological aspects of sport injury, much of this work is limited in scope. Our critical literature review shows that researchers have focused on media representations (termed first-generation media research, see Millington & Wilson, 2016) and less on the intertwining of production, representation, and consumption side of media work. Given that the dynamic media environment includes a range of media forms within which journalists, fans, sport organizations, coaches, sport psychologists, sports medicine staff, and athletes can participate to produce and change narratives and representations within them, an exploration of these blurred lines from different social agent vantage points between production, representation, and consumption is warranted. Millington and Wilson (2016) termed this media research stream "pro-sumption", whereby investigations focus on sport injury meanings, values, and/or athlete identities, in both mainstream media forms (e.g., news media, television, film) and new media forms (e.g., Instagram, Twitter, Facebook, YouTube).

Related to the above point regarding "pro-sumption" of media is that no investigations of have systematically explored how social agents (e.g., athletes, coaches, parents, sports medicine staff, sport psychology consultants) engage with and/or react to media stories about injury and athletes. Analysis of athlete injury media stories across a range of sports and contexts are absent within the literature, with the focus on contact sports as "risky spaces", primarily for concussion and CTE. Female athletes and younger athletes have also been under-researched with respect to the media and sport injury. Media representations of acute/traumatic injury or overuse injuries in relation to athlete's identities and lives across the injury experience (e.g., incurring injury, rehabilitation, recovery, retirement) could be explored to expand media research and sport injury psychology research. The findings could then be used to make suggestions toward building on second- and third-generation media research, whereby applied recommendations are made (second-generation) alongside how these might contribute toward social change (third-generation) (Millington & Wilson, 2016). In this regard, the media can be used as a concrete entry point for educating practitioners and athletes through showing them forms of "identity and sport injury talk" and/or images within various media forms (e.g., narrative or documentary film, Instagram, Facebook, Twitter). Through one-on-one or focus group discussions (see Chapter 12), various meanings can be highlighted, and data collected and analyzed concerning whether or not these align with athlete experiences, and the implications for mental health, rehabilitation, and performance. In turn, awareness can be raised as to how concrete forms of talk (rather than mental states within the person) as shown within various media forms, offer entry points of social action for researchers, consultants, and athletes, expanding narrative resources at individual and social levels.

Social media forms can also be studied in their own right as "naturalistic data" resources to learn more about how athletes view themselves, unsolicited through online forums, Instagram, Twitter, Facebook posts, or blog postings concerning sport injury–related topics (e.g., injury meaning, rehabilitation, retirement, reactions to injury stories in the media). Finally, social media data – as shown in our opening example – could also be explored intertextually in terms of how athletes mobilize the media to resist or reconfigure narratives that are less, or more, productive for psychological well-being, sport participation, and performance. The research in sport sociology concerning pain and risk culture has primarily focused on what is inherently bad and/or threatening for athlete health (Atkinson, 2019). Sport injury psychology work has shown that injuries can be repositioned by athletes for growth (Wadey et al., 2019). Studying the production, representation, and consumption aspects of sport injury in relation to growth and positivity in media forms would also expand understanding.

Conclusion

In this chapter, the value and benefits of studying the media as a cultural site to expand sport injury psychology research was outlined. Despite the potential to expand sport injury understanding in a sociocultural context, the media has been minimally "tapped" as a data resource to learn more about sport injury meanings and athlete experiences and identities. Given that media research on sport injury has developed at a slow pace, the exploration of the media in its many ubiquitous forms (e.g., Twitter, Facebook, Instagram, blogs, television, film) to study sport injury psychology topics is wide open. Qualitative research methods might be particularly advantageous to use to learn more about the sociocultural construction of sport injury regarding first-, second-, and third-wave media research.

Critical Discussion Questions

1) How might forms of media research be utilized to fill contentious issues or gaps in sport injury psychology research?

2) What new, or different, research questions can be generated by studying the intertwining of media production, representation, and consumption?

3) In what ways can social media forms be used by practitioners, social agents, and athletes, as forms of activism or sport injury reform?

References

Anderson, E., & Kian, E. M. (2012). Examining media contestation of masculinity and head trauma in the National Football League. *Men and Masculinities*, *15*(2), 152–173. doi: 10.1177/1097184X11430127

Andrews, D. L., & Jackson, S. J. (2001). Sport celebrities, public culture, and private experience. In D. L. Andrews & S. J. Jackson (Eds.), *Sport stars: The cultural politics of sporting celebrity* (pp. 1–19). London: Routledge.

Atkinson, M. A. (2019). Sport and risk culture. In K. Young (Ed.), *The suffering body in sport: Shifting thresholds of risk, pain and injury* (pp. 5–21). Bingley, UK: Emerald Publishing.

Bieler, D. (2019, April 12). 'My pain is not your entertainment': Gymnast who broke both legs wants people to stop sharing injury video. *The national post*. Retrieved from https://nationalpost.com/news/world/my-pain-is-not-your-entertainment-gymnast-who-broke-both-legs-wants-people-to-stop-sharing-injury-video

Billings, A., & Hardin, M. (2014). *Routledge handbook of sport and new media*. London: Routledge.

Bonhomme, J., Seanor, M., Schinke, R. J., & Stambulova, N. B. (2020). The career trajectories of two world champion boxers: Interpretive thematic analysis of media stories. *Sport in Society*, *23*(4), 560–576. doi: 10.1080/17430437.2018.1463727

Bundon, A. (2016). The web and digital qualitative methods: Researching online and researching the online in sport and exercise studies. In B. Smith & A. C. Sparkes (Eds.), *Routledge handbook of qualitative research in sport and exercise* (pp. 355–367). London: Routledge.

Bundon, A. (2017). *Digital qualitative research in sport and exercise*. London: Routledge.

Cosh, S., Crabb, S., & Tully, P. J. (2015). A champion out of the pool? A discursive exploration of two Australian Olympic swimmers' transition from elite sport to retirement. *Psychology of Sport and Exercise*, *19*, 33–41. doi: 10.1016/j.psychsport.2015.02.006

Furness, Z. (2016). Reframing concussions, masculinity, and NFL mythology in League of Denial. *Popular Communication*, *14*(1), 49–57. doi: 10.1080/15405702.2015.1084628

Howe, D. (2004). *Sport, professionalism and pain: Ethnographies of injury and risk*. London: Routledge.

Hughes, R., & Coakley, J. (1991). Positive deviance among athletes: The implications of over conformity to the sports ethic. *Social of Sport Journal*, *8*, 307–325. doi: 10.1123/ssj.8.4.307

McGannon, K. R., Cunningham, S. M., & Schinke, R. J. (2013). Understanding concussion in socio-cultural context: A media analysis of a National Hockey League star's concussion. *Psychology of Sport and Exercise*, *14*(6), 891–899. doi: 10.1016/j.psychsport.2013.08.003

McGannon, K. R., Gonsalves, C. A., Schinke, R. J., & Busanich, R. (2015). Negotiating motherhood and athletic identity: A qualitative analysis of Olympic athlete mother representations in media narratives. *Psychology of Sport and Exercise*, *20*, 51–59. doi: 10.1016/j.psychsport.2015.04.010

McGannon, K. R., & McMahon, J. (2016). Media representations and athlete identities: Examining benefits for sport psychology. *Qualitative Methods in Psychology Bulletin*, *22*, 43–53.

McGannon, K. R., & Smith, B. (2015). Centralizing culture in cultural sport psychology research: The potential of narrative inquiry and discursive psychology. *Psychology of Sport and Exercise, 17*, 79–87. doi: 10.1016/j.psychsport.2014.07.010

McMahon, J. A., & Barker-Ruchti, N. (2016). The media's role in transmitting a cultural ideology and the effect on the general public. *Qualitative Research in Sport, Exercise, and Health, 8*(2), 131–146. doi: 10.1080/2159676X.2015.1121912

McMahon, J. A., McGannon, K. R., & Zehntner, C. (2017). Slim to win: An ethnodrama of three elite swimmers' 'presentation of self' in relation to dominant cultural ideology. *Sociology of Sport Journal, 34*(2), 108–123. doi: 10.1123/ssj.2015-0166

Millington, B., & Wilson, B. (2016). Media research: From text to context. In B. Smith & A. Sparkes (Eds.), *Routledge international handbook of qualitative research in sport and exercise* (pp. 152–242). London: Routledge.

Nixon, H. L. (1992). A social network analysis of influences on athletes to play with pain and injuries. *Journal of Sport and Social Issues, 16*(2), 127–135. doi: 10.1177/019372359201600208

Nixon, H. L. (1993). Accepting the risks of pain and injury in sport: Mediated cultural influences on playing hurt. *Sociology of Sport Journal, 10*(2), 183–196. doi: 10.1123/ssj.10.2.183

Pedersen, P. M. (2013). *Routledge handbook of sport communication.* London: Routledge.

Roderick, M. (2006). The sociology of pain and injury in sport: Main perspectives and problems. In S. Loland, B. Skirstad & I. Waddington (Eds.), *Pain and injury in sport: Social and ethical analysis* (pp. 17–33). London: Routledge.

Sabo, D. (2009). Sports injury, the pain principle, and the promise of reform. *Journal of Intercollegiate Athletics, 2*(1), 145–152. doi: 10.1123/jis.2.1.145

Sabo, D., & Jansen, S. C. (1998). Prometheus unbound: Constructions of masculinity in the sports media. In L. A. Wenner (Ed.), *Mediasport* (pp. 202–217). London: Routledge.

Safai, P. (2003). Healing the body in the "culture of risk": Examining the negotiation of treatment between sport medicine clinicians and injured athletes in Canadian intercollegiate sport. *Sociology of Sport Journal, 20*(2), 127–146. doi: 10.1123/ssj.20.2.127

Sanderson, J., Weathers, M., Grevious, A., Tehan, M., & Warren, S. (2016). A hero or sissy? Exploring media framings of NFL quarterbacks injury decisions. *Communication and Sport, 4*(1), 3–22. doi: 10.1177/2167479514536982

Slater, M. J., Barker, J. B., Coffee, P., & Jones, M. V. (2015). Leading for gold: Social identity leadership processes at the London 2012 Olympic Games. *Qualitative Research in Sport, Exercise, and Health, 7*(2), 192–209. doi: 10.1080/2159676X.2014.936030

Ventresca, M. (2019). The curious case of CTE: Mediating materialities of traumatic brain injury. *Communication and Sport, 7*(2), 135–156. doi: 10.1177/2167479518761636

Wadey, R., Day, M., Cavallerio, F., & Martinelli, L. (2019). Multilevel model of sport injuries (MMSI): Can coaches impact and be impacted by sport injury? In R. Thelwell & M. Dicks (Eds.), *Professional advances in sports coaching: Research and practice* (pp. 540–580). London: Routledge.

Wenner, L. A. (2015). Sport and media. In R. Giulanotti (Ed.), *Routledge handbook of the sociology of sport* (pp. 377–387). London: Routledge.

Wiese-Bjornstal, D. M. (2010). Psychology and socioculture affect injury risk, response, and recovery in high-intensity athletes: A consensus statement. *Scandinavian Journal of Medicine and Science in Sports, 20* Suppl. 2, 103–111. doi: 10.1111/j.1600-0838.2010.01195.x.

Wiese-Bjornstal, D. M., Smith, A. M., Shaffer, S. M., & Morrey, M. A. (1998). An integrated model of response to sport injury: Psychological and sociological dynamics. *Journal of Applied Sport Psychology, 10*(1), 46–69. doi: 10.1080/10413209808406377

Young, K. (1993). Violence, risk, and liability in male sports culture. *Sociology of Sport Journal*, *10*(4), 373–396. doi: 10.1123/ssj.10.4.373

Young, K. (2004). Sports related pain and injury: Sociological notes. In K. Young (Ed.), *Sporting bodies, damaged selves: Sociological studies of sports-related injury* (pp. 1–25). Oxford, UK: Elsevier Press.

Young, K. (2019). An eye on SRV: The role of the media. In K. Young (Ed.), *Sport, violence and society* (2nd ed.) (pp. 231–265). London: Routledge.

Young, K., McTeer, W., & White, P. (1994). Body talk: Male athletes reflect on sport, injury, and pain. *Sociology of Sport Journal*, 11, 175–194. doi: 10.1123/ssj.11.2.175

3   Gender Matters!

How Can Sociocultural Perspectives on Pain, Injury, and the Sporting Body Benefit Future Research in Sport Injury Psychology?

Tanya Bunsell and Mark Doidge

Introduction

Despite the growing body of literature available on gender, pain, and injury within sport sociology, history, philosophy, feminism, and, more recently, cultural sport psychology, little has been disseminated and engaged with in sport injury psychology research to inform professional practice. In addition, there has been increasing inquiry into the gendered dimensions of injuries within physical performance, especially in regard to understanding "the specific risks that women face and how they may be reduced" (Theberge, 2012, p. 183). Yet the social context in which these gendered dimensions take place has frequently been overlooked in the sport injury psychology literature, despite repeated calls to explore the sociocultural context to further understand injury meanings, response, and recovery of injured athletes (Wadey, Day, Cavallerio, & Martinelli, 2018; Wiese-Bjornstal, 2010; Wiese-Bjornstal, Smith, Shaffer, & Morrey, 1998). According to Gill and Kamphoff (2010) this is due to sport psychology research mirroring the gendered boundaries of elite sport, which is a male-dominated realm which values the "hard" sciences.

To understand the gendered aspects of pain, this chapter recognizes pain as the unwanted, injurious type that disrupts and constricts one's habitual world (Leder, 1990). Pain is cultural; how we interpret it, the stories and metaphors we use to describe it, and how others react to it, are all determined by our sociocultural perspective. Yet, at the same time it clearly impacts upon our corporeal selves. As Scarry (1985) argues, pain is not an abstract, passive phenomenon, but is real – it hurts and is literally carved out of and into a fleshy, sentient body. Significant pain changes everything. The physical leans powerfully upon one's ability to meet social expectations of what one "ought to be" (Goffman, 1983). If, our identity is formed through our interactions, then this feedback will inevitably assail the foundations of our identity creating an "ontological assault" on the embodied gendered self (Shilling, 2008, p.114).

This chapter argues that our bodies are inscribed by society, that these bodies can be transformed by pain, and that pain is gendered.[1] Gender shapes our interpretations of pain, and its impact on our identity, narratives, interactions, and outlook. In particular, within sport, gender may impact upon athletes' perceptions of their identity, health, and even recovery time. It is vital that sport injury psychology researchers and practitioners, along with the wider network of sport professionals that includes coaches, physiotherapists, and strength and conditioning instructors, are aware of the gendered dimensions of pain and injury in order to provide the appropriate support to athletes. This may entail a questioning of both their own and the athletes' perceptions, biases, and practices. In order to critically review and raise awareness of the sociocultural research to inform future research in sport injury psychology, this chapter introduces the historical dimensions that led to the female body being seen as weaker. This is followed by the role sport plays in reinforcing masculinity, before focusing on how female athletes have challenged these notions through sport, and before assessing how this impacts our understandings of pain and injury. The chapter will then close with future research directions and critical discussion questions.

Women as the Weaker Sex: An Historical Overview

Traditionally, Western thought emphasized that humans are made up of "two opposed dichotomous characteristics: mind and body, thought and extension, reason and passion, psychology and biology" (Grosz, 1994, p. 3). This mind–body dualism is hierarchical, with the "higher" realm of the mind pitted against the unruly, irrational temptress of the body. Advances in neurological analysis have attempted to dismantle this dualism by arguing that the somatic body is a unified entity that changes over time through various physical, psychological, social, and neurological influences (Damasio, 1994). Developing the notion of the socialized body, Turner (1996, p. 6) argues that, "politics are expressed through the conduit of the human body". Consequently, the body becomes a site through which the power relations of gender are played out. The female reproductive system has come to symbolize women as more embodied and in need of physical protection. In contrast, male embodiment is seen as less restrictive, which has enabled men more freedom to engage in a range of activities (Shilling, 1993). Women's bodies have therefore been perceived as controlling their minds and thereby in need of protection, while men's minds have been viewed as controlling their bodies, including the ability to "overcome" pain.

Feminist analysis from the 1960s to the 1990s (labeled Second-Wave Feminism) argued that the discourses, ideologies, and practices surrounding women's bodies have been used to justify gender inequalities and in turn have been used to shape women's bodies and lives (Martin, 2001). Sex distinctions between "male" and "female" became increasingly important; they were defined in opposition to each other based on anatomical differences. These biological differences became the foundations in which the disparity between masculine and feminine identities could be understood. Femininity became synonymous, at least for the white, middle-class woman, with embodied qualities of weakness, passivity, sickliness, and fragility. This contrasts significantly with the image of the self-contained male body and the heroic masculine ideals of a "strong, stoic, resolutely independent, self-disciplined individual who holds himself erect with self-control, proud of his capacity to distance himself from his body" (Bologh, 1990, p. 17).

Scientific theories were used to justify women's exclusion from the public sphere, including sport. Females were seen as incapable of strenuous activity, which was believed to take the limited supply of energy away from, and damage, their reproductive systems, as well as making women unfeminine and unattractive (Vertinsky, 1994). Not only was sport unfeminine, due to violence and aggression, which was perceived as going against women's more caring, nurturing, and gentle nature, but women were seen as more sensitive to pain and as physically too fragile. The twentieth century, however, saw a rapid cultural shift in gender ideologies. Against the political backdrop of the women's rights movement, and the two World War's fitness drives and concerns over the health of the nation, along with the opportunities that the wars opened up for females, an increasing number of women began to participate in the realms of work and sport. With the removal of some legal barriers, new laws around sex discrimination, and the creation of a compulsory physical education curriculum within schools, the 1960s and 1970s saw a rapid expansion of females participating in sport (Theberge, 2012).

As more women took up sport, they challenged social conventions on two related but distinguishable aspects: first, the notion that femininity corresponded with weakness and masculinity equated strength, and second, the idea that female athletes were automatically masculine. Nevertheless, old ideologies lingered. Despite Violet Piercy running the marathon distance between Windsor and London in 1926, women were excluded from marathon competition. Roberta Gibbs unofficially ran the Boston Marathon in 1966, 1967, and 1968, and Katherine Switzer famously entered the race in 1967 (under the name K. V. Switzer), where a male race official attempted to rip off her number and eject her from the race. It was not until 1972 that women were officially allowed to run the Boston Marathon.

Persistent gender stereotypes meant that sports were frequently deemed either "feminine" or "masculine". Females who participated in overtly masculine activities such as rugby or bodybuilding were stigmatized as gender outlaws. In this light, sports deemed violent or dangerous, like boxing and ski-jumping, have only become Olympic sports for women since 2012 and 2014 respectively. Indeed, the London 2012 Olympics was the first Olympics when every national team and event had female athletes.[2] While men still dominate the territory of sport, and hold the larger part of professional positions, women continue to "gain ground" with an unprecedented number of women now participating in sport and physical activity (Theberge, 2006). In turn, this increase, along with the professionalism of female sports, has meant there is an increase in the risk of pain and injury. Before investigating further female athletes' relationship to pain and injury, it is worth examining the social-cultural context further, "fleshing out" how pain and injury have been associated with masculinity in sport.

"Take it Like a Man": Becoming a Man Through Sport

Historically, sports have "validated masculinity" and made possible a strong and assertive proclamation of men's strength, valor, and, above all, superiority over women (Dunning, 1999). Earlier literature on sports and masculinities focused on the ways sports define and reinforce traditional concepts of masculinity. The work of Lenskyj (1990) and Messner (1992) highlighted how team sports provide a safe and acceptable space for male bonding and intimacy, yet at the same time encourage competition and status hierarchies (Connell, 1992). Those at the top of the hierarchy embody traits of strength, power, force, dominance, capability, authority, sexual prowess, and the ability to give and endure pain and take risks, whereas those at the bottom embody traits associated with femininity such as vulnerability, softness, kindness, and showing emotion. Those demonstrating "feminine" traits were subsequently subordinated and stigmatized. Tolerance of pain thus becomes a sign of masculinity and (physical and mental) strength.

The male body is not just a physical entity but an embodied way of orientating the world. As Connell (1987, p. 297) explains: "It involves the size and shape, habits of posture and movement, particular skills and lack of others, the image of one's own body, the way it is presented to others and the ways they respond to it". Sport can be seen as a masculinizing process, where males learn to "be a man" and form male identity through the use of their body: that is, to exhibit violence, toughness, and aggression, and as a mechanism for reproducing "femphobic", homophobic, and misogynistic attitudes (Dunning, 1999). Sports operate on a spectrum, with more masculine sports being those that regularly engage in physical contact and violence, such as rugby and combat sports. Within the sporting domain, the body is often portrayed as an obstacle to be overcome, dominated and controlled by the will of the mind, or as a well-oiled machine or dangerous weapon (Messner, 1992). The plethora of violent analogies, slogans, and metaphors (cf. Medlin-Silver, Lampard, & Bunsell, 2017; Young, 2012), which are still highly visible today are a testament to the ingrained ideology of mind–body dualism.

Sport can be viewed as an institution for reproducing hegemonic masculinities and legitimizing violence in all its forms, including that of pain and injury (Young, 2012). This normalization of pain and injury within the culture of sport requires athletes to endure physical hardship leading to a high tolerance of pain (Pike, 2004). Through body pedagogies bodies become hardened. Furthermore, pain frequently becomes glorified within the sporting subculture, with injuries often being perceived as something to be to fought and not "given in" to. This hero status is often reiterated in the media (see Chapter 2), which includes narratives of male athletes who conquer their injuries and go on to compete, refusing to submit or admit defeat despite their suffering. Young, McTeer, and White (1994, p. 176) explain this attitude as part of the "machismo and fatalism of athletic culture", although the "character-building" qualities of toughness, endurance of pain, and discipline, can equally be applied to the army or other types of male-dominated institutions. Hughes and Coakley (1991) postulate that this is embedded within the "sport ethic": of striving for distinction, making sacrifices, playing through pain, and accepting few limits in the quest for success, team spirit, and status. Athletes, coaches, and other sport professionals are heavily invested in this ideology (Nixon, 1992). Roderick, Waddington, and Parker (2000, p. 7), argue that "playing with pain or when injured is a central aspect of the culture of professional football", and is regarded as a "good attitude" by managers, with physiotherapists and medical clinicians collaborating to get players on the field and keep them there (see Chapter 9). Indeed, those bodies that do not conform may be stigmatized, ignored, or inconvenienced as a result (see Chapter 6).

Kotarba (1983), however, believes the situation is more complex, with athletes making rational decisions in the presence of pain and injury, based upon its perceived severity, their age, and their career stage. Likewise, Malcolm and Sheard's (2002) work on elite rugby players suggests that far from professionalism encouraging players to sacrifice themselves there is a decreasing tolerance to playing with injury with its associated risk of longer-term physical damage. In reality, many players consider a range of complex and contradictory negotiations between competing discourses, including violence, ethics, and perhaps surprisingly, feminism (Pringle & Markula, 2005).

Since the turn of the century, research has focused more on how athletes actually experience pain and the sociocultural ramifications of pain and injury (Allen-Collinson, 2005; Atkinson, 2008; Hockey & Allen-Collinson, 2007; Howe, 2004; Loland, Skirstad, & Waddington, 2006; Sparkes & Smith, 2003; Young 1993, 2004). This small but growing body of research in this area has debunked the myth of "unfeeling" men in sport. It is well known that players with chronic, severe, and career-ending injuries may experience depression, frustration, shame, bodily betrayal, corporeal alienation/dissociation, guilt, low self-esteem, and low confidence (Sparkes & Smith, 2003; Young, 2012). Pain that interrupts athletes' embodied performances has far-reaching effects on their gendered identities, narratives, and their outlooks on their sporting selves and life trajectories (Allen-Collinson, 2005).

Although feminists were the first to point out that pain and injury in sport is a gendered and gendering practice (Young, 1993), there is a double-edged sword of taking risks and playing through pain (Messner, 1990; Sparkes & Smith, 2002). On one side, it is a sporting necessity that creates and reinforces masculinity. On the other, severe and chronic injuries can actually prevent the performance of certain masculinities (Spencer, 2012). Masculinity, like femininity, is not a fixed state, but is relative and always in a process of "becoming". Through sustained habits, intentions, interactions, and performances, a gendered body is assumed, but is never free of the precarious position that it may "fail" to perform gender (Butler, 1990). Pain and injury is one way gender identity may be interrupted. Murphy (1990, p. 94) points out that "for the male, weakening and atrophy of the body threaten all the cultural values of masculinity: strength, activeness, speed, virility, stamina and fortitude". For male athletes who have invested in sporting bodies, this loss of corporeal control may come as a particularly jarring assault to their gendered sense of self (Sparkes, 1998; Sparkes & Smith, 2002; Young, McTeer, & White, 1994); an attack that is further compounded by the pressures within athletic culture and wider society for men to remain quiet and stoic while dealing with their pain.

Pain and injury may only be a brief interruption or may force bodies to adjust to another way of being (cf. Sparkes & Smith, 2002). In the research of Spencer (2012), chronic pain, for one retired MMA fighter, acted as a constant reminder of his loss of status within the masculine hierarchy of the subculture. This is not to argue that the inability to perform violence through participation in sport entails an end to one's embodied masculinity but requires a continual reconstruction of the meanings associated with masculinity.

"We Can Do It!": Women Defying the Myth of the Fragile, Female Body

Comparatively less research has been carried out on the attitudes, experiences, and effects of pain and injury on female athletes. There has also been a lack of research comparing male and female experiences of pain and injury in the same study (Pimenta, 2019). The majority of evidence implies that females embrace the athletic attitude to pain and injury as much as their male counterparts. A masochistic attitude toward the body is encouraged by the subculture, with the omnipresent belief that in order to succeed one must suffer (Aalten, 2007). The study of Ryan (2000) graphically illustrates the psychological and physical abuse that young, female gymnastics undergo with the hope of achieving success, and the "code of silence" that keeps pain hidden. Likewise, Pike (2004) revealed that female rowers embodied similar attitudes to men, viewing the body as a machine/tool and willing to risk and endure pain and injury. Ignoring or hiding pain was normalized and female rowers confessed to training with an injury despite the risk of further damage. Malcom (2006), in her study on softball, also confirms this ethos, where athletes were expected to accept minor injuries as part and parcel of the game and to "tough it out". Females who complained were often accused of being weak or faking it and could be stigmatized.

As females are in a socially weaker position within sport, with stigma around their capabilities, less financial support, and less access to care than males, they may feel more pressure to prove themselves and push through pain and injury (Pike, 2004). For example, female athletes are more likely to subscribe to the culture of risk than their coaches and go beyond the recommended training set down by professionals (Nixon, 1994; Mosewich, Crocker, & Kowalski, 2014). In addition, Granito (2002) suggests that female athletes perceive coaches as acting far more negatively toward them following injury and believe they are taken less seriously. Interestingly, while Pimenta (2019) purports that males are more likely to express their frustrations and anger about incapacitating injuries and indeed even show masculine pride in their health-risking endeavors, Wiese-Bjornstal, Franklin, Dooley, Foster, and Winges (2015) claim that females are more likely to discuss and be open about their injuries. These competing findings not only highlight the lack of research within this sphere but provide a warning not to treat males and females as disparate, homogenous groups. Rather, it is important for sport injury psychology research to recognize the various femininities and masculinities and how they are played out within different sporting subcultures.

There is a scarcity of studies focusing on the effects of injury on female athletes. Nonetheless, research suggests that like their male counterparts, serious pain and injury creates an antagonistic relationship with the body, infringing on an athlete's sense of self, their emotions, social interactions, and how they navigate the world (Hockey & Allen-Collinson, 2007; Sparkes, 1998; Sparkes & Smith, 2003; Young, 2004); furthermore, that injury experiences may also threaten the presentation of the gendered self. Young and White (1995) were perhaps the first to note that injury impacts on a woman's sense of attractiveness and femininity; a point, that may at first view appear paradoxical given that feminine identity and athletic identity have frequently been seen as conflicting (Krane, Choi, Baird, Aimar, & Kauer, 2004). Scolnik, Nakamura, Howard, Murnaghan, and Macpherson (2018) revealed that the injured female body was frequently experienced as undesirable and unfeminine. As women no longer embodied a look which for them represented athleticism, attractiveness, and power, they felt body-conscious and flawed. In particular, dental and facial injuries may be especially harrowing for female athletes, who fail to meet the cultural imperative that females, above all else, should be heteronormatively attractive (Dashper, 2013). Nonetheless, women, it appears, regardless of the sport or level, are just as likely to take bodily risks.

Beyond the Binary?

Female athletes who show fearlessness, physical power, and assertiveness, and embody allegedly male attributes, are antithetical to traditional notions of women as weak, fragile, and soft. These women have been heralded by some feminists as reducing the physical power imbalances on which patriarchy is founded and verified (Castelnuovo & Gutherie, 1998) and creating the possibility of physical liberation (Roth & Bascow, 2004). However, Young and White (1995) argue that despite the increase of women entering the traditionally male domain of sport, rather than transforming the meaning of sport, they are complicit in its macho, violent, and health-compromising ethos. Rather than liberating either gender, it reiterates mind–body dualism by focusing on mastering the "unruly" body. This emphasis on control and invulnerability, with little attention directed to matters of health, limits bodily awareness, stifles emotional expression, and can result in self-destructive and self-loathing practices (Bordo, 1989). Ironically, these opposing views can end up reproducing the dichotomous thinking that they aim to deconstruct, and ignore the complex and competing discourses around pain and injury (cf. Kortaba, 1983; Malcolm & Sheard, 2002; Pringle & Markula, 2005). The research of Pavlidis and Fullagar (2014, p. 496) on roller derby, offers a way of exploring women's sporting corporeality beyond the binary by thinking through affect and subjectification. They concluded that pain "is not only something to simply push past in demonstrating the primacy of (masculine) mind over (female) body. Instead sport offers a relation, between toughness and vulnerability, hurting and nurturing, which enables a reimagining of women's corporeality".

The social landscape has continued to evolve over the last two decades. Within the context of neo-liberalism and its focus on "self-care" and health, there has been a rising concern over player welfare, resulting in awareness campaigns and the implementation of rules, regulations, and policies with the aim of protecting health in all its forms. In turn, this may impact upon a player's willingness and ability to play thorough pain and injury as well as attitudes within the sportsnet and coaching practices. Furthermore, reflecting the changes in society and the array of available identities increasingly seen as acceptable, work by Anderson and McGuire (2010), hints at more inclusive and "softer" masculinities within sport with more men being supportive and caring for each other when injured, with less evidence of excessive risk-taking. In addition, mindfulness-based psychological interventions (see Chapter 16) are being utilized within spor, suggesting that self-compassion may potentially be a beneficial coping strategy for athletes dealing with pain and injury (Mosewich, Crocker, & Kowalski, 2014; Smith, 2013) and could lead to an alternative approach to the body. However, Sutherland et al. (2014) highlighted that female athletes expressed concern that self-compassion would negatively affect their performance and make them "mediocre". This suggests that while there is some evidence that attitudes to pain and injury are changing, a wholesale shift appears unlikely without a dramatic change in the meaning of sport itself and the underpinning ethos that the body needs to be "overcome" in order to win. Understanding these issues, however, will help practitioners to navigate the difficult (and gendered) journey that athletes find themselves on.

Future Research Implications

The trouble with taking essentialist approaches to gender is that it ignores and marginalizes individual lived experiences and reinforces the "gender order" – that of relational female inferiority. Thus, sensitivity and reflexivity are required by practitioners and researchers in order to avoid reproducing the binary. This might include a questioning of both their own and the athlete's perceptions, biases, and practices. Studies exploring differing injury rates and types between males and females and how these can be prevented are vital, but risk, if we are not careful, reviving old ideologies surrounding the "different", more fragile, female body (cf. Theberge, 2012). The challenge lies in acknowledging the importance of sex and gender and how they shape bodily experiences and attitudes around pain and injury, but at the same time, scrutinizing the foundations of the sporting ethic in relation to traditional masculine discourse and questioning the subcultural understandings and practices around this. Although this isn't the space to undertake this analysis, recognizing the masculine foundations of modern sport will help practitioners and researchers to interrogate root traditions of the discourse around sport. Much of this discourse derives from specific nineteenth-century beliefs around masculine superiority. Reflecting on our own assumptions will help unpick these traditions as well as provide more suitable support for athletes.

Understandings of gender have been rooted in Western conceptions of male and female. Consequently, it is necessary to investigate the ways by which dominant ideologies around pain and injury are contested and negotiated, as well as accommodated and affirmed, through the traditional gender binary. But, more than this, we need to reimagine dichotomous thinking – by examining both males' and females' complex and contradictory relationships to pain, and exploring their pain communities (see Chapter 5) and painful affects – and how it creates multiple feminine and masculine subjectivities, and how sport could become a more gender-inclusive transformational cultural site (Pavlidis & Fullagar, 2014). Although this chapter has focussed on the male–female binary, it is important to recognize the lack of research on intersex, non-binary, and transgendered sporting bodies. Not all cultures conform to the Western gender binary and other cultures may recognize a plurality of genders. As pain is socioculturally learned and understood, knowledge of pain and gender needs to take into consideration these sociocultural understandings of gender in order to fully comprehend pain. Consequently, epistemologies of pain should also move beyond traditional Western conceptions of mind and body toward more embodied neurological understandings (Damasio, 1994). Recognizing pain as being sociocultural suggests that future research should take into account the various intersections of athlete identity. These should include not just gender, but also the sociocultural impact of sexuality, ethnicity, age, (dis)ability, and religion.

Finally, taking into account the diverse sociocultural and gendered understandings of pain and injury, future research is also required to understand how to put this into practice (see Chapter 14). Different sports will have their own subcultural expectations and experiences. Various professions working in sport will have their own ways of engaging with pain and injury. And ultimately, each athlete will have their own lived experience that draws upon the various activities, interactions, and understandings they have encountered. Incorporating these strands will further our sociocultural understandings of pain and injury.

Conclusion

This chapter has briefly highlighted how gender structures the attitudes, expectations, and experiences of pain and injury within sporting milieus, touching upon the ways by which injury experiences may threaten the presentation of the gendered self. The literature review supports the crucial call for a shift from primarily cerebral approaches to pain and injury toward more research into the lived experiences of enfleshed subjects. This is particularly important when considering how gender shapes the motivations, identities, interactions, and phenomenological experiences of pain and injury, so listening to lived experiences will help researchers and practitioners understand the nuances of individual athletes. This chapter has raised awareness as to how narratives around pain and injury are constructed through gender, which affects how pain is shared with coaches, other team members, stakeholders, and practitioners. It earnestly echoes the need for sport injury psychology to explore the sociocultural context to further understand injury meanings, response, and recovery of injured athletes. Most of all, the chapter argues that sport psychology can ill afford to ignore gender. Gender matters.

Critical Discussion Questions

1) What is your own attitude to gender, pain, and injury? Where has this come from? How does it impact upon your own body/life and work practice?
2) How might an athlete's pain and injury narrative be shaped through gender?
3) How can we use gender research to inform practice?

Notes

1 Emphasizing the bodily aspects of gender, which is the focus of this chapter, it is useful to define sex and gender at the outset. Most commonly, since around the 1960s, sex is understood as the categorical assignment of either "male" or "female" at birth, based upon "natural", biological anatomy/genitalia (however, as theory and research has evolved, this reductionist understanding of sex has become "problematic"). Gender on the other hand has become recognized as a social construction, based on cultural ideals of femininity and masculinity (for further reading, see Butler, 1990; Connell, 1987; Grosz, 1994; Bordo, 1989; Martin, 2001; Messner, 1992).

2 It should be noted that there is currently only one Olympic sport that is single gender: synchronized swimming (for women only).

References

Aalten, A. (2007). Listening to the dancer's body. *The Sociological Review*, *55*(1_suppl), 109–125. doi: 10.1111/j.1467-954X.2007.00696.x

Allen-Collinson, J. (2005). Emotions, interaction and the injured sporting body. *International Review for the Sociology of Sport*, *40*(2), 221–240. doi: 10.1177/1012690205057203

Anderson, E., & McGuire, R. (2010). Inclusive masculinity and the gendered politics of men's rugby. *The Journal of Gender Studies*, *19*(3), 249–261. doi: 10.1080/09589236.2010.494341

Atkinson, M. (2008). Triathlon, suffering and exciting significance. *Leisure Studies*, *27*(2), 165–180. doi: 10.1080/02614360801902216

Bologh, R. (1990). *Max Weber and masculine thinking - A feminist inquiry*. Boston, MA: Unwin Hyman.

Bordo, S. (1989). The body and the reproduction of femininity: A feminist appropriation of Foucault. In A. Jaggar & S. Bordo (Eds.), *Gender/body/knowledge: Feminist reconstructions of being and knowing* (pp. 13–33). New Brunswick, NJ: Rutgers UP.

Butler, J. (1990). *Gender trouble: Feminism and the subversion of identity*. New York: Routledge.

Castelnuovo, S., & Guthrie, S. R. (1998). *Feminism and the female body: Liberation the amazon within*. London: Lynne Rienner.

Connell, R. (1987). *Gender and power: Society, the person and sexual politics*. Cambridge: Polity Press.

Connell, R. (1992). A very straight gay: Masculinity, homosexual experience and the dynamics of gender. *American Sociological Review*, *57*(6), 735–751. doi: 10.2307/2096120

Damasio, A. (1994). *Descartes' error: Emotion, reason and the human brain*. London: Vintage.

Dashper, K. (2013). Getting better: An autoethnographic tale of recovery from sport injury. *Sociology of Sport Journal*, *30*(3), 323–339. doi: 10.1123/ssj.30.3.323

Dunning, E. (1999). *Sport matters: Sociological studies of sport, violence and civilisation*. London: Routledge.

Gill, D., & Kamphoff, C. (2010). Gender and cultural diversity. In J. M. Williams (Ed.), *Applied sport psychology* (pp. 417–439). New York: McGraw-Hill.

Goffman, E. (1983). The interaction order. *American Sociological Review, 48*(1), 1–17. doi: 10.2307/2095141

Granito, V. (2002). Psychological response to athletic injury: Gender differences. *Journal of Sport Behavior, 25*(3), 243–259.

Grosz, E. (1994). *Volatile bodies: Towards a corporeal feminism.* Bloomington, IN: Indiana University Press.

Hockey, J., & Allen-Collinson, J. (2007). Grasping the phenomenology of sporting bodies. *International Review for the Sociology of Sport, 42*(2), 115–113. doi: 10.1177/1012690207084747

Howe, D. (2004). *Sport, professionalism and pain.* London: Routledge.

Hughes, R., & Coakley, J. (1991). Positive deviance among athletes: The implications of overconformity to the sport ethic. *Sociology of Sport Journal, 8*(4), 307–325. doi: 10.1123/ssj.8.4.307

Kotarba, J. (1983). *The chronic pain.* Beverly Hills, CA: Sage.

Krane, V., Choi, P., Baird, S., Aimar, C., & Kauer, K. (2004). Living the paradox: Female athletes negotiate femininity and muscularity. *Sex Roles, 50*(5/6), 315–329. doi: 10.1023/B:SERS.0000018888.48437.4f

Leder, D. (1990). *The absent body.* Chicago, IL: University of Chicago Press.

Lenskyj, H. (1990). Power and play: Gender and sexuality issues in sport and physical activity. *International Review for the Sociology of Sport, 25*(3), 235–245. doi: 10.1177/101269029002500305

Loland, S., Skirstad, B., & Waddington, I. (2006). *Pain and injury in sport: Social and ethical analysis.* London: Routledge.

Malcolm, D., & Sheard, K. (2002). Pain in the assets: The effects of commercialization and professionalization on the management of injury in English rugby union. *Sociology of Sport Journal, 19*(2), 149–169. doi: 10.1123/ssj.19.2.149

Malcom, N. (2006). "Shaking it off" and "toughing it out": Socialization to pain and injury in girls' softball. *Journal of Contemporary Ethnography, 35*(5), 495–525. doi: 10.1177/0891241605283571

Martin, E. (2001). *The woman in the body: A cultural analysis of reproduction.* Boston, MA: Beacon Press.

Medlin-Silver, N., Lampard, P., & Bunsell, T. (2017). Strength in numbers: An explorative study into the experiences of female strength and conditioning coaches. In A. Milner & J. Braddock (Eds.), *Women in sports: Breaking barriers, facing obstacles* (pp. 125–140). Santa Barbara, CA: Praeger.

Messner, M. (1990). When bodies are weapons: Masculinity and violence in sport. *International Review for the Sociology of Sport, 25*(3), 203–220. doi: 10.1177/101269029002500303

Messner, M. (1992). *Power at play. Sports and the problem of masculinity.* Boston, MA: Beacon Press.

Mosewich, A., Crocker, P., & Kowalski, K. (2014). Managing injury and other setbacks in sport: Experiences of (and resources for) high performance women athletes. *Qualitative Research in Sport, Exercise, and Health, 6*(2), 182–204. doi: 10.1080/2159676X.2013.766810

Murphy, R. (1990). *The body silent.* New York: Henry Holt.

Nixon, H. (1992). A social network analysis of influences on athletes to play with pain and injuries. *Journal of Sport and Social Issues, 16*(2), 127–135. doi: 10.1177/019372359201600208

Nixon, H. (1994). Coaches' views of risk, pain, and injury in sport, with special reference to gender differences. *Sociology of Sport Journal, 11*(1), 79–87. doi: 10.1123/ssj.11.1.79

Pavlidis, A., & Fullagar, S. (2014). The pain and pleasure of roller derby. Thinking through affect and subjectification. *International Journal of Cultural Studies, 18*(5), 483–499. doi: 10.1177/1367877913519309

Pike, E. (2004). Risk, pain, and injury: "A Natural Thing in Rowing". In K. Young (Ed.), *Sporting bodies, damaged selves: Sociological studies of sports-related injury* (pp. 151–162). Oxford: Elsevier Press.

Pimenta, N. (2019). *Experiences of pain and injury in male and female artistic gymnastics: A figurational sociological study* (Doctoral dissertation). Retrieved from https://hdl.handle.net/2134/21784.

Pringle, R., & Makula, P. (2005). No pain is sane after all: A Foucauldian analysis of masculinities in men's experiences in rugby. *Sociology of Sport Journal, 22,* 472–497. doi: 10.1260/174795407783359641

Roderick, M., Waddington, I., & Parker, G. (2000). Playing hurt: Managing injuries in English professional football. *International Review for the Sociology of Sport, 35*(2), 165–180. doi: 10.1177/101269000035002003

Roth, A., & Basow, S. (2004). Femininity, sports, and feminism: Developing a theory of physical liberation. *Journal of Sport and Social Issues, 28*(3), 245–284. doi: 10.1177/0193723504266990

Ryan, J. (2000). *Little girls in pretty boxes: The making and breaking of elite gymnasts and figure skaters.* New York: Warner Books.

Scarry, E. (1985). *The body in pain: The making and unmaking of the world.* New York: Oxford University Press.

Scolnik, M., Nakamura, Y., Howard, A., Murnaghan, L., & Macpherson, A. (2018). A qualitative analysis of the psychosocial effects of injury in female athletes. *Graduate Journal of Sport, Exercise & Physical Education Research, 6,* 29–43.

Shilling, C. (1993). *The body and social theory.* Newbury Park, CA: Sage.

Shilling, C. (2008). *Changing bodies. Habit, crisis and creativity.* London: Sage.

Smith, B. (2013). Disability, sport, and men's narratives of health: A qualitative study. *Health Psychology, 32*(1), 110–119. doi: 10.1037/a0029187

Sparkes, A. (1998). Athletic identity: An Achilles' Heel to the survival of self. *Qualitative Health Research, 8*(5), 644–664. doi: 10.1177/104973239800800506

Sparkes, A., & Smith, B. (2002). Sport, spinal cord injury, embodied masculinities and the dilemmas of narrative identity. *Men and Masculinities, 4*(3), 258–285. doi: 10.1177/1097184X02004003003

Sparkes, A., & Smith, B. (2003). Men, sport, spinal cord injury and narrative time. *Qualitative Research, 3*(3), 295–320. doi: 10.1177/1468794103033002

Spencer, D. (2012). Narratives of despair and loss: Pain, injury and masculinity in the sport of mixed martial arts. *Qualitative Research in Sport, Exercise and Health, 4*(1), 117–137. doi: 10.1080/2159676X.2011.653499

Sutherland, L., Kowalski, K., Ferguson, L., Sabiston, C., Sedgwick, W., & Crocker, P. (2014). Narratives of young women athletes' experiences of emotional pain and self-compassion. *Qualitative Research in Sport, Exercise and Health, 6*(4), 499–516. doi: 10.1080/2159676X.2014.888587

Theberge, N. (2006). The gendering of sports injury: A look at 'progress' in women's sport through a case study of the biomedical discourse on the injured athletic body. *Sport in Society, 9*(4), 634–649. doi: 10.1080/17430430600768876

Theberge, N. (2012). Studying gender and injuries: A comparative analysis of the literature on women's injuries in sport and work. *Eronomics, 55*(2), 183–193. doi: 10.1080/00140139.2011.592602

Turner, B. (1996). *The body and society: Explorations in social theory.* London: Thousand Oaks.

Vertinsky, P. (1994). Gender relations, women's history and sport history: A decade of changing enquiry, 1983–1993. *Journal of Sport and History, 21,* 1–24. Retrieved from www.jstor.org/stable/43610594

Wadey, R., Day, M., Cavallerio, F., & Martinelli, L. (2018). The multilevel model of sport injury: Can coaches impact and be impacted by injury? In R. Thelwell & M. Dicks (Eds.), *Professional advances in sports coaching: Research and practice* (pp. 408–440). New York: Routledge.

Wiese-Bjornstal, D. M. (2010). Psychology and socioculture affect injury risk, response, and recovery in high-intensity athletes: A consensus statement. *Scandinavian Journal of Medicine and Science in Sports, 20*, 103–111. doi: 10.1111/j.1600-0838.2010.01195.x

Wiese-Bjornstal, D. M., Franklin, A. N., Dooley, T. N., Foster, M. A., & Winges, J. B. (2015). Observations about sports injury surveillance and sports medicine psychology among female athletes. *Women in Sport and Physical Activity Journal, 23*(2), 64–73. doi: 10.1123/wspaj.2014-0042

Wiese-Bjornstal, D. M., Smith, A. M., Shaffer, S. M., & Morrey, M. A. (1998). An integrated model of response to sport injury: Psychological and sociological dynamics. *Journal of Applied Sport Psychology, 10*(1), 46–69. doi: 10.1080/10413209808406377

Young, K. (1993). Violence, risk, and liability in male sports culture. *Sociology of Sport Journal, 10*(4), 373–396. doi: 10.1123/ssj.10.4.373

Young, K. (2004). *Sporting bodies, damaged selves: Sociological studies of sports-related injury*. Oxford: Elsevier.

Young, K. (2012). *Sport, violence and society*. London: Routledge.

Young, K., McTeer, W., & White, P. (1994). Body talk: Male athletes reflect on sport, injury, and pain. *Sociology of Sport Journal, 11*(2), 175–194. doi: 10.1123/ssj.11.2.175

Young, K., & White, P. (1995). Sport, physical danger, and injury: The experiences of elite women athletes. *Journal of Sport and Social Issues, 19*(1), 45–61. doi: 10.1177/019372395019001004

4 Sport-Related Concussion

Critical Reflections, Methodological Musings, and New Research Directions

Nikolaus A. Dean

Introduction

Over the last decade there has been increased research attention drawn toward the topic of concussion – which is a mild traumatic brain injury (MTBI) – and more specifically, sport-related concussion (SRC). It is currently estimated that between 1.6 and 3.8 million SRCs occur each year in the United States of America, accounting for approximately 5% to 9% of *all* sport-related injuries (Langlois, Rutland-Brown, & Wald, 2006). However, despite these alarming numbers, and increased research attention, SRC still remains one of "the most complex injuries in sports medicine to diagnose, assess and manage" (McCrory et al., 2017, p. 839). One of the reasons why this injury remains so enigmatic and difficult to diagnose is because of its often asymptomatic and invisible nature, making it difficult for both athletes and medical staff to know if one has sustained a concussion (King, Brughelli, Hume, & Gissane, 2014). In addition to the injury's invisible and silent nature, participants of sporting cultures continue to trivialize and/or downplay SRC as merely a "knock to the head" or "getting one's bell rung" (Khurana & Kaye, 2012). These particular trivialized understandings of SRC can become quite problematic when it comes to accurately reporting, diagnosing, managing, and ultimately preventing the injury, as athletes attitudes are often entrenched in ideas that support the notion of playing through the pain and injury as a way of showing one's commitment to team and/or sporting culture (Hughes & Coakley, 1991). It is this nexus between SRC and ideas about pain, injury, and risk within sporting cultures that ultimately centralizes both my own and other social scientists' interests in this medical and social phenomenon, as we try to better understand the layered complexities and health implications of this injury.

To date, SRC has been explored predominately through the disciplines of epidemiology, neurology, and sensory-motor physiology while only a small, yet burgeoning, body of literature has started to explore SRC from the disciplines of sociology, and social psychology. Through these lenses, scholars have attempted to draw attention to the various ways in which SCR is linked to and often influenced by larger social, political, and cultural factors such as race, age, gender, sporting culture, and sporting environment. However, while this mushrooming of sociological inquiry has yielded the opportunity for researchers to explore SRC from various paradigms, perspectives, and innovative methodologies, there still remain a number of avenues within SRC scholarship where both the sociology of sport and sport-related social psychology research could add tremendous empirical value. To address these gaps and research avenues, I draw upon empirical data from my own research on SRC and use literature from the sociology of sport and social psychology to help ground and support my methodological, ontological, and epistemological (re)imaginings. In what follows, I first outline the current state of the field related to SRC and note the various contributions that sociocultural and social psychological analyses have made when exploring the topic of SRC. Next, I critically draw attention to and reflect upon some of the current traditions, methods, and practices being used by researchers to explore SRC and highlight a few potential research avenues that researchers could consider moving forward. Finally, I conclude this chapter by addressing Malcolm's (2018) call for a "public sociology of SRC", and provide a few suggestions on how we, as sport sociologists, sport psychologists, and researchers studying concussion can better disseminate our research in more meaningful ways and to larger audiences (also see Chapter 14).

Sociocultural Analyses of Sport-Related Concussion

Considering the current "concussion crisis" (Carroll & Rosner, 2012) faced in sport, it is somewhat surprising to know that it was only in the most recent Concussion in Sport Group (CISG) consensus statement (McCrory et al., 2017) that psychological and sociocultural factors were identified as mediating factors to consider when experiencing/managing a MTBI such as concussion (Malcolm, 2019). This was somewhat puzzling, as the exploration of *how* sociocultural factors have influenced how one understands, experiences, interprets, and embodies sport-related injuries isn't necessarily "new" to the fields of sport sociology and social psychology and, in fact, is backed up by a well-established body of literature (see Hughes & Coakley, 1991; Messner, 1990; Nixon, 1992; Sabo, 2004; Wiese-Bjornstal, 2010; Young & White, 1995). However, when it comes to the topic of concussion in sport, sociocultural analyses still remain in what Malcolm (2019) calls the "infancies" of this medical and social phenomenon. In fact, Malcolm has even gone as far as to suggest that sociocultural investigations of concussion "have barely been born" (p. 207) within the realm of sport sociology. This is notable, as sport psychologists McGannon, Cunningham, and Schinke (2013) have also argued that "research from sport sociology [can] provide compelling evidence that psychosocial issues of sport injuries such as concussion can be further understood within the context of socio-cultural influences" (p. 891); while others sport psychologists have noted the value of what both social psychology and psychological theory can provide when describing, explaining, and predicting "human thoughts, feelings, and actions within sport concussion contexts" (Wiese-Bjornstal, White, Russell, & Smith, 2015, p. 182). However, despite these urgencies and calls to action from both the realms of sport sociology and sport psychology, only a handful of studies exist that have explored SRC within a sociocultural context.

To date, a small but mounting body of sociocultural scholarship has explored the ways in which SRC has been framed and represented in sport media (see Anderson & Kian, 2012; Brayton, Helstein, Ramsey, & Rickards, 2019; Cassilo & Sanderson, 2018; McGannon et al., 2013; Sanderson, Weathers, Grevious, Tehan, & Warren, 2016; Ventresca, 2019). For example, research from Anderson and Kian (2012) explored the media framings of National Football League quarterback Aaron Rodgers and his decision to self-withdraw after sustaining a concussion. They found that media coverage and sport reporters seemed to be shifting away from the "warrior narrative" to favor and support the idea of health over sacrifice due to increased cultural awareness about the repercussions of concussion, along with shifting away from hegemonic masculine ideals and notions that one must sacrifice one's body, and play through pain and injury for the good of the team. Moreover, Sanderson et al. (2016), built upon Anderson and Kian's earlier work to suggest that sport journalists' framings of concussion could potentially catalyze a shift in football culture norms, that again, favored one's health over pushing through injury. More recently, Ventresca (2019) examined how media discourses were sites of multiple "becomings" of chronic traumatic encephalopathy (CTE) – the degenerative brain disease linked with multiple concussions – and found that these discourses were sites where multiple actors, including journalists, scientists, sport organizations, and athletes struggled to accurately represent and conceptualize the material complexities of the disease. Through these mass-media analyses, researchers have been able to identify the various ways in which concussion has been framed and represented across media platforms and have, importantly, highlighted some of the outcomes, influences, and repercussions that these representations of concussion have had on audience members and sporting cultures.

While media analyses of concussion appear to be developing and growing within the realm of sociocultural analyses, the exploration of the lived experience of SRC still remains less developed, and only a handful of studies have explored the topic. Malcolm's (2009) earlier research on elite rugby players found that the athlete's attitudes toward concussion were shaped by ambiguous and uncertain understandings about the injury and found that these understandings informed the athlete's decision on how to manage their concussive injuries. In addition, Sanderson Weathers, Snedaker, and Gramlich (2017) explored athletes' reasons for (not) reporting a SRC. In their study, they determined that male athletes were more likely to play through and not report a concussion than female athletes and found that both male and female athletes did not report a concussion for three main reasons: (1) perceived lack of resources (i.e., lack of medical trainer on site), (2) perceived lack of severity, and (3) conformance to sporting culture norms. In more recent work, Liston, McDowell, Malcolm, Scott, and Waddington (2018) used qualitative interviews to explore and capture athletes' perceptions and attitudes toward SRC in non-elite rugby. What they found was that the athletes displayed irreverent attitudes toward concussion, which, they argued, encouraged risk-taking behaviors and ultimately led to the denial of and downplaying of SRC in rugby culture. Similarly, recent research from Dean and Bundon (2019) used qualitative interviews to explore understandings of SRC in Canadian surf culture. They found that both male and female surfers were willing to accept risks and push through their concussive symptoms as a way of showing one's commitment to the surfing subculture and found that surfers would return to surf following a suspected concussion for three reasons: (1) wave conditions, (2) limited amount of time to surf, (3) and pressure from others in the water.

Finally, using the method of autoethnography, I used my own personal narratives as a way to draw attention to the ways in which larger political, social, and cultural factors influenced how I perceived, embodied, and experienced SRC within a post-secondary sporting culture (Dean, 2019). By drawing upon and reflecting upon my own experiences of SRC, I used the method of autoethnography (see Chapter 12) not only to give a voice to SRC but also to provide a nuanced perspective of the injury. Collectively, through these studies, myself and others have contended that exploring lived experiences of SRC can help illuminate how various sociocultural factors can influence how athletes perceive, give meaning toward, and manage SRC. Considering the academic work before us, I now critically draw attention to a few different areas of interest that I believe warrant further investigation from sport sociology, sport psychology, and other academic disciplines, as we try to better understand this medical and social phenomenon.

Future Research Implications

Exploring SRC in Alternative, Individualized, and Non-Contact Sporting Cultures

To date, the majority of SRC-based research has focused on three commonalities: "traditional"[1] sport, team sport, and contact sport. In fact, the vast majority of SRC studies have explored concussion in the sports of rugby, hockey, and football. This, of course, is understandable when one considers that these three sports have consistently shown some of the highest rates of concussion within sporting cultures (Putukian, D'Alonzo, Campbell-McGovern, & Wiebe, 2019). Yet, at the same time, this overreliance on traditional, team, and contact sports has meant that a number of other sporting contexts – that do not fit this above criterion – have been left unexamined. This gap is significant, as injury-based studies have also shown that SRC in rates alternative,[2] individualized, and non-contact sports are occurring at similar, if not greater rates in some sporting contexts. For example, epidemiological studies exploring the rates of injuries in skateboarding (Shuman & Meyers, 2015), mountain biking (Becker & Moroder, 2017), and surfing (Klick, Jones, & Alder, 2016; Swinney, 2015) have all noted the regularity of head-related injuries and SRC within their sporting environments. However, despite these findings, little research attention has examined SRC within alternative sporting (sub)cultures. This academic dearth, I argue, may offer ripe areas of inquiry for both sport sociologists and sport psychologists to further investigate, and could provide nuanced understandings of SRC within alternative sporting milieus.

One of the reasons why it is important to examine SRC within alternative sporting cultures is because of the space in which these activities often take place within. For example, most traditional sports take place within regimented sporting areas that are both specifically designed for sport, and often house personnel and resources to assist an athlete in case of an injury. However, differing from these sporting contexts, alternatives sports often take place outside of traditional sporting arenas, and take place within spaces that lack regulation, supervision, and confined spatial configurations. Unlike traditional sports, alternative sports can occur within spaces such as the water and/or ocean (i.e., surfing, kite-surfing, kayaking), the mountains and in the wilderness (i.e., mountain biking, rock climbing, skiing and snowboarding), and within and around urban spaces and cityscapes (i.e., skateboarding, parkour, in-line skating). What makes these sporting landscapes unique and different from traditional sporting spaces – aside from the lack of proximal resources such as coaches, teammates trainers and/or medical staff – is the fact that these activities often take place within remote and sometimes risky and/or dangerous spaces. Stranger (2011) speaks directly to this point when discussing risk of injury in surfing, arguing that "any injury in the surf, especially a knock to the head, presents a far greater risk than the same level of injury on a [traditional] playing field" (p. 95). Further contending that unlike traditional sports – who have resources and first aid on hand – participants of alternative sports, such as surfing can be "alone and/or long distances—even days—from medical assistance" (p. 96). While Stranger speaks directly toward surfers' navigations of injury, his commentary still resonates with alternative sports more broadly, and illuminates the unique sporting environments in which alternative sports take place.

It has been suggested that participants of alternative sports often leave traditional sports due to the overbearing rules and regulations emphasized within their respected sporting cultures and seek out sporting contexts that emphasize and engender ideas of freedom, risk-taking, creativity, and individuality (Wheaton, 2013). Yet, when it comes to sport-related injuries and/or SRC within these sporting contexts, not having proximal resources available to treat a potential SRC can influence how one diagnoses, manages, and decides to return-to-play (Kroshus, Garnett, Hawrilenko, Baugh, & Calzo, 2015; Sanderson et al., 2017). This point is noteworthy, as unlike traditional sporting contexts where teams often have resources and staff to evaluate, diagnose, and treat injuries, participants of alternative sports often have to rely upon their own knowledge and/or understandings of their (damaged) body, and must subsequently take appropriate action to treat and/or manage their injuries accordingly. This navigation, however, can be a complicated process depending on where the participant is located, how much they know about their injury (and how to treat it), and how badly they are injured. However, when dealing with a SRC, these concerns can be further exacerbated by the fact that SRC frequently remains invisible or asymptomatic, which can make it that much more difficult for participants to know if they have sustained one.

Noting the rapid expansion of alternative sports worldwide, along with the fact that a number of new alternative sports (i.e., surfing, skateboarding, rock climbing) will make their Olympic debut at the Tokyo 2020 Olympic Games, it is no surprise that participation rates within alternative sports continues to grow

(Gilchrist & Wheaton, 2017). Yet, at the same time, Young (2004) notes that as participation rates grow, so inevitably will the rates of sport-related injuries. Considering both the rapid expansion of alternative sport participation, and the inevitable increase in rates of injuries that will shadow the growth of these sports, it is important to consider how SRC is understood, managed, embodied, and, importantly, being prevented within these sporting (sub)cultures. Looking ahead, future researchers could examine the virtually untouched topic of SRC in alternative, individual, and non-contact sporting cultures, and could draw attention to the various ways in which the sporting space and environment may influence how one understands, manages, and embodies SRC. Moreover, future research could also consider how a SRC may influence one's relationship with their immediate sporting environment and the spaces that they inhabit, and could explore how participants navigate, treat, and prevent SRCs within sporting contexts that lack rules, regulations, and traditional resources.

Exploring the Lived Experiences of SRC and the Expansion of Methodological Toolkits

To date, much of what is known about SRC has been derived from both positivist and post-positivist paradigms that have relied heavily upon quantitative analyses, self-report surveys, and number-driven data. Although these studies have provided valuable and foundational information about the frequencies of injury and mechanisms of injury, these studies have often failed to account for the lived experiences of SRC and the subjective nature of the injury. Considering that SRC has been described as one of the most "complex injuries" in sports medicine and has been recognized as an injury that should be treated uniquely, and on an individual, and case-by-case level (King et al., 2014; McCrory et al., 2017), it is important that researchers studying concussion also adopt and rearrange their methodologies to accurately capture, account for, and evaluate the subjective nature of this complex injury. One way for researchers to expand their methodological toolkits is to think about *how* qualitative methodologies and differing research paradigms, ontologies, and epistemologies could be used and adapted within SRC studies (see Chapter 12). As Young (2012) has stressed, qualitative methods can help "illuminate key matters such as how pain and injury are lived, reflected upon or revolved at various levels" (p. 115). Following Young's words, researchers studying concussion have started to recognize the value of using qualitative methods to explore the lived and subjective experiences of SRC (see Dean & Bundon, 2019; Dean, 2019; Liston et al., 2018; Malcolm, 2009). Through the use of interviews, participant observations, media analyses, and personal narratives, concussion researchers have started to use qualitative methods within their research to help illuminate how underlining the social, the political, and the cultural can influence the ways in which athletes come to understand, perceive, and embody SRC within various sporting cultures.

Researchers studying concussion may wish to incorporate the qualitative methods of interviews, participant observations, and other ethnographic traditions within their research, as a way to capture the nuances of their embodiments and navigations of injury. In turn, by employing qualitative methods, researchers studying concussion may be able to better understand both the subjective and affective nature of the injury, while simultaneously exploring how ideas about SRC are constructed, produced, and embodied within sporting cultures. Alternatively, by expanding our methodological toolkits to include the use of innovative qualitative methods such as photo-elicitation, story completion, autoethnography, and/or mobile or digital devices, researchers studying concussion may be able to better explore (and capture) the lived experiences of SRC and may offer the opportunity for new lines of inquiry when exploring SRC. In particular, one area where qualitative methodologies can make a substantial contribution to SRC research is through the incorporation and use of mixed methods and interdisciplinary research approaches when exploring the topic of SRC. For instance, by building upon the statistical data captured by number-driven datasets, concussion researchers could use qualitative methods to further add context and nuance to the numbers by accounting for the lived and subjective nature of the injury. Through mixed methods and interdisciplinary research (between various disciplines), researchers studying concussion would not only *speak with*, rather than *speak for* the participants within their studies, but could also use qualitative methods to further enrich and support trends and findings obtained through number-driven methods. It is this convergence between research disciplines and research methodologies that is key to moving forward, as researchers try to better understand SRC. By working between disciplines and across various methodologies, researchers studying concussion would be able to provide a much more comprehensive and holistic understanding of SRC that accounts for and recognizes both psychology and sociocultural factors when exploring SRC.

A Commitment to the Public Sociology of SRC

Reflecting upon the fact that SRC has been described as both a "medical and social problem" (Malcolm, 2018, p. 141), it is important to consider how we as sport sociologists, sport psychologists, and researchers studying concussion can engage with this *problem* in both meaningful and productive ways. Recognizing this problem, Malcolm (2018) has argued that a "public sociology of SRC" is required within the field of sport sociology and from others engaged in concussion research. Through this call, Malcolm has argued that the field of sport sociology, in particular, can help illustrate "the role of social relations in medical work" and can "illustrate how certain people in certain contexts, benefit from medical provision while others may experience medical mismanagement" (p. 146); further ascribing that sociocultural studies can "enable us to take a more holistic view of public health interventions, raising fundamental questions about equality, the legitimacy of population 'control,' and the potential for powerful commercial interests to exploit the opportunities that subsequently arise" (Malcolm, 2019, p. 205).

Noting Malcolm's call for the public sociology of SRC, I have begun to reflect upon and think about innovative ways to disseminate my own SRC-based research, not only to fellow researchers, but also to larger audiences such as parents, coaches, athletes, and sport practitioners. For example, one way I have made commitments to the public sociology of SRC has been through the method of autoethnography and the sharing of personal narratives that outlined my own experiences of/with a SRC in an attempt to create "digestible stories and findings that could be [easily] understood by athletes, coaches, parents, medical practitioners, and academics of different disciplines" (Dean, 2019, p. 28). Moreover, in my more recent research on the topic of SRC in surfing, I extended my commitment to Malcolm's call for the public sociology of SRC by disseminating findings from the research with local, national, and international media outlets (see Dart, 2019; Guesgen, 2019). With these examples in mind, it is important to remember that instead of confining our research within academic bubbles – that only a select few will actually engage with – we, as researchers studying concussion, must start to think of innovative ways to share key messages and findings from our studies with larger audiences and, importantly, the individuals dealing with this injury on a day-to-day basis.

Although, these dissemination tactics may sound mundane and/or superficial, by broadcasting this research outside of the academic bubble, I was able not only to commit myself to Malcolm's call, but also to foster and build new relationships, conversations, and practices based on my own sociological engagements within the public realm. While these are only a few examples of the ways that I have personally committed myself to the public sociology of SRC, there are many more avenues and research outputs for academics to consider. For example, researchers studying concussion may wish to put together and host workshops and/or public-talks, engage with blogs and (social) media outlets, and may also consider the use of digital methods and technologies – such as video and documentary film – to capture and illustrate findings and/or educational material to larger audience. Moreover, as Malcolm (2018) has pointed out, sport sociologists, and, I would argue, those studying concussion, are particularly well positioned to help "inform, educate and subsequently shape grassroots practices" (p. 147) and can work with external agencies and organizations to both co-construct research and implement applied practices into their sporting systems (see Chapter 14). Keeping this in mind, it is not only an expansion of methodological toolkits that is needed within concussion research, but also an expansion and revisioning of the ways in which researchers studying concussion disseminate, apply, and articulate their research findings within the public realm.

Conclusion

As the topic of SRC gains more and more traction from both researchers, media, and healthcare practitioners, it is important to critically reflect upon *how* the injury has been researched in the past, and importantly, to conceptualize and imagine how it could be explored in the future. Throughout the chapter, I critically explored the various ways that concussion and SRC have been studied and analyzed from a range of disciplines, while simultaneously outlining some of the strengthens and values of using sport sociology and sport psychology to explore SRC. In doing so, I also drew attention to a number of potential research avenues that future concussion researchers should consider moving forward. Instead of limiting our scope to more analyses of hockey, rugby, and football sporting cultures, I contended that examining SRC in alternative, individualized, and non-contact sporting environments may offer rich and insightful research endeavors for future studies to explore. In particular, future research may also want to consider how participants of these sporting (sub)cultures come to understand and embody SRC within their unique sporting contexts. For example, future studies could explore how SRC may influence one's relationship with their immediate sporting environment and the spaces that they inhabit and could investigate how participants of alternative sports navigate, manage, and understand SRCs in sporting contexts that lack rules, regulation, and traditional resources.

In addition, I have argued that future research should consider and continue to explore the lived experiences of SRC, as explorations of this topic may not only yield the potential to add a voice and substance to the numbers contrived from quantitative analyses of concussion, but could also illuminate how underlining social, political, and cultural factors influences the ways in which athletes come to understand, perceive, and embody SRC within various sporting (sub)cultures. Keeping these points in mind, I drew attention to and argued for the expansion of methodological, ontological, and epistemological approaches when exploring the topic of SRC, and highlighted some of the advantages of expanding one's methodological toolkit. Finally, I concluded this chapter by echoing Malcolm's (2018) call for "a public sociology of SRC" and offered a few different avenues and examples for *how* researchers studying concussion could (better) disseminate their research in more digestible and palpable ways.

Critical Discussion Questions

1) What are ways to destigmatize sport-related concussion within sporting (sub) cultures? Is this possible? Explain.
2) What are particular ways you could disseminate concussion knowledge and education to participants, coaches, medical staff, and/or sport organizers within your sporting community in a way that would be palpable and easily understood?
3) Reflecting upon your own involvement in sport, how could either a sport-psychology–based study or sport-sociology–based study be used to explore concussion within your sporting community? What are some of the advantages and disadvantages of these studies?

Notes

1   While I recognize that the term, "traditional" sport is often blurred and contested within the field of action sport research, I use Wheaton's (2013) discussion to refer to "traditional" sports as those that are rule-bound, competitive, institutionalized, and

often Westernized. Through this understanding, sports such as basketball, soccer (football), American Football, hockey, and rugby may be considered traditional sports.
2 Following Rinehart's (2000) suggestion, I use the term, "alternative sports" to encapsulate a range of activities that are "either ideologically or practically… alternatives to mainstream sports and to mainstream sport values" (p. 506).

References

Anderson, E., & Kian, E. M. (2012). Examining media contestation of masculinity and head trauma in the National Football League. *Men and Masculinities, 15*(2), 152–173. doi: 10.1177/1097184X11430127

Becker, J., & Moroder, P. (2017). Extreme mountain biking injuries. In F. Feletti (Ed.), *Extreme sports medicine* (pp. 139–150). Switzerland: Springer International Publishing.

Brayton, S., Helstein, M. T., Ramsey, M., & Rickards, N. (2019). Exploring the missing link between the concussion "crisis" and labor politics in professional sports. *Communication and Sport, 7*(1), 110–131. doi: 10.1177/2167479517740342

Carroll, L., & Rosner, D. (2012). *The concussion crisis: Anatomy of a silent epidemic*. New York: Simon & Schuster.

Cassilo, D., & Sanderson, J. (2018). From social isolation to becoming an advocate: Exploring athletes' grief discourse about lived concussion experiences in online forums. *Communication and Sport, 6*(1), 86–110. doi: 10.1177/2167479518790039

Dart, T. (2019, August). "My world just crumbled": The untold wreckage of concussions in surfing. *The Guardian*. Retrieved from https://www.theguardian.com/sport/2019/aug/29/surfing-concussions-mercedes-maidana

Dean, N. A. (2019). "Just act normal": Concussion and the (re)negotiation of athletic identity. *Sociology of Sport Journal, 36*(1), 22–31. doi: 10.1123/ssj.2018-0033

Dean, N. A., & Bundon, A. (2019). "You're only falling into water!": Exploring surfers' understandings of concussion in Canadian surf culture. *Qualitative Research in Sport, Exercise and Health, 12*, 579–596 doi: 10.1080/2159676X.2019.1657930

Gilchrist, P., & Wheaton, B. (2017). The social benefits of informal and lifestyle sports: A research agenda. *International Journal of Sport Policy and Politics, 9*(1), 1–10. doi: 10.1080/19406940.2017.1293132

Guesgen, M. (2019, August). Surfers off Canada's West Coast face significant risks of concussion. Retrieved from https://www.theglobeandmail.com/canada/british-columbia/article-surfers-off-canadas-west-coast-face-significant-risks-of-concussions/

Hughes, R., & Coakley, J. (1991). Positive deviance among athletes: The implications of overconformity to the sport ethic. *Sociology of Sport Journal, 8*(4), 307–325. doi: 10.1123/ssj.8.4.307

Khurana, V., & Kaye, A. (2012). An overview of concussion in sport. *Journal of Clinical Neuroscience, 19*(1), 1–11. doi: 10.1016/j.jocn.2011.08.002

King, D., Brughalli, M., Hume, P., & Gissane, C. (2014). Assessment, management and knowledge of sport-related concussion: Systematic review. *Sports Medicine, 44*(4), 449–471. doi: 10.1007/s40279-013-0134-x

Klick, C., Jones, C. M. C., & Adler, D. (2016). Surfing USA: An epidemiological study of surfing injuries presenting to US ED's 2002 to 2013. *American Journal of Emergency Medicine, 34*(8), 1491–1496. doi: 10.1016/j.ajem.2016.05.008

Kroshus, E., Garnett, B., Hawrilenko, M., Baugh, C. M., & Calzo, J. P. (2015). Concussion under-reporting and pressure from coaches, teammates, fans, and parents. *Social Science and Medicine, 134*, 66–75. doi: 10.1016/j. socscimed.2015.04.011

Langlois, J., Rutland-Brown, W., & Wald, M. (2006). The epidemiology and impact of traumatic brain injury: A brief overview. *Journal of Head Trauma Rehabilitation, 21*(5), 375–378.

Liston, K., McDowell, M., Malcolm, D., Scott-Bell, A., & Waddington, I. (2018). On being 'head strong': The pain zone and concussion in non-elite rugby union. *International Review for the Sociology of Sport, 53*(6), 668–684. doi:10.177/101269021679966

Malcolm, D. (2009). Medical uncertainty and clinical-athlete relations: The management of concussion injuries in rugby union. *Sociology of Sport Journal, 26*(2), 191–210. doi: 10.1123/ssj.26.2.19

Malcolm, D. (2018). Concussion in sport: Public, professional and critical sociologies. *Sociology of Sport Journal, 35*(2), 141–148. doi: 10.1123/ssj.2017-0113

Malcolm, D. (2019). Sociocultural aspects of concussion. In G. A Bloom & J. G Caron (Eds.), *Psychological aspects of sport-related concussions* (pp. 199–211). London, UK: Routledge.

McCrory, P., Meeuwisse, W. H., Dvorak, J., Aubry, M., Bailes, J., Broglio, S., … Vos, P. E. (2017). Consensus statement on concussion in sport. 5th international conference on concussion in sport held in Berlin, October 2016. *Consensus Statement*, 1–10. doi: 10.1136/bjsports-2017-097699

McGannon, K. R., Cunningham, S. M., & Schinke, R. J. (2013). Understanding concussion in socio-cultural context: A media analysis of a National Hockey League star's concussion. *Psychology of Sport and Exercise, 14*(6), 891–899. doi: 10.1016/j.psychsport.2013.08.003

Messner, M. A. (1990). When bodies are weapons: Masculinity and violence in sport. *International Review for the Sociology of Sport, 25*(3), 203–220. doi: 10.1177%2F101269029002500303

Nixon, H. L. (1992). A social network analysis of influences on athletes to play with pain and injury. *Journal of Sport and Social Issues, 16*(2), 127–135. doi: 10.1177/2F019372359201600208

Putukian, M., D' Alonzo, B. A., Campbell-McGovern, C. S., & Wiebe, D. J. (2019). The Ivy League-big ten epidemiology of concussion study. *The American Journal of Sports Medicine, 47*(5), 1236–1247. doi: 10.1177/0363546519830100

Rinehart, R. (2000). Emerging/arriving sport: Alternatives to formal sports. In J. Coakley & E. Dunning (Eds.), *Handbook of sports studies* (pp. 504–519). London, UK: Sage.

Sabo, D. (2004). The politics of sports injury: Hierarchy, power and the pain principle. In K. Young (Ed.), *Sporting bodies, damaged selves: Sociological studies of sport-related injury* (pp. 59–79). Amsterdam: Elsevier.

Sanderson, J., Weathers, M., Grevious, A., Tehan, M., & Warren, S. (2016). A hero or sissy? Exploring media framing of NFL quarterbacks injury decisions. *Communication and Sport, 4*(1), 3–22. doi: 10.1177/2167479514536982

Sanderson, J., Weathers, M., Snedaker, K., & Gramlich, K. (2017). "I was able to still do my job on the field and keep playing": An investigation of female and male athletes' experiences with (not) reporting concussions. *Communication and Sport, 5*(3), 267–287. doi: 10.1177/2167479515623455

Shuman, K. M., & Meyers, M. C. (2015). Skateboarding injuries: An updated review. *The Physician and Sportsmedicine, 43*(3), 317–323. doi: 10.1080/00913847.2015.1050953

Stranger, M. (2011). *Surfing life: Surface, substructure and the commodification of the sublime*. Surrey: Ashgate Publishing Company.

Swinney, C. (2015). Assessing the prevalence of traumatic head injury amongst recreational surfers in the United Sates. *Hawaii Journal of Medicine and Public Health, 74*(12), 403–405.

Ventresca, M. (2019). The curious case of CTE: Mediating materialities of traumatic brain injury. *Communication and Sport, 7*(2), 135–156. doi: 10.1177/2167479518761636

Wheaton, B. (2013). *The cultural politics of lifestyle sports*. London, UK: Routledge.

Wiese-Bjornstal, D. M. (2010). Psychology and socioculture affect injury risk, response, and recovery in high-intensity athletes: A consensus statement. *Scandinavian Journal of Medicine and Science in Sports, 20*, 103–111. doi: 10.1111/j.1600-0838.2010.01195.x

Wiese-Bjornstal, D. M., White, A. C., Russell, H. C., & Smith, A. M. (2015). Psychology of sport concussions. *Kinesiology Review, 4*(2), 169–189. doi: 10.1123/kr.2015-0012

Young, K. (2004). Sports-related pain and injury: Sociological notes. In K. Young (Ed.), *Sporting bodies, damaged selves: Sociological studies of sports-related injury* (pp. 1–28). Amsterdam: Elsevier.

Young, K. (2012). Risk, pain and injury in sport: A cause or effect of violence? In K. Young (Ed.), *Sport violence and society* (pp. 100–118). New York: Routledge.

Young, K., & White, P. (1995). Sport, physical danger, and injury: The experiences of elite women athletes. *Journal of Sport and Social Issues, 19*(1), 45–61. doi: 10.1177/2F019372395019001004

5 Pain and Injury
From the Unidimensional to the Multidimensional

Michael Atkinson

Introduction

I have immersed myself in one ethnography or another throughout my entire academic career. More often than not, my ethnographic proclivities lead me to explore physically taxing and rather dangerous physical cultures. I simply have an academic fascination with pain and suffering. During my doctoral studies at the University of Calgary, Kevin Young's teaching exposed me to the history of pain and injury research in the sociology of sport and I quickly became enamoured with the substantive area. Kevin encouraged me to pursue ethnographies of pain and suffering at a time when interviewing and surveys reigned supreme. Nearly 25 years later, I continue to study how people across diverse physical cultural landscapes develop complicated relationships with pain, injury, and suffering. From the outset it is important to acknowledge how tricky the concept of pain actually is to study in practice. The complexity of pain as a concept is due to both its definitional simplicity (i.e., pain is something "that hurts") and the sheer diversity of pain experiences among sport and physical cultural participants. In this chapter, I review mainstay conceptualizations of pain and injury in sport research and introduce a relatively new heuristic for studying pain as an injury process: the concept of a *pain community*. Here, the goal is to emphasize the multilayered and multi-leveled nature of pain and injury alongside the need for integrated theoretical and methodological approaches to their study.

Sport and Painkilling

There is certainly no shortage of empirical examples and case studies of pain and injury in sport. It is difficult to even conceive of sport without both wanted and unwanted pain (Atkinson & Young, 2008) as deeply woven into fabric of athletic performance (Young, 2012). For nearly 40 years, sociologists and psychologists of sport have attended to a wide range of pain- and injury-producing activities in sport, ranging from on-field pain and suffering, to minor and catastrophic injury and its implications, to cultural codes (e.g., gender, class, ethnicity, race, sex, religion; see Chapter 3) for understanding how people construct the meaning of pain, and to policy-driven attempts to mitigate the risk of injury in sports settings. The corpus of pain research generally attests to the phenomenological, micrological, and small group settings through which athletes develop, and come to terms with, pain and injury; and, how sport-based risk is collectively approached by a wide range of sport insiders. Researchers have played an important role in cataloging and theoretically dissecting the litany of pain and injury experiences athletes endure, and as such, underscored the physically and emotionally deleterious nature of intense competition.

More recently, the nascent "Exercise is Medicine" (EiM) movement has shifted focus toward how participation in sport, exercise, and physical activity may serve to actually mitigate non-athletic forms of personal pain, injury, and suffering (Cairney, McGannon, & Atkinson, 2018). Approached as a universal panacea for combating and treating the effects of obesity, cancer, depression, anxiety, and a spectrum of other trauma-inducing diseases or conditions, sport is studied (and promoted) as a cost-effective inoculant against disease, illnesses, and disorders. Relatedly, research on the two-decades-old "Sport for Development and Peace" (SfDP) movement underlines the potential of leveraging sport in the pursuit of alleviating the painful and injury-producing effects of poverty, social inequality, diseases like HIV/AIDS, environmental instability, war, and other forms of injustice on marginalized people (Darnell, Chawansky, Marchessault, Holmes, & Hayhurst, 2018). In the case of EiM and SfDP, sport and exercise are often uncritically regarded as a magic bullet capable of addressing, at least the manifest symptoms of, bio-hazards, social threats, and deeply structured social inequality people encounter.

In what follows, I briefly review the dominant, emergent, and yet untapped zones of pain in extant research on sport, exercise, health, and physical culture. I then turn to address the concept of a *pain community* and its potential utility in pain and injury research; in particular, as a vehicle for genuinely conducting multidisciplinary and theoretically interred research. In this process I argue pain research in sport would be enhanced through conceptual connections to pain, injury, and suffering research in wider health and illness contexts.

Critical Review: Conceptual and Theoretical Pain/Injury Zones

The word "pain" typically conjures an image in the mind of sport-related injury, or a physically noxious sensation athletes encounter as part of competition. From a very unidimensional lens, pain is a biological state of personal discomfort. Yet anyone in pain can attest to the suffocatingly limited construction of pain by biomedical experts. Still, research efforts inside and outside of the worlds of kinesiology, sport sciences, and health sciences generally uncritically validates the base biomedical directive that pain research should focus squarely on how (unwanted) pain and injury occur within self-contained athlete bodies; and how pain management is the driving force underpinning research efforts (Smith, 2008). As Smith (2018, p. 25) notes, "the extensive discussion of pain within the medical and critical health literature has, in this vein, produced a wide array of pain management methods for both acute and chronic pain sufferers" (see also Aldrich & Eccleston, 2000; Roessler, 2006). In sport and exercise faculties around the world, athletes who have suffered broken bones or torn ligaments, experience fatigue and exhaustion, or suffer from self-loss resulting from competitive failure, are studied and treated by exercise physiologists, biomechanists, sport psychologists, and others in restitutive attempts to make their pain and suffering simply "go away" (see Chapter 1).

For anyone in a multi- and interdisciplinary faculty like kinesiology, sport sciences, and health sciences, the narrow focus on biological/physical pain is both theoretically naïve and substantively misleading. People simply do not feel pain in acute ways; they experience pain as human beings in a multidimensional process. Even a cursory analysis of people's participation in sport and exercise worlds evidences the diversity of pain manifestations. In an attempt to develop a more theoretically robust and reality-congruent conceptualization of pain, Saunders (1986) acknowledged the need to attend to the psychological pain caused by physically painful illnesses (e.g., doubt, anxiety, uncertainty) alongside the social (e.g., loss of status, loss of relationships, loss of roles), spiritual (e.g., loss of faith, loss of belief in God, loss of belief in a higher power), and existential (e.g., personal authenticity, meaning of life, questions about the purpose of life) aspects of pain and suffering.

Saunders (1986) much-neglected model of "total pain" validates a core sport, exercise, and health science mantra extolling the virtues of studying sport from a "cell to society" perspective. Felt pain is clearly a matter of biology, human anatomy, and how the central nervous system is veritably wired, but is also a matter of how one learns to confront and receive pain through embodied experience and culture-specific interpretive frames acquired through socialization processes. Pain is also something individual persons do not uniquely experience as pain is culturally mediated, storied, symbolized, and interrogated by many others. While rarely addressed in reference to Saunders' (1986) model of total pain, or extracted from Young's (2012) seminal research on violence and pain in sport, the focused analysis of total pain in sport leads researchers to its deeply *relational* nature. As outlined by Elias (1978, 1991) through his articulation of "the hinge", it is difficult to conceive of a phenomenon like pain without seeing its relationally (read *totally*) interwoven physical, psychological, and social nature for any one individual experiencing pain, and how a person "in pain" is relationally connected to a set of others who attend to one's pain in a variety of ways. Strangely, however, research in the social sciences of sport (the focus of this chapter) rarely accounts for pain as a total and/or relational phenomenon, privileging instead disciplinary (and subdisciplinary) pain ontologies and epistemologies.

Dominant Pain Zones in Sport Research

The first, and perhaps most common, disciplinary cluster of research on pain in sport, health, and exercise attends to the *individual experience of pain and injury for athletes* and its implications on mental wellness, health, performance, or involvement in sport (Atkinson, 2018; Roderick, Smith, & Potrac, 2017). Largely the terrain of sport (social) psychologists, research in this analytic stream presents empirical evidence of the devastating personal effects of injury on competitive athletes, such as depression and isolation (Hughes & Leavey, 2017); the development of character, resilience, and mental toughness in the face of suffering (Crust, 2007); emotional regulation in sport (Martinent & Ferrand, 2015); the stress of competitive pain and learned personal coping mechanisms (Hunt & Day, 2018); the experience of psychological or sexual abuse by coaches and other sport insiders (Owton, 2016); the use of painkillers or performance by athletes to mask trauma (Turner, Barlow, & Ilbery, 2002); and the chilling emotional effects of retiring or leaving sport (Roderick, 2014). Sobering research on how athletes experience post-concussion syndrome (see Chapter 4) or CTE has removed the "Ozian" curtain concealing the tremendous toll of physical competition on individual athletes (Moore, Kay, & Ellemberg, 2018). Separate and collective emphasis in this category of pain research highlights the management strategies developed by individual athletes or sports experts to help people cope with sport-related pain, and pain itself is mainly positioned as a normal and yet unwanted (or needing to be controlled) psycho-emotional state.

Sociological accounts of individual confrontations with pain and injury in sport worlds have drawn on narrative (see Chapter 1) and autoethnographic methods to detail the phenomenological aspects of being an athlete in pain. Autoethnographic accounts of running and long-distance sports in particular (Allen-Collinson, 2005) provide poetic evidence of how athletes immersed in their respective physical cultures often go to great lengths to manage their involvement in pain and injury-producing activities. Personal stories or narratives about pain, which abound in the medical humanities literature (Charon, 2008), serve to humanize athletes in their grapples with and negotiations of pain in sport. This narrative approach is perhaps best and most consistently evidenced in the study of how battles with sport-related eating disorders are storied by sufferers (Papathomas & Lavallee, 2010). Deeply idiographic pain stories about problematic eating often hint at or directly explore the relational aspects of pain via detailed analytic walk-throughs of how one becomes anorexic, how anorexia is done in practice, how anorexia feels, how sport culture contributes to one's anorexia, and how one's anorexia affects others including one's teammates, coaches, friends and families (Papathomas, Smith, & Lavallee, 2015).

A second main cluster of pain and injury research documents the powerful effects of *cultural mindsets and pain traditions in specific sports cultures*. As the standard sociological analysis goes, organized sport is physically dangerous but also culturally perilous because, as a hierarchical social institution, it socializes young athletes to nearly blindly accept the risk of pain and injury inherent in sport participation. Nixon (1992, 1993) describes the existence of vast socializing networks in sport, which he termed "sportsnets", that both explicitly instruct young athletes to almost tacitly accept and extol the virtues of experiencing sports-based pain as an essential component of being involved in athletics. Echoing what Hughes and Coakley (1991) describe as a vital component of the "Sport Ethic", Nixon (1992, 1993) underscores how the tolerance of physical pain and suffering is a culturally learned and venerated edict. A flood of sociological research in the late mid-1980s and early 1990s analytically pointed in the same direction – sport cultures normalize a broad spectrum of pain as a means of producing high performance. Frey (1991), Curry (1993), Messner (1990), Sabo (1989), and Young (1993) were among the cast of central sociological characters pioneering the critical inspection of the social mechanisms by which athletes consent to a broad range of painful experiences in sport, and the cultural frameworks promulgated to reproduce these mechanisms over time.

The early 1990s could be heralded as the golden age of research on cultures of painful risk-taking in sport. Though core sociological frames of socialization, enculturation, and interpersonal learning informed dissections of how and why athletes become accepting of pain, injury, and risk as a badge of (subcultural) honour, the most pervasive sociological account within research of the golden age focused on the relationship between sports pain and achieved masculinity (see Chapter 3). Sabo's (1989) and Messner's (1990, 1992) research perhaps lit the conceptual torches in the field, and 15 years of subsequent pain and injury in sport research consistently illustrated how being injured, for example, is easily reconciled as a clever (sub)cultural tactic among male athletes for achieving and representing one's sense of (hyper)masculinity in the cultural field (Young, 2012). To this end, the ability to endure pain is a marker of one's achieved masculine strength, dominance, fearlessness, and power. Thus, risk-taking is part of proving a particular brand of masculine character in sport zones – which also, by definition, marginalizes other masculinities, femininities, and (non-hetero) sexualities (Messner, 1992). Attaching masculinity to pain has borne tremendous empirical fruit over time in the process of explaining why athletes push themselves to a range of physical, emotional, and social extremes in the name of sport. But one might argue in the contemporary era of research on pain and injury, such fruit is now rather low-hanging.

Sociological research on pain in sport points to how putting oneself in harm's way and accepting exceptionally dangerous hazards within already hazardous social fields can be overrepresented in particular sports cultures. Athletes who perform with a perceived indifference to or celebration of styles of reckless play that facilitate dominance over opponents that may produce painful injury (Young, 2004), who align such practices with hegemonic and unyielding constructions of gender, race, class, and sexuality (Kidder, 2017), who feel institutional and subcultural pressure to engage in extremely hazardous pursuits (Andreasson & Johansson, 2018), and who consent to playing while injured or in considerable pain (Madrigal & Robbins, 2017) have been widely documented in power and performance sports like rugby, American football, ice hockey, boxing, and a range of others. Amplified risk-taking in these contexts *relationally* validates one's status as an achieved athlete in the sports, and serves as an important social indicator of one's commitment to sport excellence. Safai's (2004) research on pain in sport illustrates how a network of actors inside these cultures directly encourage or implicitly suggest an athlete's long-term membership in a sport culture is contingent on an almost unreflexive acceptance of pain and injury; what Hughes and Coakley (1991) first proposed as the over-conformity to the "Sport Ethic". Young's (2012) two decades' worth of research on power and performance sport cultures draws attention to precisely what is so risky for athletes in uncompromising sport cultures: the use of the body as a weapon of performance and identity; the normalization of one's own self-objectification and self-alienation; the learned (and often times compelled) disregard for one's personal safety; the immersion in lifestyles of pain and injury; the subcultural neglect of basic human needs; and one's existence in (stereotypically) hostile social settings that stigmatize weakness and failure.

Around the more contested aspects of pain in sport revolves the idea that collective involvement in physically dangerous pursuits is a form of "edge-work" (Scott & Austin, 2016) or "symbolic play with death" (le Breton, 2000). Full emotional immersion in thrilling but physically hazardous sports like sky-diving or BASE jumping, cliff skiing, motocross, surfing, street luge, mountain biking, and others provides many participants with a means of experiencing physical, emotional, and psychological sensations of suffering and anxiety not provided in everyday life (Bunn, 2017). While most sports are unwritten by exposure to a range of hazards that risk or produce painful injury, a significant part of the allure of risk, adventure, whizz, or extreme sports is the degree to which participants place themselves in the direct path of pain for sheer pleasure. The idea of sport-related pain and injury providing a form of gritty pleasure to participants is still relatively novel in the field, and one of the least analytically explored in the social scientific analysis of sport (Wellard, 2013).

Participants may engage in sports and other physical cultural pursuits to deliberately test their (total) pain thresholds. Atkinson (2008), in the study of triathlon, accounted for how participants may seek out painful forms of physical activity in sport as a means of managing (inter)personal pains away from competition. Being hit by an opponent in a recreational ice hockey league, pushing one's body to extreme exhaustion and beyond through ultramarathon running, or being thrown to the ground in judo or hit in mixed martial arts training can be rewarding to people as painful physical pleasures in and of themselves. While the risk of long-term injury is not alluring *per se*, the hazards posed by the pursuits and the degree to which the body/mind is taxed to its limits (almost sadomasochistically) is meaningful (Pringle, Rinehart, & Caudwell, 2015) As Atkinson (2008) reminds us, immersion in such grueling physical ordeals is a way of encountering and working through liminal-existential questions regarding the self, one's agency, and one's sense of achieved identity.

The third main area of research examines how pain is approached from *institutional and policy initiatives*. Studies of how injury prevention might be better managed (Emery, Black, & Kolstad, 2017), how athletes might be protected from physical and sexual abuse at the hands of coaches (Kerr, Battaglia, & Sterling, 2019), how performance-enhancing drugs should be regulated (Engelberg & Skinner, 2016), how resources for athletes struggling with mental illness are required (Uphill, Sly, & Swain, 2016), and how within-game violence is controlled abound. Emphasis in these studies draws attention to how individuals tasked with regulatory roles in sports communities are not only primary definers of pain, but also centrally aid in the protection of others vulnerable to pain. Here, critical studies of sports medicine and physicians (Malcolm, 2017) provide insight on how pain itself is biomedically defined in athletic contexts and comes into conceptual conflict with how athletes socially construct pain.

Thinking even more broadly about total pain, a spate of nascent non-governmental organizations and private enterprises compromising the global "Sport for Development and Peace" (SfDP) movement address pains suffered in and by a range of communities outside of traditional athlete cultures. Using sports like soccer as local levers to ostensibly combat the pains of food scarcity and drought, the transmission of sexual infections and diseases, postwar trauma, child-trafficking, and poverty in the developing world (predominantly Africa and nations in the global south), SfDP research documents how sports communities are increasingly aware of and sensitive to more diffuse and complicated social pains suffered in structured non-sports communities. In a related way, the literature on corporate social responsibility or corporate citizenship in sport (Rowe, Karg, & Sherry, 2019) reviews how major sports organizations (e.g., NBA, NFL, FIFA, NBA) and sport-related corporations (e.g., athletic equipment) increasingly invest in charitable initiatives and outreach programs as a way of aiding people in need. In Canada, for example, the Canadian Tire corporation's "Jumpstart" program is a quasi customer-funded campaign designed to provide financial assistance to young people from low socioeconomic backgrounds so they may participate in organized sport (i.e., as a means of improving their physical, mental, and social health).

Finally, we might consider how sport produces one variety of pain or another for a variety of non-human actors. Non-human animals and the environment have been studied as direct recipients of pain caused as a result of sport and exercise practices (Atkinson, 2014). Without anthropomorphizing how animals are painfully abused and mistreated in an array of sports pastimes, our attention is drawn to how animal pain is both objectified and negated in sports like fishing, hunting, dog/horse racing, rodeo, and others. Similarly, studies of the environmental impact of sport on ocean life, mountain areas, woodland areas, and other green spaces attests to how ecosystems are "painfully" destroyed through sports practices such as golfing, boating, skiing, sports mega-events, and a host of others (Wilson & Millington, 2017). This final cluster of pain-related research in sport not only pushes theoretical boundaries of who, and what, are the objects and subjects of pain in sport and exercise, but also how the concept of pain itself requires expansion into new dimensions (see Young, 2012, 2019).

Future Research Implications

I competed, somewhat recreationally, as a long-distance runner and duathlete between 2004 and 2012 as part of a trans-continental ethnography (Atkinson, 2008). Over the course of the research I played around with the notion that certain sports groups can be categorized as "pain communities" (Atkinson, 2008). I felt a deep reluctance to succinctly define what constitutes a pain community in my early writing on the concept, favoring instead a preliminary empirical account of how pain serves to organize people into mutually oriented groups of actors. Here, however, I offer a sensitizing conceptual definition of a *pain community* as the following:

> A set of mutually oriented actors bound together in a practice that directly places individuals in the path of potentially painful experiences, and/or a set of actors who attend to the alleviation of pain commonly experienced by a specific population. Pain communities range from incredibly small, tight-knit, and esoteric subcultures with minimal internal differentiation (such as a local running club), to an expansive, multi-level, conglomeration of diverse and tangentially related persons (such as a hospital, or broader medical health system). Some pain communities are fleeting and temporary, seasonal, or event-based, or permanently endure over time in order to address ongoing social concerns. A pain community shares (and debates) cultural conceptualizations of pain, its dimensions, and deep relationship to the human condition. One's position in the experience of, witnessing of, care for, or regulation of pain in such communities establishes and contours one's roles and statuses held therein. Pain communities can be primary definers of broader social constructions of pain, particularly as they relate to the complicated relationships between embodiment, identity, representation, power, policy, ethics, and pain management. Finally, pain communities may come to intersect with one another tactically or functionally give their respective interests or shared expertise (e.g., runners who require medical assistance from doctors over time to treat sports injuries).

With the above definition in mind, and aided by even a minimal sociological imagination, one is able to recognize the sheer volume and diversity of pain communities across the social landscape. Organized sport, in the widest sense, is an enormous pain community in and of itself with hundreds and hundreds of smaller pain communities embedded within, and structurally differentiated by, their focal "pain concerns"; from small affiliations of recreational athletes and hobbyists, to clubs, to teams, to sports physicians and health care practitioners, to National Sports Organizations and policymakers, even to academics who collectively interrogate pain and suffering processes in sport from any range of disciplinary perspectives. How a pain community is defined, then, is partly a matter of participants' perspectives (i.e., who do we see as a part of our direct community) but also a matter of visualizing how smaller communities are nested within a relational network of others that together form an extensive pain community.

The concept of a pain community offered in this chapter is closely aligned with Elias' (1978, 1991) description of a figuration; or more simply, an historically located but fluid and dynamic network or web of mutually interdependent actors. The concept of a figuration brings awareness to the interconnections shared between people beyond proximal interaction in everyday life, while emphasizing meaningful distal connections not captured in vague concepts like institutions, culture, and society. Indeed, one might consider a pain community as a broader pain figuration of interconnected people. Duathletes and triathletes are members of a general figuration of athletes pursuing distance sport, but also are those sharing communal values of pain exploration and management (Atkinson, 2008). Triathlon *totally* hurts in a litany of ways. Riding a bike alone for hours in training, swimming during early morning sessions in heavily chlorinated cold pool water, and running in the summer heat or winter winds involve encounters with pain, injury, suffering, unpleasantness, and other forms of physical, emotional, and psychological discomfort. One is tired, hungry, sore, or in stress-producing motion nearly all of the time. Committing to the volume of training required may severely strain interpersonal relationships outside of the sport, including with one's family, detract from work responsibilities, financially tax a person, and test the limits of one's personal resolve in the face of pain. Recognizing this, athletes in these groups form very close relationships of support and mutual understanding to help one another through their multifaceted suffering both in and outside of the sport. But they also provide training, and performative and social frameworks for understanding how pains suffered actually benefit participants: from feeling excited through strenuous and gruelling physical activity, to the potential for personal growth during pain, to managing sorrow, frustration or turmoil in one's life, to how pain affirms or validates one's acquired character (e.g., strong, courageous, leader, manager, stoic, moral) and attributed identity (e.g., gender, class, ethnicity) frames (Atkinson, 2008). I came to analyze the very centrality of encountering pain as a – and, perhaps, *the* – defining element of the group. To this end, these are genuine (total) pain communities.

But not all pain communities are similar to triathletes, and certainly not all pain communities are restricted to the sporting world. Think of, for example, the sheer diversity of communities (either loosely identified or tightly protected) devoted in one way another to the exploration, management, and representation of human pain (physical, emotional, social) outside of sport. Communities as diverse as medical doctors, weight-loss experts and physical trainers, bioethicists, drugstore owners, clergy persons and spiritual healers, persons with eating disorders, aestheticians, nurses, artists, alcohol or drug recovery groups, ambulance drivers, social workers and youth counselors, philosophers, chiropractors, S&M practitioners, psychologists, law makers and lawyers, tattoo enthusiasts, animal or environmental rights activists, gang members, novelists, cancer survivors and their support groups, massage therapists, and the police are all communities of one sort or another that centrally attend to one (or more aspects) of human pain and suffering as their central mandates of existence. Rather than approach these communities as both substantively and conceptually unrelated, future research would do well to analyze their theoretical connections in the pursuit of a more robust and reality-congruent understanding of the complex, multidimensional nature of pain in the human condition and how people are bound together relationally through shared/common pain experiences.

In the more immediate context of sport, health, and physical cultural studies, the sensitizing concept of a pain community accomplishes two central organizing tasks. In the first instance, and relating back to the first section of this chapter, researchers need to appreciate pain *as a main conceptual common ground* in a vast array of studies of sport, exercise, and health communities. Future research might focus on how pain communities are differently constituted, constructed, experienced, utilized, and intersect others in sport and exercise zones. Quite simply, pain communities tend to depend on one another in sport (i.e., think of how athletes depend on trainers and vice versa), and examining how pain communities serve one another in complementary processes is important. Second, as Smith (2018, 2019) notes in her path-breaking conceptual definition of pain, sport and exercise worlds are primary places to study the multi-dimensional nature of pain itself. Considering how sport experiences expose one or place one in the path of physical pain, psychological pain, social pain, emotional pain, spiritual, and existential pain, collating and examining how the multiple dimensions of pain interlock through sport is critical for better grasping the socially organizing nature of total pain for people. In these studies, the emphasis should be on generating dialogue with other pain literatures in the hope of contributing to a broader discourse on how pain writes much of the human experience.

Conclusion

Nearly four decades of critical research on pain and injury in sport communities collectively accounts for the multidimensional nature of pain and its experience. While considerable attention is given to personal injury, pain and its devastating effects, focused research on the idea of pain as a community-level project in sport, exercise, physical culture is overdue. In this pursuit, cross-disciplinary connection to theoretical and methodological innovation in health research is warranted as part of a collaborative push toward interprofessional understandings of pain. Particularly innovative work on pain (and injury) community experiences would also stretch research boundaries to the humanities and the field of aesthetics, ergonomics, pharmacology, business studies and economics, environmental sciences, and bioethics to name only a few. Questions regarding the purpose (beyond the critique of how people become injured in sport, experience pain, and how cultural frames teach people how to understand pain) would likely emerge, revealing new ground in pain research yet to be traversed.

Saunders' (1986) heavily lauded total pain model provides an analytic springboard for considering how sport researchers might incorporate an integrated, multidimensional model of pain and injury into active research. Any given research venture in the social scientific study of sport brushes against or eclipses the boundaries of each pain category Saunders (1986) outlines. Future research might attend to all dimensions of pain rather than favoring one or two, addressing how either individuals experience each in most cases of pain experience, and how separate members of a pain community might be tasked with addressing one or more dimensions specifically as their mandate of group membership. Finally, Saunders' (1986) model provides a pathway for truly interdisciplinary research on pain as it situates pain as a phenomenon requiring theoretical and methodological diversity spanning across paradigms.

Critical Discussion Questions

1) Given the fuzzy boundaries established in this chapter regarding what actually constitutes sport-related pain and injury, think about what pain includes and excludes in the sport and exercise worlds. Is there anything missing in this chapter regarding manifestations of pain in sport and exercise practices?
2) Identify and discuss the defining features of *three* different pain communities in sport.
3) What can medical health professionals learn about pain from the study of sport-related pain?

References

Aldrich, S., & Eccleston, C. (2000). Making sense of everyday pain. *Social Science and Medicine*, *50*(11), 1631–1641. doi: 10.1016/s0277-9536(99)00391-3

Allen-Collinson, J. (2005). Emotions, interaction and the injured sporting body. *International Review for the Sociology of Sport*, *40*, 221–240. doi: 10.1177%2F1012690205057203

Andreasson, J., & Johansson, T. (2018). *Extreme sports, extreme bodies*. London, UK: Routledge.

Atkinson, M. (2008). Triathlon, suffering and exciting significance. *Leisure Studies*, *27*(2), 165–180. doi: 10.1080/02614360801902216

Atkinson, M. (2014). The terrier [men]. *Sociology of Sport Journal*, *31*(4), 420–437. doi: 10.1123/ssj.2014-0089

Atkinson, M. (2018). *Sport, mental illness, and sociology*. Amsterdam: Emerald.

Atkinson, M., & Young, K. (2008). *Sport, deviance and social control*. Champaign, IL: Human Kinetics.

Bunn, M. (2017). I'm gonna do this over and over and over forever! Overlapping fields and climbing practice. *International Review for the Sociology of Sport*, *52*, 584–597. doi: 10.1177%2F1012690215609785

Cairney, J., McGannon, K., & Atkinson, M. (2018). Exercise as medicine: Critical considerations in the qualitative research landscape. *Qualitative Research in Sport, Exercise and Health*, *10*(4), 391–399. doi: 10.1080/2159676X.2018.1476010

Charon, R. (2008). *Narrative medicine: Honoring stories of illness*. New York: Oxford University Press.

Crust, L. (2007). Mental toughness in sport: A review. *International Journal of Sport and Exercise Psychology*, *5*(3), 270–290. doi: 10.1080/1612197X.2007.9671836

Curry, T. (1993). A little pain never hurt anyone: Athletic career socialization and the normalization of sports injury. *Symbolic Interaction*, *16*(3), 273–290. doi: 10.1525/si.1993.16.3.273

Darnell, S., Chawansky, M., Marchessault, D., Holmes, M., & Hayhurst, L. (2018). The state of play: Critical sociological insights into recent 'Sport for Development and Peace' research. *International Review for the Sociology of Sport*, *53*(2), 133–151. doi: 10.1177%2F1012690216646762

Elias, N. (1978). *The civilizing process*. Oxford: Blackwell.

Elias, N. (1991). *The society of individuals*. Oxford: Blackwell.

Emery, C., Black, A., & Kolstad, A. (2017). What strategies can be used to effectively reduce the risk of concussion in sport? A systematic review. *British Journal of Sports Medicine, 51*(12), 978–984. doi: 10.1136/bjsports-2016-097452

Engelberg, T., & Skinner, J. (2016). Doing in sport: Whose problem is it? *Sport Management Review, 19*(1), 1–5. doi: 10.1016/j.smr.2015.12.001

Frey, J. (1991). Social risk and the meaning of sport. *Sociology of Sport Journal, 8*(2), 136–145. doi: 10.1123/ssj.8.2.136

Hughes, L., & Leavey, G. (2017). Setting the bar: Athletes and vulnerability to mental illness. *The British Journal of Psychiatry, 200*(2), 95–96. doi: 10.1192/bjp.bp.111.095976

Hughes, R., & Coakley, J. (1991). Positive deviance among athletes: The implications of overconformity to the Sport Ethic. *Sociology of Sport Journal, 8*(4), 307–325. doi: 10.1123/ssj.8.4.307

Hunt, E., & Day, M. (2018). Narratives of chronic pain in sport. *Journal of Clinical Sport Psychology, 13*(1), 1–16. doi: 10.1123/jcsp.2017-0003

Kerr, G., Battaglia, A., & Stirling, A. (2019). Maltreatment in youth sport: A systemic issue. *Kinesiology Review, 8*(3), 237–243. doi: 10.1123/kr.2019-0016

Kidder, J. (2017). *Parkour and the city: Risk, masculinity, and meaning in a postmodern sport*. New Brunswick, NJ: Rutgers University Press.

Le Breton, D. (2000). Playing symbolically with death in extreme sports. *Body & Society, 6*, 1–11. doi: 10.1177%2F1357034X00006001001

Madrigal, L., & Robbins, J. (2017). Roller derby: Experiences with injury and pain in players' behavioral repertoires. *Journal of Sport Behavior, 40*, 171–190.

Malcolm, D. (2017). *Sport, medicine and health: The medicalization of sport?* London: Routledge.

Martinent, G., & Ferrand, C. (2015). A field study of discrete emotions: Athletes' cognitive appraisals during competition. *Research Quarterly for Exercise and Sport, 86*(1), 51–62. doi: 10.1080/02701367.2014.975176.

Messner, M. (1990). When bodies are weapons: Masculinity and violence in Sport. *International Review for the Sociology of Sport, 25*(3), 203–218. doi: 10.1177/101269029002500303

Messner, M. (1992). *Power at play: Sports and the problem of masculinity*. Boston, MA: Beacon Press.

Moore, D., Kay, J., & Ellemberg, D. (2018). The long-term outcomes of sport-related concussion in pediatric populations. *International Journal of Psychophysiology, 132*(A), 14–24. doi: 10.1016/j.ijpsycho.2018.04.003

Nixon, H. (1992). A social network analysis of influences on athletes to play with pain and injuries. *Journal of Sport and Social Issues, 16*(2), 127–135. doi: 10.1177%2F019372359201600208

Nixon, H. (1993). Accepting the risks of pain and injury in sport: Mediated cultural influences on playing hurt. *Sociology of Sport Journal, 10*(2), 183–196. doi: 10.1123/ssj.10.2.183

Owton, H. (2016). *Sexual Abuse in Sport: A qualitative case study*. London, UK: Palgrave MacMillan.

Papathomas, A., & Lavallee, D. (2010). Athlete experiences of disordered eating in sport. *Qualitative Research in Sport and Exercise, 2*(3), 354–370. doi: 10.1080/19398441.2010.517042

Papathomas, A., Smith, B., & Lavallee, D. (2015). Family experiences of living with an eating disorder: A narrative analysis. *Journal of Health Psychology, 20*(3), 313–325. doi: 10.1177/1359105314566608

Pringle, R., Rinehart, R., & Caudwell, J. (2015). *Sport and the social significance of pleasure*. New York: Routledge.

Roderick, M. (2014). From identification to dis-identification: Case studies of job loss in professional football. *Qualitative Research in Sport, Exercise and Health*, *6*(2), 143–160. doi: 10.1080/2159676X.2013.796491

Roderick, M., Smith, A., & Potrac, P. (2017). The sociology of sports work, emotions and mental health: Scoping the field and future directions. *Sociology of Sport Journal*, *34*(2), 99–107. doi: 10.1123/ssj.2017-0082

Roessler, K. (2006). Sport and the psychology of pain. In S. Loland, B. Skirstad & I. Waddington (Eds.), *Pain and injury in sport: Social and ethical analysis* (pp. 34–48). London: Routledge.

Rowe, K., Karg, A., & Sherry, E. (2019). Community-oriented practice: Examining corporate social responsibility and development activities in professional sport. *Sport Management Review*, *23*(3), 363–378. doi: 10.1016/j.smr.2018.05.001

Sabo, D. (1989). Pigskin, patriarchy and pain. In D. Sabo & M. Messner (Eds.), *Sex, violence, and power in sports: Rethinking masculinity* (p. 82–88). Freedom, CA: The Crossing Press.

Safai, P. (2004). Negotiating with risk: Exploring the role of the sport medicine clinician. In K. Young (Ed.), *Sporting bodies, damaged selves: Sociological studies of sports-related injuries* (pp. 269–286). Oxford, UK: Elsevier.

Saunders, D. C. (1986). The nature and nurture of pain control. *Journal of Pain and Symptom Management*, *1*(4), 199–201. doi: 10.1016/s0885-3924(86)80041-0

Scott, S., & Austin, M. (2016). Edgework, fun, and identification in a recreational subculture: Street BMX riders. *Qualitative Sociology Review*, *12*, 85–99. Retrieved from http://www.qualitativesociologyreview.org

Smith, K. (2018). Total pain. In M. Atkinson (Ed.), *Sport, mental illness, and sociology* (pp. 23–43). London: Elsevier.

Smith, K. (2019). The suffering body in sport. In K. Young (Ed.), *The suffering body in sport: Shifting thresholds in pain, risk and injury* (pp. 121–140). London: Elsevier.

Smith, R. (2008). Pain in the act: The meaning of pain among professional wrestlers. *Qualitative Sociology*, *31*(2), 129–148.

Turner, A., Barlow, J., & Ilbery, B. (2002). Play hurt, live hurt: Living with and managing osteoarthritis from the perspective of ex-professional footballers. *Journal of Health Psychology*, *7*(3), 285–301. doi: 10.1177%2F1359105302007003222

Uphill, M., Sly, D., & Swain, J. (2016). From mental health to mental wealth in athletes: Looking back and moving forward. *Frontiers in Psychology*, *21*, 935. doi: 10.3389/fpsyg.2016.00935

Wellard, I. (2013). *Sport, fun and enjoyment: An embodied approach*. London, UK: Routledge.

Wilson, B., & Millington, B. (2017). Physical cultural studies, sport and the environment. In M. Silk, D. Andrews, & H. Thorpe (Eds.), *Routledge handbook of physical cultural studies* (pp. 333–343). Abingdon, UK: Routledge.

Young, K. (1993). Risk and liability in male sports culture. *Sociology of Sport Journal*, *10*(4), 373–396. doi: 10.1123/ssj.10.4.373

Young, K. (2004). *Sporting bodies, damaged selves: Sociological studies of sports-related injury*. Amsterdam: Elsevier.

Young, K. (2012). *Sport, violence, and society*. New York: Routledge.

Young, K. (2019). *The suffering body in sport: Shifting thresholds in pain, risk and injury*. London, UK: Elsevier.

6 "Slim-To-Win" to Injury

How Swimmers are Engaging
With "Health Risk" Culture Due
to Entrenched Body Ideals

Jenny McMahon and Kerry R. McGannon

Introduction

"Slim-to-win" is an entrenched ideology in swimming culture based on merito-cratic ideas whereby the "slim" and "fatless" body shape is perceived as enhancing competitive performance (Jones, Glintmeyer, & McKenzie, 2005; Lang, 2010; McGannon & McMahon, 2019; McMahon & Dinan Thompson, 2008; McMahon, Penney, & Dinan Thompson, 2012). Similar to other sporting cultures such as running and gymnastics, "slim-to-win" within swimming is part of a wider cultural discourse within sport that aligns "thin body ideals", for both male and female athletes, with certain practices to achieve such ideals (e.g., daily weigh-ins, skin folds, disordered eating, body surveillance, food monitoring, over-exercising, overuse injuries) (Busanich, McGannon, & Schinke, 2014, 2016; Cavallerio, Wadey, & Wagstaff, 2016; McGannon & McMahon, 2019; Papathomas & Lavallee, 2014). The "slim-to-win" ideology has been found to be uncritically recycled by coaches, swimmers, support staff, and parents in swimming culture. We refer to the recycling of this dominant ideology as uncritical and problematic because swimming is indeed a sport where there is no demonstrated benefit linked to thinness from a performance perspective (McMahon et al., 2012). For instance, Maglischo (1993) found no relationship between body shape and drag measured during actual swimming and established that even the most lean and tapered swimmers cannot remain streamlined enough to eliminate turbulence. Similarly, Pyne (2007) explained that while some studies in different sports associate better performance with lower skin folds and a slim body shape, there is no such supporting evidence in the sport of swimming, which is surprising given the emphasis on weight and shape by every coach. Despite these findings, the belief that the slimmer or leaner a swimmer becomes, the better s/he will perform remains a taken-for-granted notion and continues to saturate swimming culture (McMahon et al., 2012; McMahon, McGannon, & Zehntner, 2017). However, Howe (2004) warns that when competitive performance is at the forefront of cultural ideologies, practices, and expectations (as is occurring in swimming with "slim-to-win"), engaging with "risk culture" will potentially take a paramount role within an athlete's individual sporting habitus.

Within the present chapter, we aim to explore how the "slim-to-win" ideology has influenced athletes and cultural insiders to engage with "risk culture" resulting in subsequent sports injury. Moreover, we are also interested in identifying the types of risks taken and by whom within a sporting context (i.e., swimming). This is accomplished by first outlining what "risk culture" is and how it can potentially lead to sports injury and also why it occurs in sporting contexts. Two athletes' stories from previous research investigating amateur and elite swimming in Australia are also presented in order to identify how and why athletes' health and well-being are being compromised and by whom. By doing this, we hope we address what Cavallerio et al. (2016) says is lacking in sport psychology and injury research, namely, the identification of if and how sport is potentially "damaging athletes' health" (p. 100).

Critical Reflections

A number of researchers in sport injury psychology have called for sport injury researchers to explore the sociocultural context within which injury occurs (e.g., Wadey, Day, Cavallerio, & Martinelli, 2018; Wiese-Bjornstal, 2010; Wiese-Bjornstal, Smith, Shaffer, & Morrey, 1998). As Wadey et al. (2018 explains, when we consider injury through the sociocultural lens, it may inherently "help to provide a more critical, nuanced, and holistic understanding of sport injury" (p. 3). One related area of interest to explore in this regard is "risk culture", which has been shown to be prevalent in every level of sport (Howe, 2004; Safari & Malcolm, 2016). Sociocultural sport research has shown that risk culture occurs when athletes and cultural insiders (e.g., coaches, physiologists, parents; see Chapters 9, 10, and 11) are willing to take, and indeed accept risks that may compromise athletes' health and well-being in the name of competitive performance (e.g., Howe, 2004; McEwan & Young, 2011; Nixon, 1992). Engaging with risk culture is serious because it can lead to injury by affecting athletes' mental and physical health in the short term (i.e., during sport participation) and in the long term (i.e., post sport). Donnelly (2004) explains that in order to understand more about why "risk culture" is engaged with so readily in sport contexts, emphasis needs to be placed on identifying the influences on the decisions to take risks, and the types of risks taken. Once more is understood about why the "culture of risk" is taken up in specific sporting contexts, athletes and sporting insiders can be better supported through the formulation of specific interventions. Such identification may further assist in preventing subsequent injury (e.g., physical and mental) from occurring (Donnelly, 2004; Howe, 2004).

Previous research (e.g., McGannon & McMahon, 2019; McMahon et al., 2012; McMahon et al., 2017) has highlighted the powerful ways in which the "slim-to-win" ideology and associated practices can operate within Australian swimming culture, and how the ideology is disseminated and engaged with by coaches, team managers, athletes, and other cultural insiders (e.g., parents). An example of how "slim-to-win" operated within Australian swimming culture was made known by Leisel Jones, a four-time Olympian who explained within her published autobiography that swimming coaches would publicly weigh swimmers. Those female swimmers who did not make or maintain weight would be labeled as fat and with the code number 6:1:20, representing the word "fat" in terms of the order of letters in the alphabet (Zaccardi, 2015). Jones explained that if she put on weight at daily weigh-ins, she would be publicly ridiculed by coaches because her body failed to meet their expectations (Geary, 2015). Coaches also played a role in attempting to mould Jones' body to a "slim-to-win" shape for performance as they actively encouraged her to skip meals and consume only meal replacement shakes when it failed to achieve the desired "slim" shape (McGannon & McMahon, 2019; Zaccardi, 2015). Jones was not the only one affected, as she noted that other female swimmers would sob in the shower after they were weighed, weighed, and weighed again by men as old as her father who would constantly pass judgment (Zaccardi, 2015). The "slim-to-win" requirements were made clear to the Australian swimmers: in order to achieve performance they needed to have a "slim" and "fatless" body shape. Those swimmers who failed to achieve the "slim-to-win" shape were punished through disparaging comments (made publicly by coaches), excessive running (i.e., 16 km) leading in some cases to overuse injuries, and social isolation and food restriction, in some cases leading to mental health issues (Cavallerio et al., 2016; McGannon & McMahon, 2019; McMahon, 2010; McMahon et al., 2012; McMahon et al., 2017). However, as previous researchers investigating the "culture of risk" in sport (e.g., Howe, 2004; McEwan & Young, 2011; Safari & Malcolm, 2016) warn, when performance is central to cultural ideologies within sport (as is occurring with the "slim-to-win" ideology), the engagement of "risk culture" and associated practices that may harm the body and self may result. This point highlights the nexus between cultural ideologies such as "slim-to-win" and the nuanced relationship between body-self and injury.

To illustrate these points further, we draw on the voice of Julie, who is a national representative swimmer but is yet to win medals on the world stage. Her experiences were presented as part of a previous research study investigating body pedagogies in Australian swimming culture (see McMahon, 2010; McMahon et al., 2012). In an attempt to conform her body to a slim and fatless shape, Julie tried dieting, overdosing on laxative medication, and visiting a dietician. Despite trying these approaches, her swimmer body still did not measure up to her coach's expectations. Having internalized these expectations, and in an act of desperation to achieve competitive performance and conform her body to a "slim-to-win" shape, Julie decided to take methamphetamines (i.e., speed). This was a prohibited substance in her sport, which in turn led to the demise of her health and an injury (e.g., elevated heart rate, chronic fatigue syndrome). Mental health issues (e.g., anxiety, disordered eating and exercise) also resulted.

A friend of mine from school told me that she used methamphetamines to lose weight and had great success. She lost 20 kilograms in just three months! I am desperate to represent my country in my sport and my coach is constantly taunting me about how much fat I have. I am tired of him yelling at me. I am tired of him making me run 10 kilometres after training each night. I am tired of him weighing me publicly and announcing that I am a loser when I don't achieve the right weight number. I am tired of him telling other parents and swimmers (in front of me) how fat I am. If I don't lose weight, I won't get to represent my country. I have been dieting for ages and it is not enough. I know speed is a prohibited substance. I know that if I get caught taking it, I will be banned, but I am desperate. I research the effects of the drug, but it does not deter me, even though I could potentially have a heart attack. I only will take it for a few months until I get the "slim-to-win" body shape that will bring me Olympic glory. I contact a friend who I know "deals." It is not long after that before I have purchased my first-ever speed. I feel a sense of fulfilment knowing that speed is going to help me stop eating and achieve that ideal body shape that I so desperately seek and that I know will bring me success.

(McMahon, 2010)

The above example shows how Julie internalized the ideology and associated risky practices of "slim-to-win" by way of deciding to take a banned substance to manage and control her weight. According to Howe (2004), while engaging with risk culture involves the active decision-making of athletes, the practices are the result of risk culture being ingrained within sport and sporting practices by cultural insiders. In the above example, when the punishment enforced by coaches (e.g., running 10 km) and other self-control measures (e.g., seeking advice from a dietician, eating healthy) did not work for Julie, engaging with "risk culture" seemed like the next feasible option in order to achieve "slim-to-win". Julie actively decided to take methamphetamine due to "slim-to-win" and performance being at the forefront of her thinking. She engaged with risky (self) practices, which could be read as a form of self-injury, which potentially allowed her to reshape her body in terms of a "slim-to-win" body shape, in order to exhibit so-called visual indicators of performance demanded by coaches, team managers, and physiologists (Glassner 1990; McEwan & Young, 2011). Consequently, through the consumption of methamphetamines, her health became secondary to the "slim-to-win" look of her "outer body", resulting in a short-circuiting of the polarity between "looking" and "being" healthy (McEwan & Young, 2011; Monoghan, 2001) leading to injury, abuse of her physical body, and mental health issues.

Howe (2004) explains how engaging with health risk culture may be further viewed as a dome that entraps health and positive encounters with the body. The potentially health-damaging practice of "drug taking" for the purpose of "slim-to-win" blurred dualities for Julie (e.g., inner and outer body, mortality and immortality) (Monoghan, 2001). In essence then, risk consisted of Julie consciously knowing that she may suffer health side effects (e.g., heart attack, injury) but going ahead and consuming methamphetamine in spite of that knowledge. Indeed, risking her health through this form of self-injury (i.e., using an illicit and dangerous drug) became an integral and normalized component of her sporting world. Monaghan (2001) warns however, that there may be conflicting views and opinions centring on what constitutes "risk" from those involved in sport and the general public. For example, risks that appear unacceptable to those outside of sporting cultures may not be viewed as risks to those involved in sport (as shown in Julie's story). For Julie, the quest to acquire the ideal and performing body was taken for granted and entrenched within swimming culture; thus she viewed taking methamphetamines as a necessary and normal means to attain such a body and performance (Monoghan, 2001).

Julie's story also exemplifies how she had agency/choice in the decision to take methamphetamines, and that she was not simply a passive recipient of risk culture. Julie's story partly shows that she was empowered in knowing that taking methamphetamines would help her to achieve the ideal swimmer body that was perceived to enhance competitive performance (e.g., "I feel a sense of fulfilment knowing that speed is going to help me stop eating and achieve that ideal body shape"). Within her story, Julie also noted that she felt a sense of fulfilment because at the level of cultural significance, the slim and fatless body shape had popular currency and social capital as symbolic modes for transmitting values such as hard work, fitness, performance, and commitment (Bordo, 1993; McGannon & McMahon, 2019; McMahon, 2010; McMahon et al., 2012).

Others involved in sport have also been found to compromise swimmers' health and well-being, normalizing forms of "self-injury" as a result of the "slim-to-win" ideology and practices. Recent research (McMahon & McGannon, 2018) has shown that through acts of desperation, swimmers sought the assistance of medical doctors as a result of viewing their bodies as a problem that could be fixed through medical transformation (Theberge, 2007). Similar to the sporting context, the medical science context has been shown to view the sporting body as a machine (Theberge, 2007), which has resulted in medical risks being taken in order to assist athletes to achieve performance outcomes, regardless of the cost to athlete health (i.e., self-injury, physical injury) and well-being (McMahon & McGannon, 2018; Monaghan, 2001; Paraschak, 2012; Theberge, 2007). Theberge (2007) conducted an investigation in sports medicine and the culture of risk among doctors, physiotherapists, and administrators in elite Canadian sport and found that performance concerns were at the epicenter of medical practice. Due to performance being at the forefront of doctors' thinking, the boundaries between human performance and medical practice became obscured, with many doctors erring on the side of performance rather than considering athletes' long-term health (de la Pena, 2003; Magdalinski, 2009; McNamee, 2014; Scott, 2012). This finding highlights how medical practitioners are engaging with the culture of risk as a result of performance pressures placed on athletes, and also reproducing risk culture practices and norms (Theberge, 2007). Below, we draw on Jasmine's experience to exemplify these points. Jasmine is a former national representative swimmer, having competed at numerous international meets. Although she has won numerous international medals, she has missed qualifying standards for the last two national teams. In turn, coaches blame her weight and body shape for her failure to perform. In the story below, Jasmine sought the assistance of a sports medicine doctor in an attempt to conform her body to a "slim-to-win" shape after her own measures failed to work.

> I am desperate to lose weight. The next Olympics is everything that I think about. There is one thing standing in my way from achieving that dream. It is my fat body! Not only has my coach told me that I am too fat and that is why my performance has dropped off, but I also notice that I do not look like other swimmers' bodies who are doing well (e.g., no boobs, no bum, no hips, no fat). Visits to the dietician have not worked so I book an appointment with the sports medicine doctor to see if there is something medically preventing me from losing weight.

Sports doctor: "Hi, what can I help you with today?"

Jasmine: "I am a swimmer and I am in training for the Olympics. I am having trouble losing weight. My coach says that I need to lose weight if I am going to have any chance of making the next Olympic team. I have been visiting a dietician for ages and have hardly lost any weight. According to my coach, I have not done enough, and I am beyond desperate. I am hoping you can help me."

Sports doctor: "Can you jump on the scales for me?"

> Anxiety overcomes me. Why does he need to weigh me? I already get weighed by so many people and my weight number never meets their expectations.

Sports doctor: "75.3 kilograms. You can take a seat again for me. Do you have any other medical conditions or allergies? Are you taking any other medications?"

> I tell him that I do not take any medication and that I have never had an allergy. He pauses momentarily.

Sports doctor: "Ok, I am going to prescribe you some thyroxine. Thyroxine is a medication which alters your thyroid function. I realise your blood work says your thyroid function is normal, but an overactive thyroid function can assist in weight loss. Take the tablets and it will speed things up for you. You will need to take one tablet morning and night. You may experience headaches, diarrhoea, vomiting and tremors. Come back and see me in two weeks and we will see how you are going and get you to jump onto the scales again."

> The consultation takes about 10 minutes. As I walk out of the doctor's surgery, I feel content. Just like that, the sports doctor has helped me to find the answer. Now, I will lose weight and now I will make the Olympic team.

(McMahon & McGannon, 2018)

Jasmine sought the assistance of the sports medicine doctor by subscribing to and embodying the "slim-to-win" ideology. Subsequently, she viewed her body as a problem, which should be fixed through medical transformation (Theberge, 2007), rendering her bodily appearance closer to the culturally accepted and perpetuated ideal (e.g. no fat, no bum, slim) (McMahon & Barker-Ruchti, 2017; McMahon & McGannon, 2018). The pressure and desperation that Jasmine felt to conform her body to a "slim-to-win" shape was shown in her conversation with the doctor when she noted, "I am beyond desperate, and I am hoping you can help me." The conversation also exemplifies how Jasmine understood her body through the "slim-to-win" discourse, and as a result of power relations (e.g., pressures placed on her by her coach and the doctor as a facilitator of attaining a slim body) which were reproduced through body-management practices (Markula & Pringle, 2006).

Jasmine's story further shows how the sports medicine doctor accepted the "slim-to-win" ideology without question, and in so doing, became an accomplice to the normalization of the ideology and the proliferation of the same (McMahon & McGannon, 2018). As a consequence of the "slim-to-win" ideology, the sports medical doctor imposed a medical regimen onto Jasmine (e.g., prescribed thyroxin even though she had a healthy thyroid function) as a way of assisting her to achieve the culturally ideal shape (McMahon & McGannon, 2018). Jasmine's story exemplifies the power and pervasiveness of the "slim-to-win" ideology and shows how it can be extended to another site outside of sport – that of medical practice (McMahon & Barker-Ruchti, 2017; McMahon & McGannon, 2018). Howe (2004) warns that the danger of engaging with a "culture of risk", as occurred when Jasmine's doctor altered her healthy thyroid function, is that it will become a "fog" that leads to the acceptance and normalization of health risk practices and potential forms of self-injury (i.e., taking unnecessary medication) which may be viewed as necessary in order to achieve competitively.

This medical transaction also highlighted how both Jasmine and her doctor subscribed to the importance of medical treatment (Lupton, 2012) in the name of "slim-to-win". However, the sports medicine doctor created additional pressures for Jasmine through his uncritical acceptance of "slim-to-win" and his prescribed treatment as he too categorized her body as falling outside the "norm" in terms of shape and weight (McMahon & McGannon, 2018). By viewing Jasmine's body as falling outside the "norm", the doctor targeted her with a medical intervention. In so doing, Jasmine's body was viewed as a site for treatment and repair and a site for power and control (McMahon & McGannon, 2018; Rich & Evans, 2007). This power was shown when Jasmine did not question the doctor's medical regime/treatment plan and obligingly took the thyroxine even though it would cause her thyroid function to become altered, with serious side effects (e.g., tremors). However, as Lupton (2012) explains, the athlete and doctor relationship is not entirely one-sided but rather dynamic, negotiated, and renegotiated by athletes. Jasmine's story exemplifies these points as she approached the sports medicine doctor as a knowledgeable colleague rather than a superior (Lupton, 2012) that could assist her to achieve her means (e.g., "slim-to-win" shape). Indeed, after leaving the medical consultation, Jasmine felt empowered by the help of her doctor and in knowing that she could finally make her body conform, highlighting that she had agency in the medical transaction (e.g., "As I walk out of the doctor's surgery, I feel content. Just like that, the sports doctor has helped me to find the answer").

Future Research Implications

In this chapter, we have outlined how the dominant ideology of "slim-to-win", found to saturate the sport context of swimming, has led to athletes and other cultural insiders (e.g., coaches, managers, other athletes) compromising their health through forms of self-injury (i.e., taking medications) which puts their bodies at risk of physical injury and mental health issues. In the following section, suggestions are made in the spirit of sparking research that continues in the qualitative tradition of critical insights into sport injury psychology (see Chapter 12). Previous research into the "culture of risk" in sport (e.g., Howe, 2004: McEwan & Young, 2011; Safari & Malcolm, 2016) has shown that the social networks that surround elite sporting performers can positively impact whether an individual becomes entrapped within a health risk culture that can lead to potential forms of injury. Given the potential for support networks to assist athletes to critically examine dominant ideologies such as "slim-to-win" before engaging with risk culture and becoming injured, more research is needed in this regard, particularly in relation identifying interventions. We thus propose the following research question for future work: What education interventions might better assist athletes and their support networks to better consider their health and well-being over performance and dominant cultural ideologies such as "slim-to-win"?

Implementing education interventions with athletes and their support networks is one important avenue that may prevent the "culture of risk" from being taken up (see Chapter 14) and forms of injury from occurring. For example, Mountjoy et al. (2016) has highlighted the importance of education interventions to assist those involved in sport to identify normalized forms of abuse. Similarly, Nelson, Groom, and Potrac (2016), as well as McMahon and Smith (2016), also highlighted the importance of education interventions to assist with the uncritical recycling of coaching practices by coaches. Specifically, narrative pedagogy has been identified as a contemporary theory of learning, education, and social interaction that can be utilized as an education intervention in sport. Goodson and Gill (2011) were influential in the development of narrative pedagogy with their thinking and theorizing about it stemming from the idea that narratives (e.g., conversations, text-based stories, oral stories) are a successful way for people to make sense of their lives, thus becoming a process of learning and transformation (Goodson & Gill, 2011; McMahon, Knight, & McGannon, 2018; McMahon & Smith, 2016). As a result of extensive research, Goodson and Gill (2011) found that by engaging with narratives (i.e., reading a person's story of experience) and then swapping the narrative/s with another (i.e., exchanging stories about the story), pedagogic encounters (i.e., learning opportunities) arose. Indeed, the potential of narrative pedagogy was realized as those who practiced narrative pedagogy were able to move toward a deeper understanding of the topic being explored (McMahon et al., 2018) with the possibility of social action being initiated (Goodson & Gill, 2011; McMahon & Smith, 2016).

Conclusion

Within this chapter, we have outlined how the uncritical acceptance of "slim-to-win", not only by cultural insiders but also other sport professionals (e.g., sports medicine doctors), has led to the engagement with (health) risk practices (e.g., meth-amphetamine use, prescribing thyroxin to alter a healthy thyroid function). These risk practices point to sport as a problematic environment which circulates limited meanings about the body through the engagement with these health risk behaviours. For those involved in sport in this research (i.e., Julie, Jasmine, coaches, sports medicine doctor), engaging with risk culture was seen as an integral, and even necessary component of the sporting world which would assist them to achieve "slim-to-win". The "look" of the outer body was so central for the athletes that they were willing to accept adverse effects to health (e.g., heart attack, headaches, diarrhoea, vomiting, and tremors) in order to improve the appearance of the body (into a "slim-to-win" shape). Ironically, those athletes who were desperate to achieve the ideal look of the outer body ("slim-to-win") and perceived performance enhancement, engaged with risky health practices (e.g., methamphetamine use), compromising their health and physical well-being through forms of self-inflicted injury.

Critical Discussion Questions

1) What types of education interventions might assist athletes and cultural insiders to critically examine ideologies such as "slim-to-win" and associated practices that lead to injury, in order to prevent forms of injury from occurring?
2) How can narrative pedagogy assist athletes and cultural insiders to understand – and potentially transform – the culture of health risk and sports injury through telling new and different stories about athletes, bodies, and performance?
3) How can we better support cultural insiders in sport to more critically examine and consider athlete health and well-being, in order to prevent forms of self-injury (e.g., taking illicit medications, starvation, over-exercising)?

References

Bordo, S. (1993). The body and the reproduction of femininity. In S. Bordo (Ed.), *Unbearable weight: Feminism, western culture, and the body* (pp. 90–110). Los Angeles, CA: University of California Press.

Busanich, R., McGannon, K. R., & Schinke, R. (2014). Comparing elite male and female distance runner's experiences of disordered eating through narrative analysis. *Psychology of Sport and Exercise, 15*(6), 705–712. doi: 10.1016/j.psychsport.2013.10.002

Busanich, R., McGannon, K. R., & Schinke, R. (2016). Exploring disordered eating and embodiment in male distance runners through visual narrative methods. *Qualitative Research in Sport, Exercise and Health, 8*(1), 95–112. doi: 10.1080/2159676X.2015.1028093

Cavallerio, F., Wadey, R., & Wagstaff, C. (2016). Understanding overuse injuries in rhythmic gymnastics: A 12-month ethnographic study. *Psychology of Sport and Exercise, 25,* 100–109. doi: 10.1016/j.psychsport.2016.05.002

de la Pena, C. T. (2003). *The body electric: How strange machines build the modern American.* New York: New York University Press.

Donnelly, P. (2004). Sport and risk culture. In K. Young (Ed.), *Sporting bodies, damaged selves: Sociological studies of sports-related injury* (pp. 29–58). Oxford: Elsevier Science Press.

Geary, B. (2015). 'It nearly killed me': Olympic gold medalist Leisel Jones says teen years were plagued with obsessive dieting – As she reveals her battles with mental health issues. *Daily Mail.* Retrieved from https://www.dailymail.co.uk/news/article-3253729/It-nea rly-killed-Olympic-gold-medallist-Leisel-Jones-says-teen-years-plagued-obsessive-diet ing-including-banning-chocolate-year-reveals-mental-health-battles.html

Glassner, B. (1990). Fit for postmodern selfhood. In H. Becker & M. McCall (Eds.), *Symbolic interaction and cultural studies* (pp. 215–243). Chicago, IL: University of Chicago Press.

Goodson, I. F., & Gill, S. R. (2011). *Narrative pedagogy: Life history and learning.* New York: Peter Land Publishing, Inc.

Howe, D. (2004). *Sport, professionalism and pain: Ethnographies of injury and risk.* London: Routledge.

Jones, R., Glintmeyer, N., & McKenzie, A. (2005). Slim bodies, eating disorders and the coach-athlete relationship: A tale of identity creation and disruption. *International Review for the Sociology of Sport, 40*(3), 377–391. doi: 10.1177/1012690205060231

Lang, M. (2010). Surveillance and conformity in competitive youth swimming. *Sport, Education and Society Journal, 15*(1), 19–38. doi: 10.1080/13573320903461152

Lupton, D. (2012). *Medicine as culture: Illness, disease and the body.* Thousand Oaks, CA: Sage.

Magdalinski, T. (2009). *Sport, technology and the body: The nature of performance.* New York: Routledge.

Maglischo, E. (1993). *Swimming fastest: The essential reference on technique, training and program design.* Champaign, IL: Human Kinetics.

Markula, P., & Pringle, R. (2006). *Foucault, sport and exercise: Power, knowledge and transforming the self.* London: Routledge.

McEwen, K., & Young, K. (2011). Ballet and pain: Reflections on a risk-dance culture. *Qualitative Research in Sport, Exercise and Health, 3*(2), 152–173. doi: 10.1080/2159676X.2011.572181

McGannon, K. R., & McMahon, J. (2019). Understanding female athlete disordered eating and recovery through narrative turning points in autobiographies. *Psychology of Sport and Exercise, 40,* 42–50. doi: 10.1016/j.psychsport.2018.09.003

McMahon, J. (2010). *Exposure and effect: An investigation into a culture of body pedagogies* [Unpublished PhD thesis]. University of Tasmania.

McMahon, J., & Barker-Ruchti, N. (2017). Assimilating to a boy's body shape for the sake of performance: Three female athletes' body experiences in a sporting culture. *Sport, Education and Society, 22*(2), 157–174. doi: 10.1080/13573322.2015.1013463

McMahon, J., & Dinan-Thompson, M. (2008). A malleable body – Revelations from an Australian elite swimmer. *Healthy Lifestyles Journal, 55*(1), 23–28.

McMahon, J., Knight, C., & McGannon (2018). Educating parents of children in sport about abuse using narrative pedagogy. *Sociology of Sport, 35*(4), 314–323. doi: 10.1123/ ssj.2017-0186

McMahon, J., & McGannon, K. R. (2018). The athlete–doctor relationship: Power, complicity, resistance and accomplices in recycling dominant sporting ideologies. *Sport, Education and Society, 23,* 57–69. doi: 10.1080/13573322.2018.1561434.

McMahon, J., McGannon, K. R., & Zehntner, C. (2017). 'Slim to Win': An ethnodrama of three elite swimmers' 'presentation of self' in relation to a dominant cultural ideology. *Sociology of Sport Journal, 34*(2), 108–123. doi: 10.1123/ssj.2015-0166

McMahon, J., Penney, D., & Dinan-Thompson, M. (2012). Body practices – Exposure and effect of a sporting culture? Stories from three Australian swimmers. *Sport, Education and Society, 17*(2), 181–206. doi: 10.1080/13573322.2011.607949

McMahon, J., & Smith, B. (2016). Ivor Goodson, narrative pedagogy and narrative learning theory: Some implications for sport coaching. In L. Nelson, R. Groom, & P. Potrac (Eds.), *Learning in sports coaching: Theory and application* (pp. 123–134). Abingdon: Routledge. doi: 10.4324/9781315746012

McNamee, M. (2014). *Sport, medicine, ethics.* Milton Park: Routledge.

Monoghan, L. F. (2001). Looking good, feeling good: The embodied pleasures of vibrant physicality. *Sociology of Health and Illness, 23*(3), 330–356. doi: 10.1111/1467-9566.00255

Nelson, L., Groom, R., & Potrac, P. (Eds.). (2016). *Learning in sports coaching: Theory and application.* London, UK: Routledge. doi: 10.4324/9781315746012

Nixon, H. (1992). A social network analysis of influences on athletes to play with pain and injuries. *Journal of Sport and Social Issues, 16*(2), 127–135. doi: 10.1177/019372359201600208

Papathomas, A., & Lavallee, D. (2014). Self-starvation and the performance narrative in competitive sport. *Psychology of Sport and Exercise, 15*(6), 688–695. doi: 10.1016/j.psychsport.2013.10.014

Paraschak, V. (2012). Public health, elite sport and risky behaviours at the Canada Winter Games. In D. Malcolm & P. Safari (Eds.), *The social organisation of sports medicine* (pp. 126–149). New York: Routledge.

Rich, E., & Evans, J. (2007, December). Rereading voice: Young women, anorexia and performative education. *Junctures: The Journal for Thematic Dialogue.* Retrieved from http://www.junctures.org/issues.php?issue=09&title=Voice&colour=rgb(176,153,0)

Safari, P., & Malcolm, D. (2016). Sport, health and medicine. In B. Houlihan & D. Malcolm (Eds.), *Sport and society* (3rd ed.) (pp. 157–179). London: Sage.

Scott, A. (2012). Making compromises in sports medicine: An examination of the health performance nexus in British Olympic sports. In D. Malcolm & P. Safari (Eds.), *The social organisation of sports medicine: Critical sociocultural perspectives* (pp. 227–246). London: Routledge.

Theberge, N. (2007). It's not about health, it's about performance': Sport medicine, health, and the culture of risk in Canadian sport. In J. Hargreaves & P. Vertinksy (Eds.), *Physical culture, power and the body* (pp. 176–194). Milton Park: Routledge.

Wadey, R., Day, M., Cavallerio, F., & Martinelli, L. (2018). The multilevel model of sport injury: Can coaches impact and be impacted by injury? In R. Thelwell & M. Dicks (Eds.), *Professional advances in sports coaching: Research and practice* (pp. 408–440). New York: Routledge.

Wiese-Bjornstal, D. M. (2010). Psychology and socioculture affect injury risk, response, and recovery in high-intensity athletes: A consensus statement. *Scandinavian Journal of Medicine and Science in Sport, 20*, 103–111. doi: 10.1111/j.1600-0838.2010.01195.x

Wiese-Bjornstal, D. M., Smith, A. M., Shaffer, S. M., & Morrey, M. A. (1998). An integrated model of response to sport injury: Psychological and sociological dimensions. *Journal of Applied Sport Psychology, 10*(1), 46–69. doi: 10.1080/10413209808406377

Zaccardi, N. (2015). *Leisel Jones details depression in body lengths.* Retrieved from https://olympics.nbcsports.com/2015/10/05/leisel-jones-depression-swimming-book-olympics-australia-body-lengths/?iframe=true&theme_preview=true/amp/

7 "What Doesn't Kill Us, Makes Us Stronger"

Do Injured Athletes *Really* Experience Growth?

Karen Howells and Ciara Everard

Introduction

> Since 2012 I have sustained four major injuries and setbacks, which have forced me to take long periods out of the sport. Over the last six years I have missed major championships and my performance progression has slowed due to months of little training. Yet because of this I am so much stronger psychologically and physically, my pole vault technique is so much better and I feel like I have developed in many different ways as a person.
>
> (Athletics Weekly, 2019)

The above quote is from European bronze-medal–winning pole vaulter and two-time Olympian, Holly Bradshaw. Holly's story is as remarkable as it is unremarkable. On the one hand, her account is representative of the dedication, resilience, and motivation that is required, even in the face of adversity, of any elite athlete who seeks to perform at the highest level. Yet on the other hand, her story, that of the positives that can emerge from adversity, is typical. This storyline, providing a cultural script of how an athlete could potentially experience and respond to adversity (see Chapter 1), is played out over and over again on a daily basis by elite athletes who sustain injuries and who claim to come out of the experience stronger (see Howells & Fletcher, 2016).

There is little doubt that for athletes who sustain an injury, it is an undesirable occurrence, but in many cases, these athletes are able to identify positives, such as those illustrated by Holly Bradshaw, that come from that experience. However, what is unclear is whether the injured athletes' identifications of positives are authentic (i.e., real) and transformative, or whether they are illusory (i.e., self-deceptive) and constitute conformity to a culturally informed narrative that promotes a message of "what doesn't kill you makes you stronger". Researchers examining sport injury psychology have yet to critically consider this issue in depth. Accordingly, in this chapter informed by both the sport and exercise psychology and the wider psychology literature, we will critically explore the notion of growth in injured athletes. Finally, we offer two questions to practitioners, coaches, and students to stimulate reflection in order to progress the exploration of growth in injured athletes in a direction that best supports injured athletes in a supportive and facilitative environment.

Growth Following Adversity

The notion of identifying positives following adversity (e.g., injury) is commonly referred to as *growth* especially when those positives involve transformation of the individual's life and are more enduring in nature (cf. Tedeschi & Calhoun, 2004). Researchers have identified growth in participants who have experienced an extensive and diverse variety of distressing experiences such as, but not restricted to, cancer (e.g., Arpawong, Richeimer, Weinstein, Elghamrawy, & Milam, 2013; Helgeson, 2010), sexual assault (e.g., Frazier, Conlon, & Glaser, 2001), and bereavement (e.g., Currier, Mallot, Martinez, Sandy, & Neimeyer, 2013). These studies are typically informed by one of the three[1] most widely applied models or theories of growth (see Howells, Wadey, & Day, 2020; Tedeschi, Shakespeare-Finch, Taku, & Calhoun, 2018). Despite some theoretical differences between these models or theories, there is consensus that growth is a process that involves identification of positive outcomes following a traumatic or adverse experience. These positive outcomes have been referred to as stress-related growth (SRG; Park, Cohen, & Murch, 1996), post-traumatic growth (PTG; Tedeschi & Calhoun, 1996), and adversarial growth (Linley & Joseph, 2004) and may be broadly categorized across five distinct domains (cf. Tedeschi & Calhoun, 1996), namely: a greater appreciation of life and changed sense of priorities; warmer, more intimate relationships with others; a greater sense of personal strength; recognition of new possibilities or paths for one's life; and spiritual-existential change. For *real* or *actual* growth to occur, these models and theories posit that the experience must be sufficiently severe that it results in a shattering of schematic assumptions that the individual holds about themselves and/or the world (cf. Janoff-Bulman, 1992).

Despite some coherence in respect of what growth comprises, some researchers have questioned the veridicality of growth (e.g., Maercker & Zoellner; 2004; Park, 2004; Wortman, 2004; Zoellner & Maercker, 2006a). Specifically, Maercker and Zoellner (2004) suggested that growth is reminiscent of a Janus-faced character and proposed a two-component model which comprises a constructive side and an illusory side to growth. The constructive, self-transcending side of growth, which is analogous with the assumptions of the functional descriptive model of post-traumatic growth (FDM; Tedeschi & Calhoun, 2004) is positively associated with adjustment and well-being in the long term, and may be conceived as *actual growth*. However, the illusory or dysfunctional side, they argued, involves self-deception and is associated with denial, avoidance, wishful thinking, self-consolidation, and palliation, which may occur following adversity. The identification of this illusory aspect to growth has its origins in Taylor's (1983) theory of cognitive adaptation to threatening events and her theoretical explanation of positive illusions, and Filipp's (1999) identification of attentive (namely, positive illusions, self-enhancing illusions, hope) and comparative (namely, social and temporal comparisons) coping processes. As a coping mechanism the illusory side may act as a short-term palliative coping strategy that in itself neither predicts long-term negative nor long-term positive consequences. However, despite the supporting evidence of this expanding conceptualization (e.g., Howells & Fletcher, 2016), it has received limited research in sport psychology generally and sport injury psychology specifically.

Growth in Injured Athletes

Reflecting the trend in the wider literature, a wealth of research evidence from the sport and exercise psychology literature collectively points to the notion that athletes can experience growth following a variety of adversities (see for a review, Howells, Sarkar, & Fletcher, 2017). A smaller number of studies specifically identified that athletes can experience growth following sports injury (namely, Brewer, Cornelius, Van Raalte, & Tennen, 2017;[2] Roy-Davis, Wadey, & Evans, 2017; Salim & Wadey, 2018, 2019; Salim, Wadey & Diss, 2015, 2016; Udry, Gould, Bridges, & Beck, 1997; Wadey et al., 2011; Wadey, Clarke, Podlog, & McCullough, 2013; Wadey, Podlog, Galli, & Mellalieu, 2016; Wadey, Roy-Davis, Evans, Howells, Salim, & Diss, 2019). Typically, this body of research has tended to be informed by theories that have originated elsewhere in psychology, succumbing to an age-old trend in sport and exercise psychology of "borrowing theories" (Lavallee, Kremer, Moran, & Williams, 2012, p. 10). We argue that the sport environment and the experience of sport injury is unique, and in examining the prospects for growth in injured athletes we should be critical of the extent to which we are informed by non–context-specific models and theories.

Cognizant of the potential to perpetuate the ambiguity that already exists around the use of terms to describe growth and importantly, ascribing to the view that sport injuries and rehabilitative environments are unique and should be viewed contextually through a lens that is sensitive to both the process of rehabilitation and the characteristics of the athletes themselves, Roy-Davis et al. (2017) proposed the term Sport Injury-Related Growth (SIRG). The term denotes the *perceived* changes that propel injured athletes to a higher level of functioning than that which existed prior to their injury (see Wadey & Everard, 2020). The authors' development of the Theory of SIRG (T-SIRG) provided a detailed justification for the introduction of a context-specific theory and conceptualization of SIRG. The theory refers to injury as a stressor that imposes ongoing strain throughout rehabilitation and posits that when athletes have certain internal (personality, coping style, knowledge and prior experience, perceived social support) and external (cultural scripts, physical resources, free time, received social support) resources available to them they are more likely to achieve SIRG through four internal mechanisms: meta-cognition, positive reappraisal, positive emotions, and facilitative responses. Although recent research has furthered our understanding of T-SIRG, with three studies (Salim & Wadey 2018; Salim & Wadey, 2019; Wadey, Roy-Davis et al., 2019) providing insight into its applicability, there is a lack of *critical* consideration as to whether growth, irrespective of the terminology used, actually occurs in injured athletes.

Do Injured Athletes *Really* Experience Growth?

In the immediate aftermath of experiencing injury it has been advocated that athletes report heightened negative emotions (e.g., Roy-Davis et al., 2017) and destructive cognitive processing (e.g., Udry et al., 1997). The injury can lead an athlete to question their athletic identity, encounter additional adversities (e.g., non-selection to a team, enforced retirement), and experience a loss of purpose (see Salim, Wadey, & Diss, 2016). However, after a period of time that involves cognitive processing of the injury (e.g., Udry et al., 1997), seeking meaning in the experience (e.g., Wadey et al., 2011), and providing the athletes have access to social support (e.g., Wadey et al., 2011), many athletes express that they can identify positive outcomes as a consequence of that injury. These positive outcomes include, for example: personal growth (e.g., Udry et al., 1997), increased personal strength (e.g., Wadey et al., 2011), new perspectives (e.g., Udry et al., 1997), increased motivation (e.g., Wadey et al., 2013), enhanced performance (e.g., Salim et al., 2016), enhanced body-self-awareness (e.g., Wadey et al., 2013), and a greater sense of mastery (e.g., Salim et al., 2016). However, despite the authors of the aforementioned studies interpreting that because both they and their participants have identified benefits, growth has occurred, we argue that there are several theoretical, conceptual, and methodological inconsistencies with this assertion.

Despite recent attempts to contextualize growth to enhance our understanding of growth in injured athletes, many researchers thus far have overlooked whether sport injury is sufficiently traumatic to facilitate actual growth, and failed to account for more contemporary debates in the broader growth literature (i.e., that of constructive and illusory growth); both of which will now be discussed in the following subsections.

The Experience of Injury

Despite sport performance researchers (e.g., Howells & Fletcher, 2015) ascertaining that events such as non-selection to an Olympic team may be traumatic to an elite athlete, we should question whether events such as these are comparable to the traumatic experiences that have been shown to result in growth in the wider literature (e.g., sexual assault, loss of a child; Frazier, Conlon, & Glaser, 2001; Polatinsky & Esprey, 2000). Partially addressing this concern and challenging the extant theory, Johnson and Boals (2015) suggested that it may be more prudent to consider *event centrality*, that is, the extent to which the individual construes the negative experience as a core part of the identity and which may result in them fundamentally rethinking their worldview or schematic assumptions. This explanation may be particularly relevant to athletes who have a high athletic identity and therefore could be applicable to an athlete's experience of injury. Sporting injuries have the potential to have a significant detrimental impact on athletes, disrupting their training, contributing to a potentially ongoing physical weakness (Heiderscheit, Sherry, Silder, Chumanov, & Thelen, 2010), and impacting on team selection (Wadey, Day, Cavallerio, & Martinelli, 2018). Accordingly, when encountering a sporting injury, athletes may question their identity and respond by adopting adaptive or maladaptive coping (e.g., Huysmans & Clement, 2017). However, even allowing for the individual's perception of trauma, the question remains whether sporting injuries are sufficiently traumatic to enable the growth process. According to Tedeschi and Calhoun (2004), and considering the evidence-base in sport injury, we argue that sport injuries are often not traumatic enough to create the experience of transformational changes that allude to actual growth. We acknowledge that there are exceptions to this, for example, career-ending injuries, which may be sufficiently traumatic to be researched through the lens of Tedeschi and Calhoun's conceptualization of growth. Nevertheless, we argue that not all injuries are this traumatic and this lens may not be appropriate in all instances.

This issue was, in part, addressed by the development of T-SIRG (Roy-Davis et al., 2017), which differs from other theories that postulate that the predominant mechanism leading to growth is a shattering effect on a person's assumptive world (cf. Janoff-Bulman, 1992). Specifically, the T-SIRG rebuffs the notion that growth occurs following the theory of shattered assumptions; instead the theory details four distinct mechanisms (meta-cognition, positive reappraisal, positive emotions, and facilitative responses) by which athletes may experience growth from injury. In describing these mechanisms, the T-SIRG provides an alternative explanatory pathway that is appropriate in scenarios where an event (e.g., sporting injury) is not considered to be traumatic enough to pose a seismic challenge to the individual (Roy-Davis et al., 2017). Nevertheless, the T-SIRG does not distinguish between actual growth and growth that may be illusory in nature; accordingly, it fails to account for the more contemporary debates that will be discussed in the following section.

Contemporary Debates

Despite the potential contribution of T-SIRG to the literature, Roy-Davis et al. (2017), we argue, overlooked the issue of whether growth is transformative for the individual concerned (cf. Tedeschi & Calhoun, 2004). Potentially in some individuals, the identification of growth may consist of nothing more than a protective coping strategy that allows the athlete to search for "a silver lining" as a consequence of their experience (e.g., Howells & Fletcher, 2016) which arguably cannot be conceived of as actual growth. In explaining the prevalence of studies reporting growth in participants who have experienced adversity, including injury, the identification of positive outcomes may represent individuals' perceptions of change that are attributable to deprecation of past psychological status (that is, the participant remembers their psychological state as being worse than it actually was) rather than to actual changes in psychological status. This observation is not new; even a decade ago, researchers in the wider psychology literature argued that the presence of growth may be exaggerated and that reports of growth may signify the presence of motivated illusions (cf. Taylor, 1983) designed to help individuals deal with situations in which they feel threatened, or an adherence to a cultural script (e.g., Maercker & Zoellner; 2004; Park, 2004; Zoellner & Maercker, 2006a; Wortman, 2004).

Several studies in the sport psychology literature have also queried the veridicality of growth and questioned whether growth may have illusory (or illusionary[3]) features (e.g., Wadey et al., 2013; Tamminen, Holt, & Neely, 2013) and therefore may not be transformational for the athlete. To date, only one study in the sport and exercise psychology literature has explicitly focused on the notion of growth having illusory aspects as captured in a two-component or Janus-faced model (Maercker & Zoellner; 2004; Zoellner & Maercker, 2006a). In a study that explored adversarial growth in Olympic swimmers, Howells and Fletcher (2016) identified both illusory and constructive growth in athletes who had experienced adversities, including sport injuries. They provided an example of one athlete who, following an injury, recognized his unrealistic optimism indicative of the self-deceptive nature of illusory growth:

> As an elite athlete, your primary instinct is to compete at that level and believe instinctively that you can achieve what you want to achieve. … [Following a serious injury] I'd convinced myself that, despite my lack of fitness and health, I was still going to win. Now, thinking back, that's illogical.
>
> (Howells & Fletcher, 2016, p. 179)

Nevertheless, they also identified constructive growth in an athlete who, working with a psychologist, made sense of what had happened to him: "For the clavicle fracture, [working with a sport psychologist] was about removing the gremlins that were blocking me from full, relaxed, optimal, sports performance" (Howells & Fletcher, 2016, p. 181). However, the authors contended that the two types of growth were not mutually exclusive, but rather aspects of both may temporally fluctuate or even coexist. In light of these findings, we recommend that in exploring the potential for growth in injured athletes, researchers and practitioners should interrogate whether positive outcomes are truly transformational (that is significant and enduring) or the consequence of a short-lived and less permanent coping mechanism.

Future Research Implications

Methodologically, researchers across disciplines have examined growth in injured athletes using both quantitative (Brewer et al., 2017; Wadey et al., 2016; Salim et al., 2015) and qualitative (Wadey et al., 2011, 2013, 2019; Salim et al., 2019) methods. Whether the growth reported by these studies reflects a real and authentic change, however, requires critical consideration due to the studies using cross-sectional methodological research designs (for a notable exception, see Brewer et al., 2017) and the self-reported retrospective measures of growth used. In the wider growth literature, Cho and Park (2013) argued that the growth retrospectively reported by individuals may not reflect actual growth because they surmised that, informed by the internalization of a cultural script of adversity, individuals would want to demonstrate that they were coping. Furthermore, they argued, even when individuals are in a position to recognize positive changes, they cannot

accurately report them when correlated with actual change on standard personality measures (Frazier & Kahler, 2006). This issue confuses whether reports of
growth reflect actual transformational life changes or simply retrospective reat-
tribution for the trauma experienced during the recovery process. The lack of longitudinal design in studies examining growth in injured athletes further occludes
our ability to determine the authenticity of these reports.

Researchers using a quantitative methodology to measure growth in injured
athletes have tended to use either the Post-Traumatic Growth Inventory (PTGI;
Tedeschi & Calhoun, 1996) (e.g., Galli & Reel, 2012) or the Stress-Related
Growth Scale (SRGS; Park, Cohen, & Murch, 1996) (e.g., Wadey et al., 2016). By
utilizing these instruments researchers are intentionally or inadvertently situating
their conceptualizations within a nomenclature of actual growth (that is, PTG or
SRG). For researchers adopting the term PTG, the PTGI measures growth as
a multidimensional construct (i.e., providing five separate scores), with five distinct domains being measured, namely: a greater appreciation of life and changed
sense of priorities; warmer, more intimate relationships with others; a greater
sense of personal strength; recognition of new possibilities or paths for one's life;
and spiritual-existential change. For researchers interested in SRG, the SRGS
(Park et al., 1996) measures growth as a unitary phenomenon (i.e., providing one
score) with items reflecting positive changes in personal resources, social relationships, and coping skills. Despite both scales having a high internal consistency and
test-retest reliability (Park et al., 1996; Tedeschi & Calhoun, 1996), these measures were not developed for injured athletes and therefore lack face and content
validity. To align future research with these conceptualizations, we need to use
methodologies and operationalize the concept to reflect this actual growth. We
therefore recommend more pre-to-post methodological designs, and methods of
data collection that go beyond self-report questionnaires to validate participants'
claims (e.g., biological indicators of growth, behavior checklists of growth) to provide a more coherent and rigorous dataset. The completion of these standardized
instruments in injured athletes is based on the assumption that the athletes who
suffer a traumatic sport injury experience the shattering of schematic assumptions.
This assumption may be flawed as not all athletes will experience an injury that is
severe enough to shatter assumptions. Furthermore, the dimensions reflected in
these scales are not context-specific to the growth experienced by injured athletes
and therefore may not be appropriate. These issues leave sport injury researchers
in a quandary. Informed by the contemporary literature they may be inclined to
conceptualize growth in accordance with T-SIRG but in doing so are they will not
be able to utilize an appropriate corresponding measurement tool. Accordingly,
there is scope for the development of an associated measure.

In the meantime, adopting a qualitative approach may partially negate
these concerns (see Chapter 12). Qualitative researchers exploring growth in
injured athletes have identified additional context specific positive outcomes of
injury in increased physical strength and superior performance (e.g., Salim et
al., 2016; Wadey et al., 2011), and in body-awareness (e.g. Wadey et al., 2013).
Nevertheless, the use of snap-shot one-off interviewing in these studies, however,

makes it difficult to determine whether these reported positive benefits really constitute growth or whether they are reflective of a protective coping mechanism to deal with the traumatic event (cf. Zoellner & Maercker, 2006a) or adherence to a cultural script. Therefore, we recommend the use of alternative designs that may involve innovation in the qualitative traditions (e.g., narrative inquiry), the use of multiple interviews, or the use of multiple methods (e.g., interviews and observation).

Conclusion

In sum, a wide range of positive outcomes resulting from injury have been documented in the literature. The primary purpose of this chapter was to explore whether these positive outcomes could be constituted as *growth*. Although we may question whether sporting injury is traumatic enough to engage the processes of growth, the T-SIRG partially negates this need by providing us with a set of injury-specific mechanism that may result in the development of a context-specific conceptualization of sport injury–related growth. We hope future researchers will look to further embrace alternative pathways to growth. Although recent research has made significant strides in advancing our understanding of growth from injury, we addressed some of the methodological and conceptual issues that warrant serious future consideration. Indeed, as the cultural narrative of "what doesn't kill us, makes us stronger" is becoming more pervasive than ever, it is important for researchers, coaches, and practitioners to be cognizant that growth is not an inevitable outcome from injury and may place increased pressure on athletes resulting in motivated illusions which may hinder their ability to authentically grow from the experience of injury. We hope that the questions we highlight will encourage further reflection on the conceptual and practical issues concerning this phenomenon and hence assist in facilitating athletes to positively develop and grow from their adverse experiences.

Critical Discussion Questions

1) How does actual and perceived growth differ in injured athletes?
2) Should we encourage the identification of growth in injured athletes?
3) Assuming that identification of growth is desirable, how can coaches and practitioners support injured athletes to facilitate them coming out of the experience stronger?

Notes

1   The functional descriptive model of post-traumatic growth (FDM; Calhoun, Cann, & Tedeschi, 2010; Calhoun & Tedeschi, 1998; Tedeschi & Calhoun, 1995, 2004), the organismic valuing theory of growth (OVT; Joseph & Linley, 2005), and the affective cognitive processing model of PTG (ACPM; Joseph, Murphy, & Regel, 2012).
2   However, Brewer et al. did find most participants reported little or no adversarial growth.

3 Both terms – illusory and illusionary – have been used in the literature, with the term illusionary often being favored by researchers. In this chapter we adopt the terminology (i.e., illusory) adopted by Zoellner and Maercker (2006a) in their development of the Janus-faced model of PTG.

References

Arpawong, T. E., Richeimer, S. H., Weinstein, F., Elghamrawy, A., & Milam, J. E. (2013). Posttraumatic growth, quality of life, and treatment symptoms among cancer chemotherapy outpatients. *Health Psychology*, *32*(4), 397–408. doi: 10.1037/a0028223

Athletics Weekly. (2019, January 19). Research report: Holly Bradshaw on overcoming adversity. Retrieved from https://www.athleticsweekly.com/performance/research-report-holly-bradshaw-on-overcoming-adversity-1039920055/

Brewer, B. W., Cornelius, A. E., Van Raalte, J. L., & Tennen, H. (2017). Adversarial growth after anterior cruciate ligament reconstruction. *Journal of Sport and Exercise Psychology*, *39*(2), 134–144. doi: 10.1123/jsep.2016-0210

Calhoun, L. G., Cann, A., & Tedeschi, R. G. (2010). The posttraumatic growth model: Sociocultural considerations. In T. Weiss & R. Berger (Eds.), *Posttraumatic growth and culturally competent practice: Lessons learned from around the globe* (pp. 1–14). Hoboken, NJ: Wiley Online Library. doi: 10.1002/9781118270028.ch1

Calhoun, L. G., & Tedeschi, R. G. (1998). Posttraumatic growth: Future directions. In R. G. Tedeschi, C. L. Park & L. G. Calhoun (Eds.), *Posttraumatic growth: Theory and research on change in the aftermath of crisis* (pp. 215–238). Mahwah, NJ: Lawrence Erlbaum.

Cho, D., & Park, C. L. (2013). Growth following trauma: Overview and current status. *Terapia Psicologica*, *31*(1), 69–79. doi: 10.4067/S0718–48082013000100007

Currier, J. M., Mallot, J., Martinez, T. E., Sandy, C., & Neimeyer, R. A. (2013). Bereavement, religion, and posttraumatic growth: A matched control group investigation. *Psychology of Religion and Spirituality*, *5*(2), 69–77. doi: 10.1037/a0027708

Filipp, S. H. (1999). A three–stage model of coping with loss and trauma. In A. Maercker, M. Schützwohl, & Z. Solomon (Eds.), *Posttraumatic stress disorder: A lifespan developmental perspective* (pp. 43–78). Seattle, WA: Hogrefe and Huber.

Frazier, P., Conlon, A., & Glaser, T. (2001). Positive and negative life changes following sexual assault. *Journal of Consulting and Clinical Psychology*, *69*(6), 1048–1055. doi: 10.1037/0022-006X.69.6.1048

Frazier, P. A., & Kaler, M. E. (2006). Assessing the validity of self-reported stress-related growth. *Journal of Consulting and Clinical Psychology*, *74*(5), 859–869. doi: 10.1037/0022-006X.74.5.859

Galli, N., & Reel, J. J. (2012). Can good come from bad? An examination of adversarial growth in Division I NCAA athletes. *Journal of Intercollegiate Sport*, *5*(2), 199–212. doi: 10.1123/jis.5.2.199

Heiderscheit, B. C., Sherry, M. A., Silder, A., Chumanov, E. S., & Thelen, D. G. (2010). Hamstring strain injuries: Recommendations for diagnosis, rehabilitation, and injury prevention. *Journal of Orthopaedic and Sports Physical Therapy*, *40*(2), 67–81. doi: 10.2519/jospt.2010.3047

Helgeson, V. S. (2010). Corroboration of growth following breast cancer: Ten years later. *Journal of Social and Clinical Psychology*, *29*(5), 546–574. doi: 10.1521/jscp.2010.29.5.546

Howells, K., & Fletcher, D. (2015). Sink or swim: Adversity-and growth-related experiences in Olympic swimming champions. *Psychology of Sport and Exercise*, *16*, 37–48. doi: 10.1016/j.psychsport.2014.08.004

Howells, K., & Fletcher, D. (2016). Adversarial growth in Olympic swimmers: Constructive reality or illusory self-deception? *Journal of Sport and Exercise Psychology*, *38*(2), 173–186. doi: 10.1123/jsep.2015-0189

Howells, K., Sarkar, M., & Fletcher, D. (2017). Can athletes benefit from difficulty? A systematic review of growth following adversity in competitive sport. *Progress in Brain Research*, *16*, 37–48

Howells, K., Wadey, R., & Day, M. (2020). Growth following adversity: A theoretical perspective. In R. Wadey, M. Day, & K. Howells (Eds.), *Growth following adversity in sport: A mechanism to positive change* (pp. 19–33). London: Routledge.

Huysmans, Z., & Clement, D. (2017). A preliminary exploration of the application of self-compassion within the context of sport injury. *Journal of Sport and Exercise Psychology*, *39*(1), 56–66. doi: 10.1123/jsep.2016-0144

Janoff–Bulman, R. (1992). *Shattered assumptions: Towards a new psychology of trauma*. New York, NY: The Free Press.

Johnson, S. F., & Boals, A. (2015). Redefining our ability to measure post-traumatic growth. *Psychological Trauma: Theory, Research, Practice, and Policy*, *5*(5), 422–429. doi: 10.1037/tra0000013

Joseph, S., & Linley, A. (2005). Positive adjustment to threatening events: An organismic valuing theory of growth through adversity. *Review of General Psychology*, *9*(3), 262–280. doi: 10.1037/1089-2680.9.3.262

Joseph, S., Murphy, D., & Regel, S. (2012). An affective-cognitive processing model of post-traumatic growth. *Clinical Psychology and Psychotherapy*, *19*(4), 316–324. doi: 10.1002/cpp.1798

Lavallee, D., Kremer, J., Moran, A., & Williams, M. (2012). *Sport psychology: Contemporary themes*. London: Macmillan International Higher Education.

Linley, P. A., & Joseph, S. (2004). Positive change following trauma and adversity: A review. *Journal of Traumatic Stress*, *17*(1), 11–21. doi: 10.1023/B:JOTS.0000014671.27856.7e

Maercker, A., & Zoellner, T. (2004). The Janus face of self-perceived growth: Toward a two-component model of posttraumatic growth. *Psychological Inquiry*, *15*, 41–48. Retrieved from https://www.jstor.org/stable/20447200

Park, C., Cohen, L., & Murch, R. (1996). Assessment and prediction of stress-related growth. *Journal of Personality*, *64*(1), 71–105. doi: 10.1111/j.1467-6494.1996.tb00815.x

Park, C. L. (2004). The notion of growth following stressful life experiences: Problems and prospects. *Psychological Inquiry*, *15*, 69–76. Retrieved from http://www.jstor.org/stable/20447205

Polatinsky, S., & Esprey, Y. (2000). An assessment of gender differences in the perception of benefit resulting from the loss of a child. *Journal of Traumatic Stress*, *13*(4), 709–718. doi: 10.1023/A:1007870419116

Roy-Davis, K., Wadey, R., & Evans, L. (2017). A grounded theory of sport injury-related growth. *Sport, Exercise, and Performance Psychology*, *6*(1), 35–52. doi: 10.1037/spy0000080

Salim, J., & Wadey, R. (2018). Can emotional disclosure promote sport injury-related growth? *Journal of Applied Sport Psychology*, *30*(4), 367–387. doi: 10.1016/j.psychsport.2014.12.004

Salim, J., & Wadey, R. (2019). Using gratitude to promote sport injury-related growth. *Journal of Applied Sport Psychology*. doi: 10.1080/10413200.2019.1626515

Salim, J., Wadey, R., & Diss, C. (2015). Examining the relationship between hardiness and perceived stress-related growth in a sport injury context. *Psychology of Sport and Exercise*, *19*, 10–17. doi: 10.1016/j.psychsport.2014.12.004

Salim, J., Wadey, R., & Diss, C. (2016). Examining hardiness, coping and stress-related growth following sport injury. *Journal of Applied Sport Psychology*, *28*(2), 154–169. doi: 10.1080/10413200.2015.1086448

Taylor, S. E. (1983). Adjustment to threatening events: A theory of cognitive adaptation. *American Psychologist*, *38*, 1161–1173.

Tamminen, K. A., Holt, N. L., & Neely, K. C. (2013). Exploring adversity and the potential for growth among elite female athletes. *Psychology of Sport and Exercise*, *14*(1), 28–36. doi: 10.1016/j.psychsport.2012.07.002

Tedeschi, R. G., & Calhoun, L. G. (1995). *Trauma & transformation: Growing in the aftermath of suffering*. Thousand Oaks, CA: Sage.

Tedeschi, R. G., & Calhoun, L. G. (1996). The posttraumatic growth inventory: Measuring the positive legacy of trauma. *Journal of Traumatic Stress*, *9*(3), 455–471. doi: 10.10007/BF02103658

Tedeschi, R. G., & Calhoun, L. G. (2004). Posttraumatic growth: Conceptual foundations and empirical evidence. *Psychological Inquiry*, *15*(1), 1–18. doi: 10.1207/s15327965pli1501_01

Tedeschi, R. G., Shakespeare-Finch, J., Taku, K., & Calhoun, L. G. (2018). *Posttraumatic growth: Theory, research, and applications*. New York, NY: Routledge.

Udry, E., Gould, D., Bridges, D., & Beck, L. (1997). Down but not out: Athlete responses to season-ending injuries. *Journal of Sport and Exercise Psychology*, *19*(3), 229–248. doi: 10.1123/jsep.19.3.229

Wadey, R., Clark, S., Podlog, L., & McCullough, D. (2013). Coaches' perceptions of athletes' stress–related growth following sport injury. *Psychology of Sport and Exercise*, *14*(2), 125–135. doi: 10.1016/j.psychsport.2012.08.004

Wadey, R., Day, M., Cavallerio, F., & Martinelli, L. (2018). Multilevel model of sport injury (MMSI): Can coaches impact and be impacted by injury? In R. Thelwell & M. Dicks (Eds.), *Professional advances in sport coaching: Research and practice* (pp. 336–357). New York, NY: Routledge.

Wadey, R., Evans, L., Evans, K., & Mitchell, I. (2011). Perceived benefits following sport injury: A qualitative examination of their antecedents and underlying mechanisms. *Journal of Applied Sport Psychology*, *23*(2), 142–158. doi: 10.1080/10413200.2010.543119

Wadey, R., Evans, L., Hanton, S., Sarkar, M., & Oliver, H. (2019). Can preinjury adversity affect postinjury responses? A 5-year prospective, multi-study analysis. *Frontiers in Psychology*, *10*, 1–13. doi: 10.3389/fpsyg.2019.01411

Wadey, R., & Everard, C. (2020). Sport Injury-Related Growth: A conceptual foundation. In R. Wadey, M. Day & K. Howells (Eds.), *Growth following adversity in sport: A mechanism to positive change* (pp. 189–203). London: Routledge.

Wadey, R., Podlog, L., Galli, N., & Mellalieu, S. D. (2016). Stress-related growth following sport injury: Examining the applicability of the organismic valuing theory. *Scandinavian Journal of Medicine and Science in Sports*, *26*(10), 1132–1139. doi: 10.1111/sms.12579

Wadey, R., Roy-Davis, K., Evans, L., Howells, K., Salim, J., & Diss, C. (2019). Sport psychology consultants' perspectives on facilitating sport injury-related growth. *The Sport Psychologist*, *33*(3), 244–255. doi: 10.1123/tsp.2018-0110

Wortman, C. B. (2004). Posttraumatic growth: Progress and problems. *Psychological Inquiry*, *15*, 81–90. Retrieved from http://www.jstor.org/stable/20447207

Zoellner, T., & Maercker, A. (2006a). Posttraumatic growth in clinical psychology - A critical review and introduction of a two-component model. *Clinical Psychology Review*, *26*(5), 626–653. doi: 10.1016/j.cpr.2006.01.008

8 Time to Re-Examine Injured Athletes' Emotional Responses

Katherine A. Tamminen, Rachel Dunn, and Sarah Gairdner

Introduction

The study of emotions among injured athletes has been an important area of inquiry in the field of sport injury psychology. While efforts to understand the features of athletes' emotional experiences have contributed valuable information to the literature, in this chapter we suggest there are some empirical and theoretical gaps in the literature regarding the conceptualization of emotions, our understanding of how athletes' emotions are experienced, the interpersonal processes influencing emotional experiences, and ways of helping athletes process their emotions. We also view this as an important opportunity to draw on research and theory from other related disciplines to aid in the development of more complex and nuanced conversations about emotional responses to injury in sport.

Researchers investigating injured athletes' emotional experiences have found that athletes experience several emotions in response to sport-related injuries, including fear, sadness, anger, and anxiety (Appaneal & Habif, 2013). Injured athletes have also reported other affective states such as feeling helpless, frustrated, irritated, and confused about their identity as an athlete (Collinson, 2005; Ruddock-Hudson, O'Halloran, & Murphy, 2012; Tracey, 2003). While it appears common for many athletes to report negative emotions when injured, enduring or pervasive negative emotions can be problematic for athletes' recovery. For example, Crombez, Vlaeyen, Heuts, and Lysens (1999) found that when athletes worried excessively about experiencing pain, they rated their injury as worse and took longer to return to sport. Others have found that increased emotional distress in response to injury can negatively impact an athlete's well-being and rehabilitation, sometimes extending the time athletes spend away from competitive sport (Appaneal & Habif, 2013). Clearly, injuries are emotionally laden experiences and have consequences for athletes' injury and rehabilitation back into sport participation and competition.

Athletes' emotional responses also change as they navigate the process of injury rehabilitation. Hsu, Meierbachtol, and George (2016) conducted a literature review of athletes' rehabilitation process in relation to their emotional fear of reinjury, concluding that fear, frustration, and anxiety were most intense immediately following injury and reduced as athletes navigated their rehabilitation program.

Furthermore, there also appear to be differences in athletes' emotional responses to injury depending on the type of injury sustained; one study by Hutchison, Mainwaring, Comper, Richards, and Bisschop (2009) found that concussed athletes demonstrated emotional responses such as fatigue and decreased vigor, while athletes with musculoskeletal injuries tended to display emotional anger (Hutchison et al., 2009). Thus, emotions are varied and change over time, and there also appear to be differences in the ways that athletes experience different types of injuries.

Critical Review

There is no shortage of evidence documenting the importance of emotions and emotional responses in athletes' injury experiences. However, a critical review of this body of literature suggests some areas that could benefit from further attention. Below, we outline several research and theoretical issues that may help to advance this body of literature, followed by a summary of implications for future research.

Research Considerations

One limitation to the body of literature on emotions among injured athletes is that researchers have typically adopted nomothetic, group-level approaches to studying athletes' emotional responses to injury (e.g., Covassin et al., 2014; Hutchison et al., 2009; Ruddock-Hudson et al., 2012). However, adopting idiographic, individual-level approaches would be valuable to advance understanding of the intricacies of athletes' emotional experiences, for example by examining how athletes' emotional responses may be shaped by their previous injury experiences, career stage, achievement expectations, not to mention their pre-injury emotional tendencies (e.g., emotional expressivity, emotion regulation, support-seeking). Some examples of qualitative research that have combined idiographic and nomothetic approaches to understand the similarities and differences in athletes' emotions during periods of injury and rehabilitation include work by Clement, Arvinen-Barrow, and Fetty (2015), Ruddock-Hudson, O'Halloran, and Murphy (2012), and Tracey (2003). Evidence from these studies indicates that there were variations in the severity and types of emotions that athletes reported over the course of their injuries. Athletes reported that knowing the severity of their injuries affected their emotional experiences, either worsening or alleviating their initial negative emotional responses, and during the return to sport activities, athletes described a variety of emotional experiences including anxiety, relief, and excitement (Clement et al., 2015; Ruddock-Hudson et al., 2012).

Another example of research detailing the idiosyncratic emotional experiences of injured athletes was reported by Collinson (2005), who described an autoethnographic examination of emotions among two long-distance runners who experienced long-term knee injuries. In this work, Collinson draws attention to the different ways that athletes understand and make meaning about their injuries over an extended period of time, and the variations in the different emotions that fluctuated over the course of injury and rehabilitation, including vacillations between alarm, anxiety, and fear; optimism, relief, and doubt; faith, hope, and disappointment; despair, anger, and blame; anger, empowerment, and momentum. An important aspect of Collinson's study was the conceptualization of emotions as "self-feelings as an embodied form of consciousness" (p. 222); this approach, informed by biological, social, and sociological perspectives, is now gaining popularity in contemporary theories of emotion in the broader field of psychology (see later for work by Barrett, 2017). Collinson's work also centers on the relational and interactional dimensions of emotions and draws attention to the ways that running partners, doctors, and athletic therapists influence emotional experiences (see also Nixon, 1992). Collectively, these examples of idiographic approaches to understanding athletes' emotional experiences during periods of injury are valuable for highlighting the nuanced and idiosyncratic nature of emotions, as well as the various sources of influence on emotions (e.g., athletic therapists, knowledge of injury severity). We encourage further qualitative work in this area (see Chapter 12), although idiographic investigations of athletes' emotions need not be restricted to qualitative research approaches: n-of-1 studies using quantitative approaches can be used to prospectively study athletes' emotional experiences over time, as well as to evaluate interventions for helping injured athletes manage their emotions (cf. Kwasnicka, & Naughton, 2019; see also Chapter 14).

The need to study emotional change before and after injury points to another necessary avenue for future research: namely, longitudinal designs should continue to be used to assess how athletes' emotional responses evolve throughout their injury experience. Some longitudinal research has been conducted; for example, Hutchinson et al. (2009) studied the different responses of athletes with concussions compared to musculoskeletal injuries over a 29-day period. Another recent contribution to this area was a study by Wadey, Evans, Hanton, Sarkar, and Oliver (2019), who examined athletes' psychological responses to injury over a five-year period while also accounting for their pre-injury levels of adversity (e.g., prior negative major life events). Athletes with moderate pre-injury adversity reported better responses following their injuries (e.g., less devastation, dispiritedness, and restlessness) compared to athletes with lower or higher pre-injury adversity, and they also used greater problem- and emotion-focused coping strategies to deal with their injuries. Follow-up interviews with the athletes elaborated on the distinctions between groups of athletes, suggesting that individual differences in appraisals of the injury experience, available social support, and perceptions of having the appropriate coping resources to deal with their injury were important features that shaped the athletes' injury experiences. As injury recovery can often span months, there is a need to understand how athletes' emotional responses change over time and the ways that athletes experience and manage their emotions.

By studying athletes over longer periods, researchers would also be able to address other poignant questions, such as how emotional reactions vary in response to repeated injury occurrences, rehabilitation set-backs, as well as comparing chronic versus acute injury experiences. In doing so, it may also be useful to consider how injuries may be precipitating events that can trigger more severe emotional distress and periods of depression. Researchers may consider drawing on models proposed by Monroe, Anderson, and Harkness (2019) to understand whether athletes' emotional responses to injury can be better predicted in advance of occurrence, and to investigate how intervention approaches can predict and buffer against the onset of more severe emotional distress.

Theoretical Considerations

Although researchers have documented a variety of emotional responses to injury, one limitation across this body of research pertains to the way emotions have been conceptualized and studied, and the range of emotions that have been investigated. It is understandable that researchers have focused primarily on negatively toned or unpleasant affective experiences, although researchers have tended to focus on a narrow set of descriptive terms when asking athletes about the emotions they experience (e.g., anxious, depressed, sad, angry). This narrow and static approach restricts the cognitive and linguistic access that athletes have when attempting to fully and accurately reconstitute their injury experiences. There also appears to be a bias toward negative emotions, neglecting the potentially positively valenced emotions, such as relief, which are less acceptable feelings in relation to an injury. An expansion of emotional descriptive terms could also be useful in helping researchers and stakeholders better understand the vast array of intra and interpersonal emotions that athletes experience in relation to their injuries (see Roy-Davis, Wadey, & Evans, 2017 for further consideration of positive emotions and growth following injury).

A second major theoretical issue pertains to the inconsistency in conceptualizing and measuring emotions and related affective phenomena. For example, some studies assess athletes' emotions using the Profile of Mood States (POMS) questionnaire, which asks athletes to report their experiences of six mood states (tension, depression, anger, vigor, fatigue, confusion; McNair, Lorr, & Droppleman, 1971), while other studies have used the Emotional Responses to Athletic Injury Questionnaire, which asks athletes to report the extent to which they are experiencing 12 emotions, with a higher score reflecting greater emotional disturbance (e.g., Langford, Webster, & Feller, 2009). Other researchers have used measures of psychological readiness to return to sport that include items assessing emotions (e.g., nervous, frustrated, afraid), confidence, and risk appraisals, with a higher score indicating greater psychological readiness to return to sport (Webster, Feller, & Lambros, 2008). Furthermore, in some studies emotional responses have been considered within athletes' broader experiences of psychological stress, depression, or anxiety (Andersen & Williams, 1988). Thus, it is challenging to assess the literature on emotions among injured athletes due to the variety of ways that emotions are conceptualized and measured; such variation in the conceptualization and measurement of emotions makes it difficult for researchers to summarize and review the existing literature focusing on athletes' injury-related emotional experiences. Furthermore, the inclusion of different emotions and affective terms in measures of athletes' responses to injury reflects different theoretical bases and understandings of what emotions are and how they are linked to other outcomes. Inconsistencies in the conceptualization and measurement of emotions can also lead to difficulties in designing interventions or counseling approaches for helping athletes manage their emotional responses to injury. For example, the types of strategies and support provided to athletes for managing anger or sadness would differ from those provided to athletes managing fear of reinjury, or for athletes experiencing clinically diagnosed depression or anxiety.

Researchers investigating athletes' responses to injury should carefully deline-ate between the concepts they are investigating, and the way that emotions are measured should reflect the theoretical basis underlying how emotions are con-ceptualized. Although the terms "emotion", "mood", and "mood states" are often used interchangeably when referring to affective phenomena, they have different definitions. The term "mood" refers to more diffuse, global, longer-lasting affec-tive experiences, whereas the term "emotion" refers to a brief episode consisting of a complex set of co-occurring physiological, behavioral, cognitive, neural, and endocrine components that are "elicited *by* something, are reactions *to* something, and are generally *about* something" (Ekkekakis, 2013, p. 43). It is also important to distinguish between emotions and related behaviors and cognitions when investi-gating athletes' injury responses.

Considering that the experience of injury for an athlete is replete with indi-vidual meanings and consequences, it may be helpful to draw on theoretical per-spectives that consider the ways that athletes construct their emotions through the interpretations of their bodily experiences. Barrett (2017) offers a valuable per-spective from which to consider these experiences in her Theory of Constructed Emotions (TCE). This contemporary perspective challenges essentialist models of emotion and posits that emotions are constructed as the individual makes sense of their bodily experiences (core affect) within their immediate circumstances or situation. The TCE describes emotions as functional states that serve to com-municate meanings and messages to others, and emotions are viewed as a source of social influence (Barrett, 2012). According to this perspective, sensations from the environment are combined with bodily sensations and are categorized as the experience or perception of emotion through the addition of past information or experiences. The synthesis of sensations and categorization of experience as emotion is a quick, unconscious, and ongoing process that enables a meaningful and efficient guide for action. There is mounting evidence for the utility of the TCE (see Feldman-Barett, 2017 for an overview), and applying this perspective to injured athletes presents a unique opportunity to explore the holistic, embodied nature of emotions.

Interpersonal Perspectives

The study of emotional phenomena in sport has recently demonstrated an "interpersonal turn" whereby researchers have amassed evidence regarding the interpersonal or social aspects of emotions in sport. To date, however, there is limited work specifically examining the interpersonal processes at play surrounding emotions among injured athletes. However, there is some initial evidence that highlights the importance of social relationships and interpersonal influence on injured athletes' emotional experiences. For example, Anghel (2010) found that strong cohesion between rugby team members was associated with non-injured athletes experiencing feelings similar to an injured teammate, as well as experiencing more physical trauma themselves. In their review of sports injury research, Christakou and Lavallee (2009) noted that injured athletes' emotional responses to rehabilitation can be influenced by medical practitioners' expectations for their rehabilitation adherence, meaning that how others in sports organizations perceive and respond to injured athletes play a role in athletes' emotional responses to their injury. Athletes have also reported that their emotions were influenced by the expressions on their athletic therapists' faces when discussing and diagnosing injuries, and that they experienced feelings of loneliness, alienation, and sadness due to being isolated and removed from practice (Tracey, 2003). These studies highlight the need to consider athletes' responses to injury as part of their social network and sports organization (see also Mankad, Gordon, & Wallman, 2009).

Researchers examining emotions among injured athletes may benefit from considering theoretical perspectives that explicitly position emotions as social phenomena and that consider the interpersonal processes related to emotional experiences, emotion regulation, and emotion socialization. Thus, adopting social-functional approaches to emotion would be valuable. Social-functional approaches refer to a variety of models and theoretical perspectives that share common assumptions that emotions help to coordinate social interactions and that emotions influence the individual expressing them as well as others around them.

A social-functional approach to understanding the experiences and effects of emotions among injured athletes could draw on work by Keltner and Haidt (1999), who outlined the social functions of emotions at four levels. At the individual level, emotions inform the person about their social environment and provide information about actions or changes that may be necessary in a given situation. At the dyadic level, emotional expressions help to coordinate social interactions between people by helping others to know what one is experiencing, what their beliefs are within the current situation, and what their actions or intentions are. Emotions also signal affiliative and distancing functions between individuals (see also Fisher & Manstead, 2016). For example, an athlete's expressions of sadness or distress when injured can serve to elicit support or empathy from others, signaling that support is needed to help them deal with the demands of their injury. At the group level, emotions are thought to function by regulating individuals' roles and behaviors within groups, defining group boundaries, and by helping group members to deal with group problems or stressors (e.g., communal coping; see Tamminen et al., 2016; Leprince, D'Arripe-Longueville, & Doron, 2018). Finally, at the cultural level of analysis, the cultural norms and scripts surrounding emotions are considered. Thus, at the cultural level, emotions are thought to help individuals learn the norms and values of their (sport) culture, and they also serve to "reify and perpetuate cultural ideologies and power structures" (Keltner & Haidt, 1999, p. 514).

In advancing research on the interpersonal processes influencing emotions among injured athletes, researchers could look to investigate how athletes' emotions are socialized or constrained through interactions with teammates, coaches, and athletic therapists. Analyzing emotions among injured athletes at the group or cultural levels may reveal whether athletes who occupy different roles on teams (e.g., leaders, team captains, rookies) are "allowed" to express particular types of emotions around their teammates and coaches such as uncertainty, sadness, or despair, as opposed to suppressing these types of emotions and instead expressing hope, optimism, and stoicism during their injury and rehabilitation.

Helping Injured Athletes With Their Emotions

An additional area of inquiry focusing on injured athletes' emotional responses concerns the examination of how to best help athletes manage and process their emotions. The tendency to disclose thoughts and emotions in relation to a stressful, traumatic, or significant life event is a normal part of the coping process; however, competitive and elite athletes often struggle with disclosure and often opt for suppression and inhibition as their chosen methods of coping (Howe, 2004). Research and treatment approaches rooted in psychology and psychotherapy that encourage emotional disclosure, rather than inhibition and suppression of negative emotions, are potentially fruitful in understanding emotional reactions in injured athletes. For example, Pennebaker's written disclosure paradigm highlights how individuals can use expressive writing to narrate their emotional experiences with a traumatic event, such as an injury (Pennebaker, 1989). Mankad and Gordon (2010) used Pennebaker's approach to explore the grief process associated with athletic injury and identified that while there is a strongly held belief that athletes independently overcome damaging emotions during the early stages of their rehabilitation process, athletes were still struggling with negative emotion even months after the injury had occurred. Greenberg, Wortman, and Stone (1996), and Mankad and Gordon (2010) both illustrate that writing about trauma is not necessarily about revisiting the trauma itself, but instead about increasing the sense of control over one's emotions through improved self-regulatory processes. Thus, future research could attempt to utilize methods, such as written, verbal, and expressive arts disclosure paradigms, which may encourage more open, nuanced, and raw athlete reactions to injury highlighting the untold emotional responses to injury (see also Salim & Wadey, 2018).

Additional research examining the types of training that therapists and coaches can draw on to help athletes process their negative emotions surrounding their injuries would be valuable for improving applied practice in this area. While there is evidence that athletic therapists believe sport psychology education is helpful for working with injured athletes and use basic psychological strategies such as goal setting and positive affirmation with athletes (Zakrajsek, Fisher, & Martin, 2017), there is limited research that has examined the development of interpersonal counseling skills for athletic therapists and trainers to assist athletes in processing their emotions. Furthermore, athletic trainers have reported feeling inadequately trained to assist athletes with mental health issues (Moulton, Molstad, & Turner, 1997). Because athletic therapists and trainers are often the "front line" in responding to athletes' injuries and spend a considerable amount of time with athletes throughout the recovery process, future research may examine whether providing augmented training for therapists to help them deal with athletes' emotions is helpful for athletes' recovery and emotional processing.

Although the majority of athletes sustaining injuries in sport do successfully recover and return to competition, some sporting injuries are more severe or traumatic to the individual involved (and occasionally to the bystanders who witness the injury; Martinelli, Day, & Lowry, 2017). In a study by Kennedy and Evans (2001) in which they examined new spinal cord injured (SCI) patients, they outlined that in a small, but significant, portion of individuals who sustained partial or complete spinal lesions, high levels of trauma-related distress were reported. In light of the observation that athletes can, at times, be involved in collisions, falls, and violent conflicts which are incredibly physically intense, with the additional emotional trauma of the lost athletic body/self, it is important to highlight that post-traumatic distress may very well exist in many athletes. When conceptualizing athletic injury, especially in the case of career-ending injuries, SCIs, or traumatic brain injuries, there is an opportunity to draw on the broader trauma literature, which highlights long-term consequences, coping styles, and psychotherapeutic interventions related to trauma and post-traumatic stress disorder (PTSD). A relevant example by Marusak, Martin, Etkin, and Thomason (2015) details how childhood trauma exposure disrupts autonomic regulation of emotional processing, and increases sensitivity to emotional conflict. Their findings also highlight the correlation between disrupted autonomic regulation as increased risk for psychopathology following trauma. These data provide a compelling rationale for exploring the ways in which traumatic athletic injury may have long term implications for both autonomic regulatory functioning and also leave athletes at increased risk for long-term emotional pathology.

Other research among veterans diagnosed with PTSD demonstrated that adopting a distanced perspective when describing traumatic experiences protected individuals against increased physiological reactivity (such as increased heart rate and skin conductance reactivity) as they relived their trauma experiences (Wisco et al., 2015). Implementing this approach to analyzing past traumatic experiences within the sporting context could potentially mitigate negative responses to relived traumatic memories, and has particular utility in this population in light of the fact that athletes have the mental skills to manipulate their internal visualizations. Additionally, "trauma-informed care" has been proposed as an approach to medical care that aims to address distress, provide emotional support, and encourage positive coping, all while attempting to mitigate negative consequences associated with trauma (Marsac et al., 2016). There is a plethora of new and novel research in the psychotherapeutic, psychological, and medical literature surrounding trauma-based investigations which may be applied to athletic injuries and may allow for fruitful and insightful research avenues and interventional strategies.

Future Research Implications

Based on the topics outline in this chapter, we propose several areas for future research to advance the literature on emotions among injured athletes. First, we suggest that greater clarity is needed in the conceptualization of emotions and related phenomena; work by Ekkekakis (2013) in the field of exercise and physical activity would be a useful resource, as well as work by Barrett (2017) and an overview of emotions in sport by Wagstaff and Tamminen (in press). Researchers should not be constrained to a narrow set of unpleasant emotions or affective experiences and they should consider a broader array of emotional experiences that athletes may have during their injury. The continued use of idiographic and longitudinal designs would yield rich insights into the complexity of athletes' injury experiences as well as the idiosyncratic nature of injury, recovery, re-injury, and so on. Theoretically, the field of research on emotional responses in injured athletes has started to embrace interpersonal or social perspectives of emotions; adopting social-functional perspectives would contribute greatly to our understanding of how emotions function in social interactions between athletes and their teammates, coaches, and athletic therapists (see also Chapters 9 and 10). Finally, continued work examining the use of disclosure paradigms and trauma-informed approaches will help to provide practical applications for individuals working with injured athletes to help them process their emotions during the injury and recovery experience.

Conclusion

Investigating emotions among injured athletes is important for helping individuals maintain their psychological well-being and to understand how to best help athletes navigate their injury experience. Building on the current research examining athletes' responses to injuries, we foresee several opportunities for advances in this field. Greater precision in the use of terms describing affective phenomena such as emotion, mood, stress will help to bring greater clarity to the literature in this area. At the same time, we encourage researchers to consider contemporary perspectives such as the Theory of Constructed Emotion (Barrett, 2017), as well as interpersonal and social-functional perspectives of emotion that challenge current individualistic and essentialist views of emotions. Furthermore, attending to athletes' emotional processing using disclosure paradigms and trauma-informed approaches to care will broaden our understanding of how emotions can best be managed and processed across the trajectory of athletes' injury experiences.

Critical Discussion Questions

1) What repertoire of emotions do athletes draw on when they experience injuries? How are athletes' emotional responses during injury shaped and constrained by their linguistic resources, as well as by the discourses surrounding injury in sport?

2) Drawing on interpersonal and social perspectives of emotions, how do athletic therapists and clinicians respond to the emotional expressions of injured athletes? What is the impact of different ways of responding to injured athletes' emotional disclosure?

3) How can therapists, trainers, and clinicians respond in ways that are most effective for helping athletes process their emotions surrounding their injuries?

Acknowledgment:

We would like to thank Kyle Farwell for his assistance with this chapter.

References

Andersen, M. B., & Williams, J. M. (1988). A model of stress and athletic injury: Prediction and prevention. *Journal of Sport and Exercise Psychology*, *10*(3), 294–306. doi: 10.1123/jsep.10.3.294

Anghel, A. (2010). Emotional contagion in a cohesive rugby team. *Sport Science Review*, *19*(3), 165–178. doi: 10.2478/v10237-011-0024-9

Appaneal, R. N., & Habif, S. (2013). Psychological antecedents to sport injury. In N. L. Arvinen-Barrow & N. Walker (Eds.), *The psychology of sport injury and rehabilitation* (pp. 6–22). New York: Routledge.

Barrett, L. F. (2012). Emotions are real. *Emotion*, *12*(3), 413–429. doi: 10.1037/a0027555

Barrett, L. F. (2017). The theory of constructed emotion: An active inference account of interception and categorization. *Social Cognitive and Affective Neuroscience*, *12*(1), 1–23. doi: 10.1093/scan/nsw154

Christakou, A., & Lavallee, D. (2009). Rehabilitation from sports injuries: From theory to practice. *Perspectives in Public Health*, *129*(3), 120–126. doi: 10.1177/1466424008094802

Clement, D., Arvinen-Barrow, M., & Fetty, T. (2015). Psychosocial responses during different phases of sport-injury rehabilitation: A qualitative study. *Journal of Athletic Training*, *50*(1), 95–104. doi: 10.4085/1062-6050-49.3.52

Collinson, J. A. (2005). Emotions, interaction and the injured sporting body. *International Review for the Sociology of Sport*, *40*(2), 221–240. doi: 10.1177/1012690205057203

Covassin, T., Crutcher, B., Bleecker, A., Heiden, E., Dailey, A., & Yang, J. (2014). Postinjury anxiety and social support among collegiate athletes: A comparison between orthopaedic injuries and concussions. *Journal of Athletic Training*, *49*(4), 462–468. doi: 10.4085/1062-6059-49.2.03.

Crombez, G., Vlaeyen, J. W. S., Heuts, P. H. T. G., & Lysens, R. (1999). Pain-related fear is more disabling than pain itself: Evidence on the role of pain-related fear in chronic back pain disability. *Pain*, *80*(1–2), 329–339. doi: 10.1016/S0304-3959(98)00229-2

Ekkekakis, P. (2013). *The measurement of affect, mood, and emotion*. New York: Cambridge University Press.

Greenberg, M. A., Wortman, C. B., & Stone, A. A. (1996). Emotional expression and physical health: Revising traumatic memories or fostering self-regulation? *Journal of Personality and Social Psychology, 71*(3), 588–602. doi: 10.1037//0022-3514.71.3.588

Fischer, A. H., & Manstead, A. S. R. (2016). Social functions of emotion and emotion regulation. In M. Lewis, J. Haviland, & L. Feldman Barrett (Eds.), *Handbook of emotion* (4th ed., pp. 456–469). New York, NY: Guilford.

Howe, P. D. (2004). *Sport, professionalism and pain.* London, Routledge.

Hsu, C.-J., Meierbachtol, A., & George, S. Z. (2016). Fear of reinjury in athletes: Implications for rehabilitation. *Sports Health, 9*(2), 162–167. doi: 10.1177/1941738116666813.

Hutchison, M., Mainwaring, L. M., Comper, P., Richards, D. W., & Bisschop, S. M. (2009). Differential emotional responses of varsity athletes to concussion and musculoskeletal injuries. *Clinical Journal of Sport Medicine, 19*(1), 13–19. doi: 10.1097/JSM.0b013e318190ba06

Keltner, D., & Haidt, J. (1999). Social functions of emotions at four levels of analysis. *Cognition and Emotion, 13*(5), 505–521. doi: 10.1080/026999399379168

Kennedy, P., & Evans, M. J. (2001). Evaluation of post traumatic distress in the first 6 months following SCI. *Spinal Cord, 39*(7), 381–386. doi: 10.1038/sj.sc.3101172

Kwasnicka, D., & Naughton, F. (2019). N-of-1 methods: A practical guide to exploring trajectories of behaviour change and designing precision behaviour change interventions. *Psychology of Sport and Exercise.* doi: 10.1016/j.psychsport.2019.101570

Langford, J. L., Webster, K. E., & Feller, J. A. (2009). A prospective longitudinal study to assess psychological changes following anterior cruciate ligament reconstruction surgery. *British Journal of Sports Medicine, 43*(5), 377–378. doi: 10.1136/bjsm.2007.044818

Leprince, C., D'Arripe-Longueville, F., & Doron, J. (2018). Coping in teams: Exploring athletes' communal coping strategies to deal with shared stressors. *Frontiers in Psychology, 9*, 1908. doi: 10.3389/fpsyg.2018.01908

Mankad, A., & Gordon, S. (2010). Psycholinguistic changes in athletes' grief response to injury after written emotional disclosure. *Journal of Sport Rehabilitation, 19*(3), 328–342. doi: 10.1123/jsr.19.3.328

Mankad, A., Gordon, S., & Wallman, K. (2009). Perceptions of emotional climate among injured athletes. *Journal of Clinical Sport Psychology, 3*(1), 1–14. doi: 10.1123/jcsp.3.1.1

Marsac, M. L., Kassam-Adams, N., Hildenbrand, A. K., Nicholls, E., Winston, F. K., Leff, S. S., & Fein, J. (2016). Implementing a trauma-informed approach in pediatric health care networks. *JAMA Pediatrics, 170*(1), 70–77. doi: 10.1001/jamapediatrics.2015.2206

Martinelli, L. A., Day, M. C., & Lowry, R. (2017). Sport coaches' experiences of athlete injury: The development and regulation of guilt. *Sports Coaching Review, 6*(2), 162–178. doi: 10.1080/21640629.2016.1195550

Marusak, H. A., Martin, K. R., Etkin, A., & Thomason, M. E. (2015). Childhood trauma exposure disrupts the automatic regulation of emotional processing. *Neuropsychopharmacology, 40*(5), 1250–1258. doi: 10.1038/npp.2014.311

McNair, D. M., Lorr, M., & Droppleman, L. F. (1971). *Manual for the profile of mood states (POMS).* San Diego, CA: Educational and Industrial Testing Service.

Monroe, S. M., Anderson, S. F., & Harkness, K. L. (2019). Life stress and major depression: The mysteries of recurrences. *Psychological Review, 126,* 791–816. doi: 10.1037/rev0000157

Moulton, M. A., Molstad, S., & Turner, A. (1997). The role of athletic trainers in counseling collegiate athletes. *Journal of Athletic Training, 32*(2), 148–150. Retrieved from https://natajournals.org/loi/attr

Nixon, H. L. (1992). A social network analyses of influences on athletes to play with pain and injuries. *Journal of Sport and Social Issues, 16*(2), 127–135. doi: 10.1177/019372359201600208

Pennebaker, J. W. (1989). Confession, inhibition, and disease. In L. Berkowitz (Ed.), *Advances in experimental social psychology* (Vol. 22, pp. 211–244). San Diego, CA: Academic Press. doi: 10.1016/S0065-2601(08)60309-3

Roy-Davis, K., Wadey, R., & Evans, L. (2017). A grounded theory of sport injury-related growth. *Sport, Exercise, and Performance Psychology, 6*(1), 35–52. doi: 10.1037/spy0000080

Ruddock-Hudson, M., O'Halloran, P., & Murphy, G. (2012). Exploring psychological reactions to injury in the Australian Football League (AFL). *Journal of Applied Sport Psychology, 24*(4), 375–390. doi: 10.1080/10413200.2011.654172

Salim, J., & Wadey, R. (2018). Can emotional disclosure promote sport injury-related growth? *Journal of Applied Sport Psychology, 30*(4), 367–387. doi: 10.1080/10413200.2017.1417338

Tamminen, K. A., Palmateer, T. M., Denton, M., Sabiston, C., Crocker, P. R., Eys, M., & Smith, B. (2016). Exploring emotions as social phenomena among Canadian varsity athletes. *Psychology of Sport and Exercise, 27*, 28–38. doi: 10.1016/j.psychsport.2016.07.010

Tracey, J. (2003). The emotional response to the injury and rehabilitation process. *Journal of Applied Sport Psychology, 15*(4), 279–293. doi: 10.1080/714044197

Wadey, R., Evans, L., Hanton, S., Sarkar, M., & Oliver, H. (2019). Can preinjury adversity affect postinjury responses? A 5-year prospective, multi-study analysis. *Frontiers in Psychology, 10*, 1411. doi: 10.3389/fpsyg.2019.01411

Wagstaff, C., & Tamminen, K. A. [in press]. Emotion. In R. Arnold & D. Fletcher (Eds.), *Stress, well-being, and performance in sport*. New York: Routledge.

Webster, K. E., Feller, J. A., & Lambros, C. (2008). Development and preliminary validation of a scale to measure psychological impact of returning to sport following anterior cruciate ligament reconstruction surgery. *Physical Therapy in Sport, 9*(1), 9–15. doi: 10.1016/j.ptsp.2007.09.003

Wisco, B. E., Marx, B. P., Sloan, D. M., Gorman, K. R., Kulish, A. L., & Pineles, S. L. (2015). Self-distancing from trauma memories reduces physiological but not subjective emotional reactivity among veterans with posttraumatic stress disorder. *Clinical Psychological Science, 3*(6), 956–963. doi: 10.1177/2167702614560745

Zakrajsek, R. A., Fisher, L. A., & Martin, S. B. (2017). Certified athletic trainers' understanding and use of sport psychology in their practice. *Journal of Applied Sport Psychology, 29*(2), 215–233. doi: 10.1080/10413200.2016.1231722

9 Physiotherapist–Injured-Athlete Relationship

Toward a Cultural and Relational Understanding

Sunita Kerai

Introduction

Over the past 50 years, researchers in sport injury psychology have explored and examined the psychological impact of sport injuries, which has resulted in a large evidence base to support how practitioners work with injured athletes (Brewer & Redmond, 2017). It has been identified that sport injuries can have severe consequences, not only affecting the physical health of the athlete but also their psychological and emotional well-being. Throughout their rehabilitation and recovery from injury, athletes can experience physical pain (see Chapter 5) in addition to feelings of anger, frustration, anxiety or fear of reinjury, and depression (see Chapter 8). These psychological and emotional responses can negatively influence athletes' rehabilitation behavior (e.g., adherence) and rehabilitation outcomes (e.g., recovery time, reinjury; Brewer & Redmond, 2017). However, despite the merits of this body of research in helping to provide an evidence base to support injured athletes' recovery, a critical appraisal of the literature soon reveals that sport injury psychology researchers have predominately focused on the impact of injury on the athlete and how members of the multidisciplinary team can come together to support the athlete (e.g., Arvinen-Barrow & Clement, 2019). For example, researchers have explored how physiotherapists can help injured athletes with their psychological, emotional, and behavioral responses to injury (Clement, Arvinen-Barrow, & Fetty, 2015) and their adherence to rehabilitation programs (Zakrajsek, Fisher, & Martin, 2018). However, Wiese-Bjornstal (2009) reported, "Injury affects more than the injured; it often also holds health-related consequences for the network of family, friends, teammates, coaching staff and even the larger communities" (pp. 64–65). Therefore, although physiotherapists have been identified as important individuals in the injured athlete's support network (e.g., Bianco, 2001; Tracy, 2008), there has been limited consideration of physiotherapists themselves (e.g., their needs, challenges faced), a more dyadic understanding of the relationship between physiotherapists and injured athletes, and the influence of the broader social-cultural-organizational environment.

In this chapter, I put forward an agenda for a more cultural and relational understanding of the physiotherapist–injured-athlete relationship or dyad. This agenda is not to detract from the study of injured athletes and physiotherapists at an intrapersonal level, quite the contrary, but to recognize and account for the social-organizational-cultural factors that have by and large been ignored to date. Given the salient role physiotherapists play in the rehabilitation of injured athletes (see Taylor & Taylor, 1997), I believe this represents an exciting and timely area for future research. Specifically, in this chapter I pose three knowledge gaps that need to be addressed: (a) the physiotherapist as a "performer" in their own right, (b) appreciation of a more dyadic understanding of the relationship, and (c) accounting for how the wider sporting culture influences transactions between physiotherapists and injured athletes. Given recent calls to examine the social-organizational-cultural factors in sport injury psychology (e.g., Wadey, Day, Cavallerio, & Martinelli, 2018), the study of the physiotherapist–injured-athlete relationship within the broader environment in sport needs to be addressed to transform sport injury psychology into a more cultural and relational discourse. The chapter closes with specific avenues for future research as well as critical questions to encourage discussion and reflection.

"What About Me?" Giving Physiotherapists a Voice

By and large, the sport psychology literature has predominantly focused on the experiences of injured athletes and how to offer them help (Brewer & Redmond, 2017). While some contemporary researchers have examined the potential effects that a serious injury could have on a witness to the injury, including teammates (e.g., O'Neill, 2008), coaches (see Chapter 10), and parents (see Chapter 11), these studies have been few and far between. In addition, the needs and challenges of being a physiotherapist working in sport has largely been ignored in the sport injury psychology literature, which seems peculiar given the critical role they have in supporting injured athletes in their rehabilitation from injury. To address this knowledge gap, Kerai, Wadey, and Salim (2019) recently interviewed ten sport physiotherapists about the stressors (i.e., environmental demands) and consequences (e.g., emotions, outcomes) experienced while working in elite sport and, following a thematic analysis, five themes were identified. First, "I Am Not a Machine" provided insight into the sport physiotherapists' workload and working hours (e.g., "working 24/7", "working beyond contractual hours", "too much work"). For example, one physiotherapist reported:

> You can end up working seven-day weeks. Plus, Christmas Day, Boxing Day, New Year's Eve, and New Year's Day. Your life revolves around a fixture list [upcoming matches] … It's a difficult profession. You can't plan ahead because everything can change. Games can get rescheduled. You could do well in a Cup run and have extra games. You could have a cluster of injuries. The manager can decide to suddenly take the team abroad. You have no real control over your own time, your own life. You're pulled in different directions and that brings with it stress and anxiety; a feeling of letting people down all the time. It's okay for a while but it can become overwhelming.

Second, "This Is Sport" reflected the demands of being a physiotherapist working in a performance- and risk-orientated culture (e.g., "ruthless pursuit of success", "sport comes first", "play through injury"). Third, "Relationships Are Messy" considered the conflicts of working with injured athletes and the multidisciplinary team. Fourth, "Under the Microscope" contemplates physiotherapists having to make the "right" decision under intense external pressures. Finally, "Beyond One's Remit" reflected the moral and ethical conflicts imposed upon physiotherapists. Consequences of these demands included: psychological strain (e.g., burnout, anger, devastation when athletes get reinjured, fear of getting it wrong, feeling alone); physical strain (e.g., fatigued and tired, racing heart rate, sweating profusely); job insecurity (e.g., if I do not do this I may be fired); relationship breakdowns (e.g., loss of trust, having no one to turn to); and engaging in emotional labor (e.g., playing the part, feelings of inauthenticity, emotional exhaustion). For example, one physiotherapist reported:

> I've always been a pretty caring and compassionate person. It's why I joined the profession in the first place. I wanted to help athletes … But, the workload is horrendous. It changed me. I became far less caring. Some days, I didn't recognize myself. I didn't like who I was becoming. The way I interacted with injured athletes. I just repaired them. Like a machine that needed to be fixed; a mechanic rather than a physio. The time demands I was under didn't allow the time to nurture them back to full health. They want everything yesterday! … I got to the point where I just didn't want to do the job anymore. They'd literally taken everything from me that I had to give, and they were still asking for more. If this is what it's like to work in elite sport, I don't want to be a part of it; it's not for me. I am *not* a machine.

Taken together, these findings give voice to physiotherapists working in sport, and illustrate how their health, welfare, and well-being is being compromised in elite sport and indicate the critical need for a duty of care to support them. However, far more research is needed to build upon this preliminary study to inform policy and practice. Interestingly, some of the aforementioned consequences of the stressors experienced by physiotherapists have been observed in contexts outside of sport literature (e.g., private practice), which has shown that often practitioners engage in emotional labor to cope with the demands of their role (Foster & Sayers, 2012). Emotional labor has been defined as, "emotion regulation performed in response to job-based emotional requirements in order to produce emotion toward and to evoke emotion from another person to achieve organizational goals" (Grandey, Diefendorff, & Rupp, 2013, p.18). Physiotherapists will do this in order to circumvent a variety of challenging situations by producing or evoking the desired emotions and behaviors within their sociocultural working environments (Foster & Sayers, 2012). However, Hings, Wagstaff, Thelwell, Gilmore, and Anderson's (2018) findings have suggested that engaging with emotional labor can be detrimental for physiotherapists, both personally (e.g., practitioner well-being) and professionally (e.g., physiotherapists feel constrained to react toward injured athletes in a certain way to safeguard their role).

Furthermore, enacting methods of emotional labor (e.g., surface acting, deep acting) have been predicted to have increased psychological repercussions, including emotional exhaustion, emotional dissonance, and feelings of inauthenticity (Lee & Chelladurai, 2016). Therefore, there is a need for future research to identify effective coping strategies that sport physiotherapists can use and, perhaps more importantly, how policies and practices can change in sport to support the health, welfare, and well-being of physiotherapists. Toward this end, it is important that future researchers give sport physiotherapists a voice to understand their experiences and co-construct positive change that builds upon the preliminary findings in this under-researched area of research (e.g., Kerai et al., 2019). Indeed, the duty of care toward physiotherapists within elite sport has been identified as a major concern (Wagstaff, 2019). However, to provide a more nuanced and critical understanding of physiotherapists' working practices in sport, it is important that sport injury researchers also consider taking a more relational approach, especially given the complex web of relations they have with significant others (e.g., injured athletes, coaches, performance directors, parents; Kerai et al., 2019).

"What About Us?" From an Individualistic to a Relational Understanding of the Physiotherapist–Injured-Athlete Relationship

This section is interested in moving the focus beyond the perceptions and actions of either the injured athlete or the physiotherapist toward the relationship itself. Until now, several researchers have examined how physiotherapists can strengthen their relationship with injured athletes, including establishing and building rapport (e.g., Bejar, Raabe, Zakraisek, Fisher, & Clement, 2019; Tracey, 2008), educating athletes about their injury and rehabilitation process (e.g., Clement, Arvinen-Barrow, & Fetty, 2015), and being a primary source of social support (e.g., Bianco, 2001). Yet, despite the merits of these studies and the identification of relational qualities needed to build, maintain, and strengthen this relationship, they remain individualistic in their methodology (i.e., they only consider one perspective). This reiterates a concern reported by Bianco and Eklund (2001) in their review and critique of the social support literature in sport injury psychology nearly 20 years ago, where they reported that the literature has focused primarily on the instrumental factors (e.g., what can physiotherapists offer athletes' needs) rather than the relational dimensions between, for example, the physiotherapist and the injured athlete. Thus, what has largely been ignored is a dyadic understanding of relationships from both perspectives.

Drawing from the field of interpersonal relationships, three diversifying units of analysis that might be of interest toward developing a relational understanding of the physiotherapist–injured-athlete relationship could be, for example, care, conflict, and compatibility (see Poczwardowski, Barott, & Jowett, 2006). For example, *care* has been identified as being incredibly important in patient–therapist interactions in contexts outside of sport, especially considering that individualized patient-centered care is advocated to achieve quality therapeutic relationships and positive outcomes (O'Keefe et al., 2016). To expand, the concept of a "working alliance" is often been used to describe relationships in which physiotherapists and athletes mutually collaborate to help athletes manage their injuries; by creating an environment of trust, working toward a common goal, forging an emotional bond between physiotherapist and athlete, and mutually agreeing upon goals and treatment options (Petitpas & Cornelius, 2004). However, the conceptualization of this approach has yet to be empirically tested in sport settings and there is a dearth of information on how physiotherapists can develop the "soft skills" needed to adapt a working alliance within their clinical practice (Babatunde, MacDermid, & MacIntyre, 2017). Importantly, there also needs to be consideration for how the impact of organizational factors can influence the formation of this type of relationship and the subsequent relational outcomes (O'Keefe et al., 2016).

Another concept in studying this relationship that might be of interest within the physiotherapist–injured-athlete relationship is *interpersonal conflict*. Wachsmuth, Jowett, and Harwood (2017) defined it as "a situation in which relationship partners perceive a disagreement about, for example, values, needs, opinions or objectives that is manifested through negative cognitive, affective and behavioral reactions" (p. 88); with conflict often divided into task (i.e., specific aspects of sport) and social (i.e., relational issues, such as clashing personalities or *incompatibility*), both of which were found to be dysfunctional for relationships (cf. Jehn, 1997). While there is no research on the determinants and outcomes of conflict in physiotherapist–injured-athlete relationships, there are limited studies that have looked at interpersonal conflict in other dyads in sport (Mellalieu, Shearer, & Shearer, 2013; Wachsmuth, Jowett, & Harwood, 2018). One area of conflict might be the power relations between physiotherapists and injured athletes. For example, in sports medicine research the healthcare-provider–patient dyad usually relies on physiotherapists using their knowledge to initiate treatment plans that patients follow; thus there is an inherent power imbalance tipped firmly in favor of the physiotherapist (Scott, 2012). However, in sport settings, many athletes will "bargain" with their physiotherapist about treatment options and are able to choose whether to follow the advice provided or seek help elsewhere (cf. Kerai et al., 2019); therefore, tipping the balance back toward the athlete. Thus, the physiotherapist's role as an injury "expert" is perhaps sometimes undermined, with the physiotherapists autonomy over treatment plans compromised (Scott, 2012). This negotiation of treatment and athlete power can lead to physiotherapists providing "quick-fix" treatments which they may not be entirely comfortable with, leading to conflict within the relationship and potential detrimental intrapersonal and relational outcomes (Scott, 2012). Yet, despite these insights drawn from other fields of research (e.g., sports medicine, sociology of sport), there is a dearth of research about interpersonal conflict within the physiotherapist–injured-athlete dyad in sport injury psychology.

Although some researchers have started to allude to relational concepts (e.g., rapport, social support, conflict, bargaining, care) in other fields of research, there remains a limitation of this research as it still only considers one perspective (e.g., patient *or* practitioner). Focusing on one individual within a relationship at a time is, I would argue, problematic because it may miss out or misrepresent some of the more complex, dynamic, and multifaceted factors that are intrinsically present in the physiotherapist–injured-athlete relationship. Drawing from the applied sport psychology literature, a good example of how this might be done by future researchers is to perhaps consider drawing upon the coach–athlete relationship literature that has rapidly grown since 2007, when Sophia Jowett developed her 3+1Cs model. The model is concerned with coaches' and athletes' closeness (e.g., trust, respect, feeling valued), commitment (e.g., maintaining a close relationship over time), complementarity (e.g., mutual distribution of power and control relative to cooperation), and co-orientation (e.g., mutual understanding). Interestingly, this model has recently been extended to understand the athlete–athlete dyad (Poczwardowski, Lamphere, Allen, Marican, & Haberl, 2019), which included the aforementioned four concepts, with the addition of compatibility (e.g., the chemistry between members). Thus, researchers could look towards coach–athlete and athlete–athlete dyads as starting points to identifying a conceptual model to expand our understanding of the physiotherapist–injured-athlete dyad, as well as other relationships (e.g., physiotherapist–coach relationship) or triadic relationships (e.g., physiotherapist–coach–athlete relationship).

Context Matters: Toward a Cultural Understanding of the Physiotherapist–Injured-Athlete Relationship

Another limitation of sport injury psychology research is that the social-organizational-cultural context is often not accounted for. When examining interpersonal relationships, Poczwardowski et al. (2006) stated the broader environment needs to be considered in order to contextualize the ever-changing understanding of dyadic relationships in a more multifaceted and highly influential nexus with other significant members of the sport environment (e.g., coaches, parents, support staff, performance directors). Toward this end, sport injury psychology researchers would do well to consider and learn from other sport-related or social science disciplines (e.g., social psychology of sport, sociology of sport, organizational psychology), which allude to concepts that can impact human behavior and interpersonal relationships (e.g., social norms and values, organizational hierarchy). Drawing upon sociology of sport research, for example, athletes have accepted risk, pain, and injury to be part and parcel of participating in sport (Hughes & Coakley, 1991). However, researchers have identified this acceptance often comes from "sportsnets" and the broader culture, which have been reported to influence athletes to rationalize and normalize pain and injury in sport and accept them as a part of the game (Curry, 1993; Nixon, 1992). Indeed, the physiotherapist–injured-athlete relationship is surrounded by a number of different sport networks and dyads (e.g., coach–athlete, parent–athlete) which can impact on the quality of the physiotherapist–injured-athlete relationship (Nixon, 1992). In 2019, Steinmann, Jaitner, and Himmelseher explored coaches' perceptions of the role of physiotherapists, and they identified that physiotherapists often found themselves in professional dilemmas between risk and precaution by being forced to work with performance-dominant coaches that have input into the injury management of their athletes.

The term "culture of risk" within sport refers to an athlete's "over-conformity to the sports ethic" (Hughes & Coakley, 1991). Put another way, it is the extent to which the culture and interpersonal messages encourage athletes to accept risk in sport and keep playing as long as possible with pain and injuries or even to return to play as quickly as possible (Nixon, 1992). With physiotherapists often finding themselves caught between the performance- and risk-orientated philosophy of the sport environment and the long-term health-focused approach of their profession (Collier, 2017; Kerai et al., 2019). To expand, Safai (2003) examined the negotiation of treatment between sport medicine clinicians and injured athletes in Canadian intercollegiate sport and found that athletes did operate within this "culture of risk" environment; where experiences included hiding or concealing their injuries, playing through injuries especially if they knew the season was coming to an end, pushing the limits of their bodies, and in some cases looking toward their teammates to judge if they should seek medical help. Furthermore, the clinician's responses indicated that they too are influenced by, and influence, a "culture of risk" and therefore negotiate with athletes within that social context. However, some operated within the "culture of precaution", where physiotherapists try to mitigate the influences of the "culture of risk" and promote long-term athlete health and judge the boundaries of sensible risks after careful consideration; however this is often inferior to short-term athlete aspirations.

In 2012, Scott interviewed 14 physiotherapists and 14 doctors and explored how they balanced the concerns about athlete health and performance. Factors that influenced treatment negotiations included pressure from athletes, the consumer-focused model of medical care within sport, athletes seeking second opinions, pressure from coaches, and impacts on decision-making and clinical autonomy. Given the hierarchy in elite sport, physiotherapists are often in a "weaker" position than that of the athlete or the coach, so given their lack of autonomy relative to these individuals they need to be able to assert their professional status and remain respected. Thus, often physiotherapists conform to the desires of those in a more powerful position over what may be "medically" correct, which could grant them social validation and security in their role and ensure that their interdependent relationships with coaches and athletes continue (cf. Kerai et al., 2019). However, it is also important to acknowledge that physiotherapists have personal agency and do not have to conform to the broader norms and power relations although this "defiance" can have potential consequences (e.g., losing one's job; Kerai et al., 2019).

Furthermore, Scott (2012) found that while doctors erred on the side of the long-term health of the athlete, physiotherapists were more performance-orientated. Codes of practice in sport physiotherapy that are less clear about helping athletes to be "healthy" allows for greater freedom in their practice and they can more easily embrace the performance motivations and demands of their "employers" or "customers". Physiotherapists are often being employed full time as part of the sport medicine team and are at the 'front-line" of athletes' health care, allowing them to be enmeshed into the social-organizational-cultural context and more ready to internalize the culture, which can impact on their behavior, actions, and decision-making (Nixon, 1992; Scott 2012). In the sociology of sport literature there seems to be a debate around health versus performance, and more research is needed as to why they are polarizing ends of a spectrum and whether or not physiotherapists can truly incorporate both into their practice without fear of scrutiny. It is important to note that while physiotherapists might err on the side of performance to appease the athlete and coach, they may be liable against legal claims by athletes who may have experienced injuries (through overuse or otherwise), where investigations will be based on whether duty of care has been breached (Friesen, Saul, Kearns, Bachynski, & Caplan, 2018).

Future Research Implications

This chapter has critically reviewed research in sport injury psychology on the physiotherapist–injured-athlete relationship. By doing so, and drawing from other fields of research (e.g., sociology of sport, sports medicine), three main knowledge gaps have been identified: (a) the physiotherapist as a "performer" in their own right, (b) appreciation of a more dyadic understanding of the relationship, and (c) accounting for how the wider sporting culture influences transactions between physiotherapists and injured athletes. Thus, three avenues of research are proposed here. First, building upon initial research in this area (e.g., Kerai et al., 2019), future studies should look at physiotherapists' own experiences, using longitudinal methodologies to investigate physiotherapists experiences of working in sport over a significant period of time (e.g., during a season or Olympic cycle). This will give researchers a better insight into the current challenges that physiotherapists are experiencing and ways which they can be better supported in working more effectively, especially given the timely and critical importance of duty of care toward physiotherapists (Wagstaff, 2019).

Second, future researchers in sport injury psychology needs to start think more dyadically rather than focusing on one group (e.g., physiotherapists *or* injured athletes), so there needs to be research surrounding what influences each relationship member exerts on the other, as a relationship is a product and process shared between two individuals (Poczwardowski et al., 2006). Research in sport injury psychology has yet to account for both athletes and physiotherapists experiences in the same study (over time or in "real time"), therefore ignoring complex, multifaceted dynamics, and creating an incomplete picture of this nuanced relationship. By looking at research on the coach–athlete relationship (e.g., Jowett, 2007; Wachsmuth et al., 2018; Yang & Jowett, 2016), future researchers could, for example, develop a specific model or theory of the physiotherapist–injured-athlete relationship to help inform subsequent programs of research and professional practice. One qualitative tradition that might be particularly well-suited to this research question is grounded theory, which is an approach that helps researchers understand psychological and social processes by developing concepts and theories to understand human action and interaction (Charmaz, 2006). This could be extremely useful when looking at the physiotherapist–injured-athlete relationship and how it unfolds throughout the rehabilitation and recovery process.

Finally, future researchers should account for the social context in their research and how this affects experiences and transactions within the physiotherapist–injured-athlete dyad. Here, researchers would do well to embrace interdisciplinary research, integrating sport injury psychology with other fields of research (e.g., sociology of sport, organizational psychology, social and personal relationships). Researchers in these disciplines have developed understandings of relational concepts to account for interpersonal behavior in dyads and among groups. Using an ethnographic approach, the researcher can immerse themselves in the environment to better understand how the wider social context is impacting on physiotherapist–injured-athlete relationships. Furthermore, Hess, Gnacinski, and Meyer (2019) recently called for more research into the medium level of abstraction which includes the approaches used by professionals in practice (i.e., lone practitioner, team-based approaches). If physiotherapists are drawing from the biopsychosocial paradigm which describes injury as multifaceted and requires a team-based approach to rehabilitation and interventions, future researchers could look at how other disciplines can work more effectively together. Other, perhaps more novel, areas of research that need to be taken into consideration include diversifying the phenomena under study (e.g., working with injured disabled athletes, differences in cultural environments, sexual or physical abuse). Furthermore, a broader representation of the physiotherapist–injured-athlete relationship will provide more nuanced understanding, including: gender structure of the relationship (e.g., female physiotherapist–male athlete, male physiotherapist–female athlete); ethnicity, age, maturity, skill level of both physiotherapists and athletes; types of relationships (typical vs. atypical, successful vs. unsuccessful).

Conclusion

The emergence and development of sport injury psychology over the past five decades has established a field of research that aims to support injured athletes' recovery following injury. However, much of the research has been conducted at the intrapersonal level, for example, understanding an athlete's psychological responses to and rehabilitation from injury. However, more research needs to be conducted at the interpersonal level of analysis which focuses on the dyadic interactions and researching both athletes and physiotherapists within the same study and the broader culture of sport. While there is a growing need for more knowledge on interpersonal relationships in sport, this chapter has shown where the research is currently at, what some of the major issues that need to be considered by researchers are, and potential avenues for promising research that are both exciting and necessary to expand our understanding of different dyads within sport.

Critical Discussion Questions

- What psychological challenges are physiotherapists likely to experience work- ing in sport and how might we best support them?
- Considering the critical importance of the physiotherapist–athlete dyad, what strategies would we use to help build and maintain this relationship over time?
- The health versus performance nexus is a dilemma that many physiothera- pists experience in elite sport. Instead of making them polarizing concepts (e.g., choosing one or the other), should physiotherapists try to find a balance? If so, what might this look like?

References

Arvinen-Barrow, M., & Clement, D. (2019). A case for interprofessional care. In M. Arvinen-Barrow & D. Clement (Eds.), *The psychology of sport and performance injury: An interprofessional case-based approach* (pp. 1–9). London: Routledge.

Babatunde, F., MacDermid, J., & MacIntyre, N. (2017). Characteristics of therapeutic alliance in musculoskeletal physiotherapy and occupational therapy practice: A scoping review of the literature. *BMC Health Services Research, 17*(1), 1–23. doi: 10.1186/s12913-017-2311-3

Bejar, M. P., Raabe, J., Zakrajsek, R. A., Fisher, L. A., & Clement, D. (2019). Athletic trainers' influence on national collegiate athletic association division I athletes' basic psychological needs during sport injury rehabilitation. *Journal of Athletic Training, 54*(3), 245–254. doi: 10.4085/1062-6050-112-18

Bianco, T. (2001). Social support and recovery from sport injury: Elite skiers share their experiences. *Research Quarterly for Exercise and Sport, 72*(4), 376–388. doi: 10.1080/02701367.2001.10608974

Bianco, T., & Eklund, R. C. (2001). Conceptual considerations for social support research in sport and exercise settings: The case of sport injury. *Journal of Sport and Exercise Psychology, 23*(2), 85–107. doi: 10.1123/jsep.23.2.85

Brewer, B. W., & Redmond, C. (2017). *Psychology of sport injury.* Champaign, IL: Human Kinetics Publishers.

Charmaz, K. (2006). *Constructing grounded theory: A practical guide through qualitative analysis.* London: Sage Publications.

Clement, D., Arvinen-Barrow, M., & Fetty, T. (2015). Psychosocial responses during different phases of sport-injury rehabilitation: A qualitative study. *Journal of Athletic Training, 50*(1), 95–104. doi: 10.4085/1062-6050-49.3.52

Collier, R. (2017). Competing interests. *Canadian Medical Association Journal, 189*(4), 179–181. doi: 10.1503/cmaj.1095377

Curry, T. J. (1993). A little pain never hurt anyone: Athletic career socialization and the normalization of sports injury. *Symbolic Interaction, 16*(3), 273–290. doi: 10.1525/si.1993.16.3.273

Foster, C., & Sayers, J. (2012). Exploring physiotherapists' emotion work in private practice. *New Zealand and Journal of Physiotherapy, 40*, 17–23.

Friesen, P., Saul, B., Kearns, L., Bachynski, K., & Caplan, A. (2018). Overuse injuries in youth sports: Legal and social responsibility. *Journal of Legal Aspects of Sport, 28*(2), 151–169. doi: 10.18060/22569

Grandey, A., Diefendorff, J., & Rupp, D. E. (Eds.). (2013). *Emotional labor in the 21st century: Diverse perspectives on emotion regulation at work.* East Sussex: Routledge.

Hess, C. W., Gnacinski, S. L., & Meyer, B. B. (2019). A review of the sport-injury and-rehabilitation literature: From abstraction to application. *The Sport Psychologist, 33*(3), 232–243. doi: 10.1123/tsp.2018-0043

Hings, R. F., Wagstaff, C. R., Thelwell, R. C., Gilmore, S., & Anderson, V. (2018). Emotional labor and professional practice in sports medicine and science. *Scandinavian Journal of Medicine and Science in Sports, 28*(2), 704–716. doi: 10.1111/sms.12941

Hughes, R., & Coakley, J. (1991). Positive deviance among athletes: The implications of overconformity to the sport ethic. *Sociology of Sport Journal, 8*(4), 307–325. doi: 10.1123/ssj.8.4.307

Jehn, K. A. (1997). A qualitative analysis of conflict types and dimensions in organizational groups. *Administrative Science Quarterly, 42*(3), 530–557. doi: 10.2307/2393737

Jowett, S. (2007). Interdependence analysis and the 3 + 1Cs model in the coach–athlete relationship. In S. Jowett & D. Lavallee (Eds.), *Social psychology in sport* (pp. 15–27). Champaign, IL: Human Kinetics.

Kerai, S., Wadey, R., & Salim, J. (2019). Stressors experienced in elite sport by physiotherapists. *Sport, Exercise, and Performance Psychology, 8*(3), 255–272. doi: 10.1037/spy0000154

Lee, Y. H., & Chelladurai, P. (2016). Affectivity, emotional labor, emotional exhaustion, and emotional intelligence in coaching. *Journal of Applied Sport Psychology, 28*(2), 170–184. doi: 10.1080/10413200.2015.1092481

Mellalieu, S., Shearer, D. A., & Shearer, C. (2013). A preliminary survey of interpersonal conflict at major games and championships. *The Sport Psychologist, 27*(2), 120–129. doi: 10.1123/tsp.27.2.120

Nixon, H. L. (1992). A social network analysis of influences on athletes to play with pain and injuries. *Journal of Sport and Social Issues, 16*(2), 127–135. doi: 10.1177/019372359201600208

O'Keeffe, M., Cullinane, P., Hurley, J., Leahy, I., Bunzli, S., O'Sullivan, P. B., & O'Sullivan, K. (2016). What influences patient-therapist interactions in musculoskeletal physical therapy? Qualitative systematic review and meta-synthesis. *Physical Therapy, 96*(5), 609–622. doi: 10.2522/ptj.20150240

O'Neill, D. F. (2008). Injury contagion in alpine ski racing: The effect of injury on teammates' performance. *Journal of Clinical Sport Psychology, 2*(3), 278–292. doi: 10.1123/jcsp.2.3.278

Petitpas, A., & Cornelius, A. (2004). Practitioner-client relationships: Building working alliances. In G. S. Kolt & M. B. Andersen (Eds.), *Psychology in the physical and manual therapies* (pp. 57–70). Edinburgh: Churchill Livingstone.

Poczwardowski, A., Barott, J. E., & Jowett, S. (2006). Diversifying approaches to research on athlete–coach relationships. *Psychology of Sport and Exercise, 7*(2), 125–142. doi: 10.1016/j.psychsport.2005.08.002

Poczwardowski, A., Lamphere, B., Allen, K., Marican, R., & Haberl, P. (2019). The 5C's model of successful partnerships in elite beach volleyball dyads. *Journal of Applied Sport Psychology*, 1–19. doi: 10.1080/10413200.2019.1573205

Safai, P. (2003). Healing the body in the "culture of risk": Examining the negotiation of treatment between sport medicine clinicians and injured athletes in Canadian intercollegiate sport. *Sociology of Sport Journal, 20*(2), 127–146. doi: 10.1123/ssj.20.2.127

Scott, A. (2012). Making compromises in sports medicine: An examination of the health performance nexus in British Olympic sports. In D. Malcolm & P. Safari (Eds.), *The social organisation of sports medicine: Critical sociocultural perspectives* (pp. 227–246). London: Routledge.

Steinmann, A., Jaitner, D., & Himmelseher, N. (2019). "One aspect of the coaching business." Function and role of sports physiotherapists from the perspective of coaches in German elite athletics. *Sports Coaching Review*, 1–20. doi: 10.1080/21640629.2019.1657680

Taylor, J., & Taylor, S. (1997). *Psychological approaches to sport injury rehabilitation*. Gaithersburg, MD: Aspen Publishers

Tracey, J. (2008). Inside the clinic: Health professionals' role in their clients' psychological rehabilitation. *Journal of Sport Rehabilitation*, *17*(4), 413–431. doi: 10.1123/jsr.17.4.413

Wachsmuth, S., Jowett, S., & Harwood, C. G. (2017). Conflict among athletes and their coaches: What is the theory and research so far? *International Review of Sport and Exercise Psychology*, *10*(1), 84–107. doi: 10.1080/1750984X.2016.1184698

Wachsmuth, S., Jowett, S., & Harwood, C. G. (2018). On understanding the nature of interpersonal conflict between coaches and athletes. *Journal of Sports Sciences*, *36*(17), 1955–1962. doi: 10.1080/02640414.2018.1428882

Wadey, R., Day, M., Cavallerio, F., & Martinelli, L. (2018). Multilevel Model of Sport Injury (MMSI): Can coaches impact and be impacted by injury? In R. Thelwell & M. Dicks (Eds.), *Professional advances in sports coaching: Research and practice* (pp. 336–357). London: Routledge.

Wagstaff, C. R. (2019). A commentary and reflections on the field of organizational sport psychology. *Journal of Applied Sport Psychology*, *31*(1), 134–146. doi: 10.1080/10413200.2018.1539885

Wiese-Bjornstal, D. M. (2009). Sport injury and college athlete health across the lifespan. *Journal of Intercollegiate Sport*, *2*(1), 64–80. doi: 10.1123/jis.2.1.64

Yang, S. X., & Jowett, S. (2016). Understanding and enhancing coach–athlete relationships through the 3+ 1Cs model. In R. Thelwell, C. Harwood & I. Greenlees (Eds.), *The psychology of sports coaching: Research and practice* (pp. 54–67). Abingdon: Routledge.

Zakrajsek, R. A., Fisher, L. A., & Martin, S. B. (2018). Certified athletic trainers' experiences with and perceptions of sport psychology services for student-athletes. *The Sport Psychologist*, *32*(4), 300–310. doi: 10.1123/tsp.2017-0119

10 Guilt Experienced by Coaches Following Athlete Injury

Laura Martinelli and Melissa Day

Introduction

Given the routine presence of the coach during training and competition, it is unsurprising that coaches are prime candidates for vicarious exposure to injury. A person may be categorized as vicariously exposed to an athlete's injury if they have witnessed the incident or listened to third-person narratives of the injury event (Day, 2012). In the case of a coach witnessing an athlete's injury, there may be close physical contact with the injury stimuli, because the coach is duty bound to provide first aid until medical professionals arrive on the scene (Cunningham, 2002; Sports Coach UK, 2012). Indeed, the achievement of a first-aid certificate is recommended, if not required, prior to, or delivered as part of, minimum sport coach qualifications; thus coaches are expected to be willing and able to provide first aid if the injury necessitates it. It has also been recognized that the coach plays an important social support role in facilitating the injured athlete's psychological and physical recovery (Bianco, 2001; Podlog & Dionigi, 2010; Udry, 2001). It is during these interactions that the coach may also be further vicariously exposed to the injury as they hear and learn about the athlete's experiences. Hence, by way of the coach adopting more of a counseling role (Buceta, 1993; Ellickson & Brown, 1990; Smith, 1992), it is possible that a coach may be vicariously exposed to the aversive details of the injury event as they allow the injured athlete to share related memories, thoughts, and feelings.

Having established that the coach is in a prime position for vicarious exposure to injury, it is then logical to question what these experiences mean for the coach. For example, what is it like for coaches to witness or hear of their athletes' injuries; what are the repercussions of these vicarious exposures and how might coaches cope? The current chapter provides some answers to these questions and identifies pathways for future research.

Injury as a Meaningful or Traumatic Experience for the Coach

For some readers, the proposition that injury could be conceptualized as a traumatic event for coaches may be unconvincing given that injury can be a regular and perhaps normalized part of working life as a sports coach, which injury rates attest to (Frisch et al., 2009; Mattila, Parkkari, Koivusilta, Kannus, & Rimpelä, 2009; Nicholl, Coleman, & Williams, 1995). However, in line with a schema-based theoretical perspective toward psychological trauma (Janoff-Bulman, 1992; Joseph & Linley, 2005; Park, 2010), an event may be traumatic because it has posed a meaningful threat to a person's individualized yet global beliefs and goals. For example, even where a coach appears knowledgeable of the risk of injury in sport, such an event can be psychologically traumatic because it has deeply contradicted existing understandings about why and how such injuries happen, as well as impacting on the individual's self-perceptions in terms of the extent to which they believed themselves to be a good, moral, willing, and/or capable coach. This suggests that the traumatic meaning of athlete injury resides not in an objective assessment of severity and prevalence, but in the coach's subjective appraisal of the event and the way in which it contradicts their expectations about the occurrence of injury and the self (Gabert-Quillen, Fallon, & Delahanty, 2011). Essentially the more the coach's initial appraisal of the event is discrepant with his or her pre-existing beliefs and goals connected to injury in sport, the greater the level of distress and possibly trauma will follow. Such a perspective encourages us to take a more idiosyncratic and relative approach when we consider what types of injuries could have meaningful consequences for the coach.

In a study that was the first of its kind, Day, Bond, and Smith (2013) evidenced the possibility that an athlete's injury could be a traumatic experience for the coach. Day et al. utilized life history interviews to explore vicarious injury among two national-level trampoline coaches from the same club, who were both present during a training session in which one of their athletes sustained an open leg fracture. Key insights gained through a narrative analysis of the interview transcripts found that both coaches recalled episodes of involuntarily re-experiencing the athlete's injury (i.e., intrusions) that were triggered upon re-entering the environment in which the incident had occurred and having contact with the injured athlete; hence there was considerable effort exerted by the coaches to avoid conversations about the injury within the training environment. By suggesting that the two coaches had experienced intrusions and avoidance in the aftermath of witnessing an athlete's injury, Day et al. construed a link with hallmark symptoms of post-traumatic stress (Brewin & Holmes, 2003; McNally, 2004). Indeed, the oscillation between intrusions (e.g., involuntarily re-experiencing the event) and behavioral as well as cognitive avoidance of event-related stimuli after witnessing an injury is recognized by the Diagnostic and Statistical Manual of Mental Disorders (DSM-5) as part of a constellation of post-traumatic stress symptoms (APA, 2013; Friedman, 2013). These symptoms become clinically significant if they persist for more than six months, thereby permitting a diagnosis of Post-Traumatic Stress Disorder (PTSD).

What Do We Mean by Guilt and Why Is it a Relevant Emotion?

Building upon the work by Day et al. (2013), Martinell, Day, and Lowry (2017) used semi-structured interviews and narrative analysis techniques to examine the emotional responses experienced by a variety of coaches in the aftermath of vicarious exposure to their athletes' injuries. Guilt was identified as a key and commonplace experience after witnessing or learning about athletic injury. For example, one coach was quoted as saying:

> whether the coach is responsible or not, he [sic] is a definite part of any of injury because it is most likely that he would have been there when his athlete got injured and he will have had thoughts or feelings somewhere down the line [pauses] about guilt.
>
> (p. 7)

Similarly, another coach stated:

> you can even feel guilty about people that you coach who injure themselves when it's nothing to do with you. So, it's not in your session, and it's not in your [yard], but because you've taught them and they go out and do something else, and then they get injured, there is a little creeping feeling of guilt.
>
> (Martinelli et al., p. 10)

Guilt is defined as an intense and unpleasant affective state accompanied by beliefs that one should have thought, felt, or acted differently (Blum, 2008; Pugh, Taylor & Berry, 2015). Guilt is therefore a multidimensional construct composed of an affective component characterized by emotional distress and a cognitive component composed of "a set of interrelated beliefs about one's role in a negative event" (Kubany & Watson, 2003, p. 53).

As part of an effort to understand why coaches conveyed guilt as an inevitable feature of their response to an athlete's injury, Martinelli et al. (2017) utilized models of trauma-related guilt (Kubany & Manke, 1995; Kubany & Watson, 2003) to further explore the coaches' accounts of athlete injury. In doing so, it was possible to recognize several specific cognitions or beliefs within the coaches' recollections of athlete injury that underpinned and magnified their experience of guilt. These included an exaggerated sense of personal responsibility (i.e., inaccurate thoughts about social position and power at the time of the event), faulty beliefs about the foreseeability and preventability of the injury (i.e., hindsight bias), when they are unable to find sufficient justification for the way they acted (i.e., unable to find a suitable reason for what they did or did not do), and when they believe they have behaved in ways that violates personal values and standards (i.e., heightened sense of wrongdoing). Martinelli et al. therefore illustrated the subjectivity of the guilt felt by these coaches and offered specific examples of thinking patterns that could prompt a coach to experience an athlete's injury as distressing because of the guilt-related meanings.

It is also important to consider the role that the wider social context played in predisposing coaches to experience guilt. As argued by Wadey, Day, Cavallerio, and Martinelli (2018), it is useful to move beyond intrapersonal and interpersonal levels of analysis, and to consider what might be happening at an institutional level as a way to make sense of how individuals respond to athlete injury. Accordingly, Hardman and Jones (2013) recognize that the moral and ethical worlds of sport coaches are increasingly defined from a deontological perspective, hence our understanding of what it means to be a sports coach typically centers on the coach's duties or obligations and their sports participants' entitlements. This is evidenced by the development of the code of practice for sports coaches by Sports Coach UK (2005) which details a host of actions that characterize good coaching practice in the context of sport, some of which are specifically related to the possibility or actual occurrence of athletic injury. For example, this code of practice states that individuals with good coaching practice are those who "ensure that the environment is as safe as possible, taking into account and minimising possible risks", and who "accept responsibility for their actions" (Sports Coach UK, 2005, p. 3).

Such institutional messages therefore place injury at the center of the way we determine the goodness of a coach. Furthermore, this message encourages a seemingly inseparable connection between the coach and the physical integrity of an athlete; hence the coach is inevitably implicated by the occurrence of an injury. Indeed, for McNamee (2011), these codes of practice "franchise 'blameability' [sic] and consequently 'punishability' [sic] to their respective organisations" (p. 25), with the sports coach acting as the face of the organization. This deontological climate to coaching is further compounded by an atmosphere of uncertainty. According to Partington (2014, p. 236), the standard duty of care that all individuals acting as sport coaches must continuously champion is "nebulous and woolly" in nature, whereby, in practice, it fails to offer clear authority as to when the occurrence of an injury unequivocally does or does not infer a breach in the coach's obligated conduct. Such ambiguity may encourage coaches to more readily interpret an instance of injury as indicative of the coach somehow failing to fulfill standards adjunct to his or her sporting role. Given that a departure or violation of values and standards are conceptualized as a cognitive determinant of guilt (Kubany & Watson, 2003; Lee, Scragg, & Turner, 2001), it may therefore be that the experience of guilt among coaches in the aftermath of athletic injury is more widespread than currently recognized, at least within the literature on sport injury and sport coaching.

What Might a Coach Initially Do in Response to Their Experience of Guilt?

Although the experience of guilt following trauma has been a point of some theoretical and empirical interest, there is a lack of consensus regarding the consequences of this emotion (Tilghman-Osbourne, Cole, & Felton, 2010) For example, Lee et al. (2001) argued that guilt may be a disabling emotional response to a traumatic event because it signals that the self is being experienced in a negative way, and Blum (2008) portrays guilt as a maladaptive emotion underpinning psychopathologies. Conversely, others address the more adaptive qualities of this emotion. In this regard, Baumeister, Stillwell, and Heatherton (1994) argued that guilt is a social emotion that serves to strengthen relationships by reducing the frequency of transgressions against others. Similarly, Carnì, Petrocchi, Del Miglio, Mancini, and Couyoumdjian (2013) described guilt as a moral emotion that helps individuals adjust to, and adopt, cultural norms for the purpose of social survival. There is also a lack of clarity over the precise relationship between guilt and the development of post-traumatic stress. Whereas the DSM-5 (APA, 2013) situates guilt as one of a constellation of post-traumatic stress symptoms, Lee et al. (2001) and Kubany and Watson (2003) have forwarded models of trauma-related guilt that conceptualize the emotion as constitutive of a type of post-traumatic response that drives other symptoms of post-traumatic stress (Browne, Trim, Myers, & Norman, 2015).

Given the different trajectories that guilt might have, Martinelli et al. (2017) also examined the ways that coaches tried to cope with their initial experience of guilt. It was reported that for some coaches, avoiding the injured athlete was key to gaining some immediate relief from the guilt. In such scenarios, coaches were reluctant to be in close physical proximity with the injured athlete, typically exemplified by refraining to visit the injured athlete in hospital. As one coach stated:

> I didn't even want to go to the hospital because I felt that much guilt. If it was professional, I would have gone straight to the hospital … I would have been there straight away after the game with Ashley … I just couldn't go, with it being a bit more personal, I felt I must get out of this.
>
> (Martinelli et al., p. 10)

This corroborates Kubany and Watson's (2003) multidimensional model of guilt in which avoidance signifies one's need for short-term respite from the emotion. Similarly, Baumeister et al. (1994) attest that the transgressor's avoidance of their victim is a commonplace consequence of guilt. However, Martinelli et al. indicated that avoidance of the injured athlete was eventually problematic for the coaches, whereby it contradicted usual standards of coaching behavior in response to injury. Essentially, by avoiding the injured athlete, coaches experienced personal discontinuity that brought about a second wave of guilt. Again, this is consistent with hypotheses made by Lee et al. (2001) and Kubany and Watson (2003) that a departure from a valued way of acting is a determinant of guilt. Martinelli et al. subsequently reported that, for these coaches, keeping a contactable distance from the injured individual became a better way to regulate their feelings of guilt to tolerable levels. Examples of this included speaking with the injured athlete on the phone or over text message, sending gifts, or offering practical assistance with respect to other stressors in the athlete's life.

Unique to one coach's story of guilt detailed by Martinelli et al. (2017) was the desire for the injured athlete to take legal action, otherwise described as seeking reparation through punishment. The use of punishment has been recognized as an extreme guilt-regulating strategy that acts as an unequivocal social signal of remorse and desire for reparation, serving to restore the transgressor's relationship with the harmed individual (Nelissen, 2012). Yet, given the compensation culture said to currently exist within sport where injured athletes readily seek claims of negligence (James, 2013), the possibility of an athlete taking legal action in the aftermath of injury is no doubt more routinely perceived as a threat by coaches and perhaps motivates them to deny their feelings of guilt. Indeed, the findings published by Martinelli et al. are derived from a more extensive research programme[1] (Martinelli, 2016) that has collected accounts by coaches attesting to just this. For example, one coach said:

> but sometimes the most traumatic things about an injury is not the person who's lying there, although that sounds awful, but it's did I do something wrong, and you have to bring up the real the real spectre of being sued … they might be your best friend in the whole world and they might love you as a coach and if something goes wrong and they think that they can claim on your insurance, bomph, they'll be straight in there … and to be able to get a claim on your insurance they have to say that you were negligent and oh they can be mean.
>
> (Martinelli, 2016, p. 120)

It is therefore clear that although some coaches view the possibility of legal action as an avenue through which they may alleviate guilt, for others it is a scenario that incites distress.

The Enduring Effects of Guilt

The experiences presented and discussed thus far have addressed the coaches' more immediate responses to potential or actual ensuing guilt. However, Martinelli (2016) found that some coaches elaborated upon the longstanding implications of experiencing guilt after a vicarious exposure to injury. For some coaches, guilt-related thinking would inevitably lead them to question their suitability to be a coach, prompting thoughts about terminating their involvement in sport. As one coach said:

> you just question yourself which is a bad thing to do, in the extent that you question, "Am I a good coach? Can I do this? Am I cut out to do this?" … I think that a lot of people, like, when they question themselves, a lot of people drop out, and be like no I can't do this, I'm not a coach.
>
> (Martinelli, 2016, p. 125)

What is also interesting about this interview excerpt is the coach's focus on their goodness as a coach in general. Guilt is conceptualized as an emotional phenomenon concerned with a specific but unstable and thus changeable aspect of the person being construed as responsible for the occurrence of a negative event. Yet, it has been argued that in reality it may be difficult for the individual to not see his or her thinking, feeling, and acting errors as stemming from more enduring qualities of the self (Blum, 2008). As such, it may be that, in entertaining guilt-related meanings, the coach is in danger of concluding that these seemingly discrete errors actually signify one's more general deficiencies in the skills, abilities, and character otherwise required to perform the coaching role. Consequently, these coaches may quickly traverse from guilt into the emotional territory of shame, the latter of which involves a more global condemnation of the self whereby pervasive qualities of the person are deemed responsible for the occurrence of a negative event (Blum, 2008; Joseph, 1999; Teroni & Deonna, 2008). Kubany and Watson (2003) support the possibility of this shift from guilt to shame to the extent that their model depicts a pathway from guilt-related cognitions to the experience of shame, yet this is poorly explained, and research by Robinaugh and McNally (2010) demonstrated that guilt was positively related to post-traumatic stress symptoms when in the presence of high levels of shame, but negatively related to post-traumatic stress symptoms when in the presence of low levels of shame. Given the potentially thin line between guilt and shame, and the detrimental consequences of shame, efforts to debrief coaches and encourage reflection after athlete injury may do well to keep the coaches focused on distinct changeable behaviors and to be cautious of coaches construing more general and potentially damaging self-perceptions that could lead to role termination.

The suggestion that the coach may construe negative meanings of athletic injury in the form of one's unsuitability for the coaching role resonates with schema-based understandings of post-traumatic responses. Accordingly, where an experience is construed to convey threatening information about the self, individuals who incorporate these negative meanings into their understanding of the self are said to have engaged in the process of negative accommodation whereby the experience is deemed as wholly representative of the self and world, often leading to goal abandonment (Joseph & Linley, 2005; Park, 2010). However, Martinelli (2016) also collected accounts of more positive meanings that could be construed over time (see Chapter 12). The suggestion that the coach may eventually benefit from an adverse event such as athletic injury resonates with the process of positive accommodation put forward by schema-based understandings of post-traumatic responses. In order to positively accommodate the experience, Joseph and Linley (2005) argue that the individual must move beyond deliberations that attempt to explain why the event happened, otherwise referred to as meaning-as-comprehensibility, to address the value or worth of an experience for one's life in particular, otherwise termed meaning-as-significance (Janoff-Bulman & McPherson Frantz, 1997). Meaning-as-significance is consequently said to underpin the experience of Post-Traumatic Growth (PTG), a concept that is representative of the beneficial changes in people's perceptions of themselves, in addition to their relationships with others and the life philosophy that a person can experience in the aftermath of trauma (Joseph & Linley, 2005; Tedeschi & Calhoun, 2004).

For those coaches who found it possible to harness something constructive from the sense of wrongdoing that underpinned their experience of guilt, this was in the form of lessons learned from mistakes. As an example of lessons learned, Martinelli (2016) detailed a series of quotations taken from an interview with an equestrian coach who was recounting one of her vicarious injuries as a coach:

> it's that little first one that really sticks with you but then I felt that I learned a lot from it as well. … I know having looked back on it, that was one of the things that made me much better at dealing with parents … if you don't think

the pony is suitable for the child, as an instructor or as a coach you have to [pauses] you have to make your feelings clear … if I'm not happy to teach that child on that pony I as a professional, I have to be able to say, I have to be brave enough to say "I'm sorry that is a totally unsuitable pony" and that can be one of the most difficult things to do … you have to go with your gut even if it doesn't make you particularly popular.

(p. 128)

These comments highlight that coaches may be able to work with their feelings of guilt, perhaps owing to the way that guilt can eventually be an adaptive emotion following adverse events (Blum, 2008; Tilghman-Obsbourne et al., 2010). Yet this may be dependent upon the individual having the time and space to construe such positive meanings. Indeed, this same equestrian coach noted:

I think if I had to go and teach pony club lesson the next day that might have been a very different situation … I probably thought for a short time I would never do pony club again [laughs] but, you know, but, I thought "oh my god no this teaching lark isn't for me".

(Martinelli, 2016, p. 129)

Although the experience of guilt may be initially interpreted negatively, with time and no doubt the right kind of support it can be harnessed in a more positive and productive way that concludes with perceptions of enhanced coaching practice.

Future Research Implications

Research addressing the way that athlete injury implicates the coach's well-being is sparse, hence there is considerable scope for more research to be done that continues to provide in-depth descriptive accounts of the meaning of injury for coaches. The area may benefit from ethnographic methodologies that utilize observations and interviews in the field to provide real-time first- and third-person perspectives about the way that coaches respond to injuries they witness or learn about. There is also a need for research that explores debriefing and reflective practices following injury and the impact that these may have on the coach's propensity to experience guilt and subsequent use of coping strategies. Furthermore, there are no empirical examples of psychology professionals providing support to coaches in the aftermath of athlete injury, yet such accounts may also further our understanding of how we can help coaches navigate potentially distressing experiences, such as guilt, in constructive ways.

Conclusion

The current chapter has discussed and evidenced some of the ways that athlete injury can be a meaningful event for the coach. By placing a spotlight on the guilt that can be experienced by coaches, insights have been offered as to why this emotion may be a routine part of the coach's response to athlete injury, in addition to empirical examples of the short- and long-term consequences of guilt. While this chapter has reported and explained the negative, unpleasant experiences of guilt, it has also detailed the possibility that more positive meanings can be construed from injury events that initially invoked guilt. It is hoped that further research will create spaces for more conversation, reflection, and understanding about the way that athlete injury implicates the coach's well-being.

Critical Discussion Questions

1) What factors might increase the coach's likelihood of experiencing guilt in response to athlete injury?
2) Given the guilt and avoidance tendencies that a coach may experience in the aftermath of athlete injury, how might we best engage coaches in a discussion about the injury in order to determine the need for psychological support?
3) What might be the social environmental conditions that support and facilitate coaches to construe positive meanings from their experience of guilt after injury?

Note

1   For details regarding the methodology (i.e., participant characteristics, data collection, and analysis methods) of Martinelli (2016), please see Martinelli, Day, and Lowry (2017).

References

American Psychiatric Association. (2013). *Diagnostic and statistical manual of mental disorders* (5th ed.). Arlington, VA: Author.

Baumeister, R. F., Stillwell, A. M., & Heatherton, T. F. (1994). Guilt: An interpersonal approach. *Psychological Bulletin, 115*(2), 243. doi: 10.1037%2F0033-2909.115.2.24

Bianco, T. (2001). Social support and recovery from athletic injury: Elite skiers share their experiences. *Research Quarterly for Exercise and Sport, 72*(4), 376–388. doi: 10.1080/02701367.2001.10608974

Brewin, C. R., & Holmes, E. A. (2003). Psychological theories of posttraumatic stress disorder. *Clinical Psychology Review, 23*(3), 339–376. doi: 10.1016/S0272-7358(03)00033-3

Browne, K. C., Trim, R. S., Myers, U. S., & Norman, S. B. (2015). Trauma-related guilt: Conceptual development and relationship with posttraumatic stress and depressive symptoms. *Journal of Traumatic Stress, 28*(2), 134–141. doi: 10.1002/jts.21999

Buceta, J. M. (1993). The sport psychologist/athletic coach dual role: Advantages, difficulties, and ethical considerations. *Journal of Applied Sport Psychology, 5*(1), 64–77. doi: 10.1080/10413209308411305

Carnì, S., Petrocchi, N., Del Miglio, C., Mancini, F., & Couyoumdjian, A. (2013). Intrapsychic and interpersonal guilt: A critical review of the recent literature. *Cognitive Processing, 14*(4), 333–346. doi: 10.1007/s10339-013-0570-4

Cunningham, A. (2002). An audit of first aid qualifications and knowledge among team officials in two English youth football leagues: A preliminary study. *British Journal of Sports Medicine, 36*(4), 295–300. doi: 10.1136/bjsm.36.4.295

Day, M. C. (2012). Coping with trauma in sport. In J. Thatcher, M. Jones & D. Lavallee (Eds.), *Coping and emotion in sport* (2nd ed., pp. 62–78). London: Routledge.

Day, M., Bond, K., & Smith, B. (2013). Holding it together: Coping with vicarious trauma in sport. *Psychology of Sport and Exercise, 14*(1), 1–11. doi: 10.1016/j.psychsport.2012.06.001

Ellickson, K. A., & Brown, D. R. (1990). Ethical considerations in dual relationships: The sport psychologist-coach. *Journal of Applied Sport Psychology, 2*(2), 186–190. doi: 10.1080/10413209008406429

Friedman, M. J. (2013). Finalizing PTSD in DSM-5: Getting here from there and where to go next. *Journal of Traumatic Stress, 26*(5), 548–556. doi: 10.1002/jts.21840

Frisch, A., Croisier, J. L., Urhausen, A., Seil, R., & Theisen, D. (2009). Injuries, risk factors and prevention initiatives in youth sport. *British Medical Bulletin, 92*(1), 95–121. doi: 10.1093/bmb/ldp034

Gabert-Quillen, C. A., Fallon, W., & Delahanty, D. L. (2011). PTSD after traumatic injury: An investigation of the impact of injury severity and peritraumatic moderators. *Journal of Health Psychology, 16*, 678–687. doi: 10.1177%2F1359105310386823

Hardman, A., & Jones, C. (2013). Philosophy for coaches. In R. L. Jones & K. Kingston (Eds.), *An introduction to sport coaching: Connecting theory to practice* (pp. 99–111). Abingdon: Routledge.

James, M. (2013). *Sports law* (2nd ed.). Basingstoke: Palgrave MacMillan.

Janoff-Bulman, R. (1992). *Shattered assumptions. Towards a new psychology of trauma.* New York: The Free Press.

Janoff-Bulman, R., & McPherson Frantz, C. (1997). The impact of trauma on meaning: From meaningless world to meaningful life. In M. Power & C. R. Brewin (Eds.), *The transformation of meaning in psychological therapies* (pp. 91–106). Hoboken, NJ: John Wiley & Sons.

Joseph, A., & Linley, P. A. (2005). Positive adjustment to threatening events: An organismic valuing theory of growth through adversity. *Review of General Psychology, 9*(3), 262–280. doi: 10.1037/1089-2680.9.3.262

Joseph, S. (1999). Attributional processes, coping and post-traumatic stress disorders. In W. Yule (Ed.), *Post-traumatic stress disorders: Concepts and therapy* (pp. 51–70). Hoboken, NJ: John Wiley & Sons.

Kubany, E. S., & Manke, F. P. (1995). Cognitive therapy for trauma-related guilt: Conceptual bases and treatment outlines. *Cognitive and Behavioral Practice, 2*(1), 27–61. doi: 10.1016/S1077-7229(05)80004-5

Kubany, E. S., & Watson, S. B. (2003). Guilt: Elaboration of a multidimensional model. *The Psychological Record, 53*(1), 51–90.

Lee, D. A., Scragg, P., & Turner, S. (2001). The role of shame and guilt in traumatic events: A clinical model of shame-based and guilt-based PTSD. *British Journal of Medical Psychology, 74*(4), 451–466. doi: 10.1348/000711201161109

Martinelli, L. A. (2016). *Understanding sport coaches' experiences of athletic injury* (Unpublished Doctoral thesis). University of Southampton, Chichester.

Martinelli, L. A., Day, M. C., & Lowry, R. (2017). Sport coaches' experiences of athlete injury: The development and regulation of guilt. *Sports Coaching Review, 6*(2), 162–178. doi: 10.1080/21640629.2016.1195550

Mattila, V. M., Parkkari, J., Koivusilta, L., Kannus, P., & Rimpelä, A. (2009). Participation in sports clubs is a strong predictor of injury hospitalization: A prospective cohort study. *Scandinavian Journal of Medicine and Science in Sports, 19*(2), 267–273. doi: 10.1111/j.1600-0838.2008.00800.x

McNally, R. J. (2004). Conceptual problems with the DSM-IV criteria for posttraumatic stress disorder. In G. M. Rosen (Ed.), *Posttraumatic stress disorder: Issues and controversies* (pp. 1–14). Hoboken, NJ: John Wiley & Sons.

McNamee, M. (2011). Celebrating trust, virtues and rules in the ethical conduct of sport coaches. In A. R. Hardman & C. Jones (Eds.), *The ethics of sport coaching* (pp. 23–41). Abingdon: Routledge.

Nelissen, R. M. (2012). Guilt-induced self-punishment as a sign of remorse. *Social Psychological and Personality Science, 3*(2), 139–144. doi: 10.1177/1948550611411520

Nicholl, J. P., Coleman, P., & Williams, B. T. (1995). The epidemiology of sports and exercise related injury in the United Kingdom. *British Journal of Sports Medicine, 29*(4), 232–238. doi: 10.1136/bjsm.29.4.232

Park, C. (2010). Making sense of the meaning literature: An integrated review of meaning making and its effects on adjustment to stressful life events. *Psychological Bulletin, 136*(2), 257–301. doi: 10.1037/a0018301

Partington, N. (2014). Legal liability of coaches: A UK perspective. *The International Sports Law Journal, 14*(3–4), 232–241. doi: 10.1007/s40318-014-0056-2

Podlog, L., & Dionigi, R. (2010). Coach strategies for addressing psychosocial challenges during the return to sport from injury. *Journal of Sports Sciences, 28*(11), 1197–1208. doi: 10.1080/02640414.2010.487873

Pugh, L. R., Taylor, P. J., & Berry, K. (2015). The role of guilt in the development of post-traumatic stress disorder: A systematic review. *Journal of Affective Disorders, 182*, 138–150. doi: 10.1016/j.jad.2015.04.026

Robinaugh, D. J., & McNally, R. J. (2010). Autobiographical memory for shame or guilt provoking events: Association with psychological symptoms. *Behaviour Research and Therapy, 48*(7), 646–652. doi: 10.1016/j.brat.2010.03.017

Smith, D. (1992). The coach as sport psychologist: An alternate view. *Journal of Applied Sport Psychology, 4*(1), 56–62. doi: 10.1080/10413209208406449

Sports Coach, U. K. (2005). *Codes of practice for sports coaches.* Leeds: The National Coaching Foundation.

Sports Coach, U. K. (2012). *UKCC level 1 guide.* Retrieved from https://www.sportscoachuk .org/sites/default/files/UKCC-Level-Guide.pdf

Tedeschi, R. G., & Calhoun, L. G. (2004). Posttraumatic growth: Conceptual foundations and empirical evidence. *Psychological Inquiry, 15*(1), 1–18. doi: 10.1207/s15327965pli1501_01

Teroni, F., & Deonna, J. A. (2008). Differentiating shame from guilt. *Consciousness and Cognition, 17*(3), 725–740. doi: 10.1016/j.concog.2008.02.002

Tilghman-Osborne, C., Cole, D. A., & Felton, J. W. (2010). Definition and measurement of guilt: Implications for clinical research and practice. *Clinical Psychology Review, 30*(5), 536–546. doi: 10.1016/j.cpr.2010.03.007

Udry, E. (2001). The role of significant others: Social support during injuries. In J. Crossman (Ed.), *Coping with sports injuries: Psychological strategies for rehabilitation* (pp. 148–161). Oxford: Oxford University Press.

Wadey, R., Day, M., Cavallerio, F., & Martinelli, L. (2018). The multi-level model of sport injury: Can coaches impact and be impacted by injury? In R. Thelwell & M. Dicks (Eds.), *Professional advances in sports coaching: Research and Practice* (pp. 408–440). London: Routledge.

11 My Daughter's Injured Again!

I Just Don't Know What to Do Anymore

*Francesca Cavallerio, Nicole Kimpton,
and Camilla J. Knight*

Introduction

If, or, perhaps more accurately, when, athletes get injured, their access to social support can play an important role in both their psychological and physical recovery. Although the support networks athletes have access to may vary in size and make-up, in most instances arguably one of the most important sources of support are parents.[1] Unfortunately, despite the importance of parents, little research attention is given to the experiences or influences of parents when their children are injured. Therefore, the aim of this chapter is to provide readers with a critical review of current understanding of the role of parents in relation to injury. Specifically, this chapter seeks to examine three questions: (a) how are parents impacted by their child's sport-related injuries? (b) what role do parents play in injury development? and (c) how can sport psychologists support parents of injured athletes? To answer these questions, a review of existing work is presented, combined with critical reflections taken from Nicole's autoethnographic extracts to encourage readers to critically appraise existing knowledge by considering existing gaps between research and real life. The points raised through the critical review will be used to illuminate future research implications to improve support provision for sport parents.

Critical Review and Reflections

Over the last 40 years there has been an increasing interest in psychological research on sports injury, which has addressed two main objectives (Brewer, 2001). On the one hand, sports injury research focused on developing an understanding of the factors that can help predict and prevent sport-related injuries; on the other, it examined athletes' responses to injury to provide functional psychological strategies to support their rehabilitation and return to sport (Wadey, Day, Cavallerio, & Martinelli, 2018). Such research has been extremely beneficial in advancing understanding of sport injuries; however, a critical pursual of the research soon reveals an almost exclusive focus on the athlete (cf. Wadey et al., 2018). Although this might appear logical, it can become limiting when, for example, one realizes the amount of studies that have highlighted the substantial role of social support for a positive recovery from injury (e.g., Mitchell, Evans, Rees, & Hardy, 2014). Only a dearth of studies that have focused on injury have adopted a level of analysis that looks beyond the athlete (e.g., Cavallerio, Wadey, & Wagstaff, 2016; Martinelli, Day, & Lowry, 2016). Chapters 9 (i.e., physiotherapists) and 10 (i.e., coaches) also provide additional perspectives on the social influence of injury.

What about sport parents, though? They are referred to in the literature as being of fundamental importance to enable participation and positive experiences in sport (e.g., Holt, Tamminen, Black, Sehn, & Wall, 2008; Knight & Holt, 2014), but there is limited research examining their role in relation to sport injury. Podlog, Kleinert, Dimmock, Miller, and Shipherd (2012) investigated parents' perspectives on their children's rehabilitation from injury, as well as the impact of injury on parents themselves. The themes highlighted by the study's participants mainly related to the financial burden of surgeries and specialist support, also linked to unpleasant feelings of uncertainty with regard to the injury's seriousness (Podlog et al., 2012). Similarly, research examining parents' experiences in sport have commonly identified injury as a substantial stressor for parents to manage (Knight & Harwood, 2009) but one which they often feel ill-equipped to cope with (Burgess, Knight, & Mellalieu, 2016). Consequently, parents are often found searching for guidance and information pertaining to how best to support their children when they are injured (cf. Burgess et al., 2016; Knight & Holt, 2014) and note that worries around injury can impact upon their behaviors and involvement with respect to their child's sport (e.g., Knight, Dorsch, Osai, Haderlie, & Sellars, 2016). The following subsections will draw from different disciplines (e.g., sociology, legal studies, psychology) to illuminate the dual role of parents during their children's sport injuries, first as "victims" of the situation, and second as potential "main characters".

How Are Parents Impacted by Injury?

Beyond studies identifying children's injury as a stressor for parents (e.g., Harwood, Drew, & Knight, 2010; Knight & Harwood, 2009), one of the few studies that focused on parents' experience in depth was Lally and Kerr's (2008) work examining the effects of gymnasts' retirement on parents. In this study, parents frequently discussed the pain their daughters were still experiencing even following retirement, and expressed lingering doubts about their daughters' physical health, highlighting feelings of helplessness and lack of knowledge. This lack of knowledge was reflected in an almost blind trust that the coach had their daughters' best interests at heart, as highlighted in recent studies (cf. Smits, Jakobs, & Knoppers, 2017; Tynan & McEvily, 2017), although on reflection they realized that perhaps they did not. As parents were socialized into the culture of gymnastics, the unwavering trust in coaches and a lack of awareness of the negative consequences of unhealthy behaviors toward pain and injury (e.g., training despite pain, not allowing complaints to be voiced) resulted in the normalization of such behaviors (Smits et al., 2017). For the parents interviewed by Lally and Kerr (2008), doubts about such behaviors, which were deemed "normal" in the gymnasium, only surfaced after retirement and detachment from the world of gymnastics.

Extending this study, Kerr and Stirling (2012) interviewed parents of retired elite athletes to explore their reflections of their child's experiences of emotionally abusive coaching practices. Reflections were categorized according to five consecutive phases of socialization into the elite sport culture: an initial "honeymoon phase", followed by decreased control over the young athletes, growing concerns being silenced, and a resultant acceptance of cultural norms. Finally, parents moved into a phase of guilt once their child retired from sport. Although this study focused explicitly upon emotional abuse, the process shared by parents closely resembles the thoughts reported in Lally and Kerr's (2008) earlier work, pointing to the similarities between experiences of emotional abuse and of injuries, particularly if they accrue as a result of physical abuse. Physical abuse is defined as causing physical harm or injury to a child on purpose, and in sport can be manifested when the intensity of training and competition exceeds a child's developmental stage, through physical punishment, or training while injured or ill (National Society for the Prevention of Cruelty to Children, 2017).

So, what is it like for the parent of a young artistic gymnast who finds themselves in this situation? To help us gain insight into the complexities of the pain–injury nexus from a parental perspective Nicole shares two scenarios with us involving her daughter Willow. We invite you to become co-participants – to engage with the reflections, think with the story, and actively consider the quandary parents of elite child athletes may face.

> **Nicole:** Waiting, waiting, waiting. I feel as though I have been waiting a lifetime for the call. My daughter, Willow had a Magnetic Resonance Imaging scan on Friday morning and the consultant said he would call this afternoon after speaking with the medical advisor from [National Governing Body]. I have been on tenterhooks since waking this morning and have had my phone within reach all day, after waiting out what felt like the longest weekend ever.
>
> The pain had started in her lower back about three weeks previously, at first just a niggle doing certain skills, then more frequently during the training sessions. She was now at the point that although she was avoiding training any skills that caused her acute pain, there was a constant dull ache that was bad enough for her to wake at night. I glance at the phone to see if I have somehow missed a call. Still nothing. I am due to pick her up from school and go to training in less than half an hour, the outcome from the meeting will determine how tonight's session will pan out. I have an uneasy feeling in my stomach with slight waves of nausea, so much is riding on this phone call. Willow has been selected to represent [Country] in a few weeks, her participation in this event all hinges on the conversation. Waiting, watching, wrestling with my thoughts – what do I actually want to hear? I really don't know. Before I fall further into the ever-widening crevasse of my conflicting cognitions, the phone rings causing me to fumble in my haste to answer.

"The scan is clear, there is no anatomical reason for Willow's pain". A million, minute bursts of electricity explode in my mind. I grapple with the information bestowed upon me. A wave of nausea hits a crescendo as the doctor states there is no clear reason why my daughter is in pain each day. I thank him for his time and slump back into the chair on which I am perched. How can this be? We were so certain it was a stress fracture that had been causing her to take painkillers on a regular basis. A cocktail of non-prescription drugs has been the only way for her to make it through even a reduced-load training session.

"She's weak ... she's lying ... she's lazy", words reverberate around my mind, mocking me, reminding me of past interactions with previous coaches. The fear of them not believing Willow haunts me; too many coaches have labeled her with the same moniker, "not tough enough". I fear her new coach will now be of the same opinion; experience informs me that no physical abnormality on a scan equals crying wolf in a coach's mind. If it can't be seen it's not a real problem. I am devastated ... devastated for Willow who will now, more than likely, be expected to train through the pain. I had secretly hoped the scan would show a problem: a disk bulge, a stress fracture, something tangible that could be rested, treated, and rehabilitated. I pick up her kit bag and head out the door to break the bad news to her ... "your back is fine".

How Might Parents Impact upon Injury?

Consideration of how parents might impact upon youth athletes' experience of injury is limited within sport injury psychology literature but has been considered from a sociological perspective. For instance, sport sociologists Grenfell and Rinehart (2003) provided an analysis of those aspects of the parent–child relationship that have an impact on young athletes' approach to intensive involvement in the sport, influencing behaviors of pain normalization and risk glorification (Hughes & Coakley, 1991). Grenfell and Rinehart (2003) suggested that children are used as a means for displaying parenting skills and therefore, "if children are only seen for their use-value, then it follows that whatever means it takes to achieve success (by whomever) could be deemed appropriate behavior" (p. 87). The authors identify what they call "conspicuous parenting" (p. 87) as a non-altruistic behavior, which, in ways that might be conscious or unconscious, aims to display the parents' own excellence. Tofler, Knapp, and Lardon (2005) analyzed this type of parental behavior from a clinical perspective, associating it with achievement-by-proxy distortion, supporting the idea that such a distorted view would warrant abuse on the child.

Drawing on a social and legal perspective, Friesen, Saul, Kearns, Bachynski, and Caplan (2018) recently examined the specific relationship between parents involved in their child's sporting lives and overuse injuries. These authors highlighted the potential damaging role of parents on their children's experience in sport, pointing out the disconnect existing between parents' and children's experiences (e.g., amount of pressure from parents). By citing the "whatever it takes" attitude toward the achievement of their child's goals (Dorsch, Smith & McDonough, 2009, p. 459), Friesen et al. drew attention toward a potential breach of fulfilling duty of care with regard to overuse injuries. They compared youth elite sport programs to child labor situations, governmental organization, and laws, and concluded that except for those cases of gross negligence and child abuse, parental ignorance is what has an effect on overuse injuries. While ignorance is not something punishable from a legal perspective, a lack of knowledge and understanding of risks is an aspect shared with studies from other fields of sport (e.g., Cavallerio, Wadey, & Wagstaff, in preparation; Smits et al., 2017). However, whether it is ignorance *per se* or, as Smits et al. (2017) described, the enactment of an environment with "a code of silence surrounding pain and injuries" (p. 75), it warrants further consideration.

Recognizing the impact of cultural and structural factors, Coakley (2006) provided a slightly more moderate reflection on why and how parents, specifically fathers, are involved in children's sporting lives and consequently may influence injury development. First, he suggested that based on a combination of cultural and structural factors, parents tend to feel that they are meeting their responsibilities as parents when their children play sport. In addition, Coakley suggested that fathers feel accountable for their children's achievements and failures within an organized sport setting and experience guilt if developmental expectations are not met, especially in the highly visible competitive arena of sport. Coakley's study highlighted how the involvement in an organized sport setting can be experienced by parents as an opportunity to provide their child not only with safe developmental opportunities, but also with a competent version of themselves. More recently, work by Pynn et al. (2019) and Watchman and Spencer-Cavaliere (2017) also pointed out how parents' perspectives toward children's sport have evolved over time. Pynn et al.'s study stressed the role of social media in creating a culture where parents feel constantly judged and questioning their own parenting skills, therefore trying to ensure their children do not miss out on opportunities. Watchman and Spencer-Cavaliere illuminated the prioritizing role given to organized sport over free play, with the former considered as a better opportunity for children to develop important life skills. Parents in the study also discussed the role played by sport organizations in forcing early specialization, which often is perceived as a non-choice on the parts of families (Watchman & Spencer-Cavaliere, 2017). Once involved in the competitive sport environment though, the accepted cultural norms are so strong that even the parents who might not be fully convinced, once in the process – as stated by Kerr and Stirling (2012) – often end up as acceptant and acquiescent beings. In their new role, parents feel depleted of their voice due to lack of sport-specific knowledge and the desire to ensure they are supporting their children's dreams (Smits et al., 2017). Nicole's extract provides a glimpse of the internal struggle of a mother who faces the silencing and belittling of a sport environment that disempowers parents, rather than supporting them to ensure the well-being of young athletes.

Nicole: "Every kid in this gym has something that hurts, it's part of the job, it comes with the sport". I look around as the coach waves his arm to highlight his point: "Look at the lump on my wrist, that came from pommel work when I was a gymnast. It hurt to train, but I learned to deal with it – Willow needs to toughen up if she wants to get anywhere." Yada yada … here we go again. Let's bash the kid when she's injured, let's make it her fault she can't, or should I say "won't" train properly, the inference being it's a choice rather than an inability. Another meeting to inform me of the inadequacies of my daughter's character.

This wrist injury has been problematic for almost a year. Willow has already had three Cortisone injections and has been warned she must look after herself as she has hit the limit for steroid shots. Each time she returns to training the medical advice is to build back up slowly and step back when the "ache" lasts for more than 12 hours. Willow insists she's been keeping to the plan, but I have my doubts. The gym is closed off to parents, so I am unable to track the number of repetitions she is doing, and today's conversation leads me to believe the medical advice is not being adhered to. I know Willow is concerned she will not be ready to compete at the National Championships in a few months and she is all too aware her place on the National Team as well as her financial and medical funding are dependent on a good performance. I fear the combination of Willow's desire to train and being pushed by the coaches to ignore the pain is going to drown out the voice of reason. I can only remind her of the medical advice and enquire how she is doing; I have no say in her training plan and know any interference will result in me being labeled a "difficult parent" and Willow will bear the brunt of my actions in the training hall.

I leave the gym feeling as though I have failed my child: I have not demanded to watch the sessions, I have not stated we will be taking our business elsewhere if they do not conform to the medical advice, I have not asked them to treat my child with the respect she deserves. My parental instincts to protect my child from harm have been whittled away over the years. I have been conditioned to accept pain and injury as par for the course and accept the coaches are experts in their field. I have been pushed into the shadows of my daughter's life. Why have I let this happen?

Future Research Implications

Given the limited literature focused on understanding and supporting parents of injured athletes, there are several avenues for future research. A recent review of the existing sport psychology literature on sport parents illuminated various aspects that need investigating, but one of the main limitations highlighted by the authors is the oversimplification of parenting and parental involvement in sport (Harwood, Knight, Thrower, & Berrow, 2019). Harwood et al. (2019) suggested that "when we talk about pressure or support, we might actually be making reference to a range of different practices that may make their own unique contribution to children's sport experiences and developmental outcomes" (p. 68). Attitudes toward parents and sport injuries appear to suffer from this oversimplified view of a situation that – as portrayed through Nicole's autoethnographic extracts as the mother of a young elite gymnast – goes beyond the binary version of pressure versus support. There is a need for researchers to illuminate the nexus between performance and health (Scott, 2012), to unveil its complexity and understand how to better support sport parents in managing their child being in pain and/ or injured. This section aims to address two main points: first, it will reflect on how we can – as sport psychology researchers – reach a better understanding of parents' experiences of managing injuries in youth sport. Second, it will suggest future implications for research to allow us to provide better informed and more effective psychological support to parents of young athletes.

How Can we Better Understand Parents' Experiences?

Research examining parents' experiences of injury in sport should consider looking beyond injury models focused on the individual and instead focus upon exploring theories and models that encourage examination at other levels (e.g., interpersonal, cultural). Wadey et al. (2018) and Wiese-Bjornstal (2019) provide recent examples of models that look at the different systems that surround, influence, and are influenced by the injured athlete (i.e., parents and the broader family network). Knight and Holt's (2014) grounded theory of optimal parental involvement in youth tennis also shows the importance of adopting theories that take relationships into consideration. Moreover, adopting more interdisciplinary approaches to study, for instance combining psychological and sociological approaches, may be particularly useful in unpacking the complexity of this experience (cf. Cavallerio et al., 2016).

The parent–coach relationship, which appears to play such a key influence on parents' experiences of injuries, would also benefit from further examination, particularly considering concepts such as coercive persuasion. Tourish, Collinson, and Barker (2009) define this as a behavior that "encourages subjects to internalize dominant cultural norms as their own, subsequently producing individuals deemed to be 'appropriate' by the ruling group while disguising many of the elements of compulsion that are involved, even from those directly affected" (p. 363). Coercive behaviors in leaders (i.e., coaches, recognized as the experts) become reflected in unquestioning conformity in followers (i.e., parents), which has been reported as having potential harmful consequences (Hogg, 2001). Sport psychology scholars could explore the effect of coercive behaviors between coaches and parents, but also strive to understand how these behaviors could be prevented and/or decreased to foster a more collaborative and trustful environment.

How Can We Better Support Parents (and, in Turn, Athletes)?

The present chapters highlighted a need to develop a specific understanding of sport situations that encourage or facilitate physical abuse. Although knowledge stemming from research on emotional and sexual abuse in the sport psychology literature has often been shown to be transferable to physical abuse (e.g., Kerr & Stirling, 2012), we need to examine what other aspects might be at play in cases of physical abuse. Building on this understanding then, we could work to support parents to recognize physically abusive behaviors that are normalized in the sport environment. Research should also look into how we can empower parents, as well as coaches, to stand up against these behaviors, rather than falling into the process of acceptance and acquiescence.

Finally, when working with parents, there is a need to provide different ways to allow them to express, discuss, and reflect on their own lived experiences, as well as those gained through witnessing other parents. Knight and Newport (2017) encouraged practitioners to develop engaging and effective interventions when working with parents, and researchers and practitioners should consider how to disseminate knowledge in ways that are creative and accessible (e.g., McMahon, Knight, & McGannon, 2018). Creative analytical practices (CAP) (e.g., creative nonfiction, ethnodrama, poetry; Richardson, 2000) allow vivid representations of research findings that make them available to non-academic audiences (Smith, McGannon, & Williams, 2015) by evoking emotions, fostering reflection, and potentially encouraging change (McMahon, 2017). Representing research findings using CAP, then, will provide practitioners with the engaging "tools" suggested by Knight and Newport (2017), increasing the potential for effective interventions to support sport parents.

Conclusion

The aim of this chapter was to review the literature related to the experience of parents in relation to injuries in sport. Existing research has almost exclusively focused on examining injuries from athletes' perspectives, and as a result little is known regarding how parents are impacted by or impact upon injury. A review of current work highlighted the need for much more research in this area, particularly exploring aspects related to the parent–coach relationship and the sport environment and culture. Autoethnographic experiences of one sport parent served to highlight the complexity of the situations that parents have to deal with and, given such complexity, far more insights and parent voices are needed to stimulate action in this important and under-researched area.

Critical Discussion Questions

1) How can we give voice to parents' experiences of injuries in sport?
2) How can we critically examine and appraise an environment and resultant parent behaviors, if the culture requires strict adhere and limited reflection?
3) How can we support parents from "being pushed into the shadows", while also building a positive and trustful relationship with their young children's coaches?

Note

1 For the purpose of this chapter, parent(s) refers to parents, step-parents, guardians, and main caregivers.

References

Brewer, B. W. (2001). Psychology of sport injury rehabilitation. In R. N. Singer, H. A. Hausenblas & C. M. Janelle (Eds.), *Handbook of sport psychology* (pp. 787–809). New York: John Willey and Sons. doi: 10.1002/9781118270011.ch18

Burgess, N. S., Knight, C. J., & Mellalieu, S. D. (2016). Parental stress and coping in elite youth gymnastics: An interpretative phenomenological analysis. *Qualitative Research in Sport, Exercise and Health, 8*(3), 237–256. doi: 10.1080/2159676X.2015.1134633

Cavallerio, F., Wadey, R., & Wagstaff, C. R. D. (2016). Understanding overuse injuries in rhythmic gymnastics: A 12-month ethnography. *Psychology of Sport and Exercise, 25,* 100–109. doi: 10.1016/j.psychsport.2016.05.002

Cavallerio, F., Wadey, R., & Wagstaff, C. R. D. (under review). *"When do I stop her?" Overuse injuries through the eyes of young gymnasts' parents: An ethnodrama.*

Coakley, J. (2006). The good father: Parental expectations and youth sports. *Leisure Studies, 25*(2), 153–163. doi: 10.1080/02614360500467735

Dorsch, T. E., Smith, A. L., & McDonough, M. H. (2009). Parents' perceptions of child-to-parent socialization in organized youth sport. *Journal of Sport and Exercise Psychology, 31*(4), 444–468. doi: 10.1123/jsep.31.4.444

Friesen, P., Saul, B., Kearns, L., Bachynski, K., & Caplan, A. (2018). Overuse injuries in youth sports: Legal and social responsibility. *Journal of Legal Aspects of Sport, 28*(2), 151–169. doi: 10.18060/22569

Grenfell, C. C., & Rinehart, R. E. (2003). Skating on thin ice: Human rights in youth figure skating. *International Review for the Sociology of Sport, 38*(1), 79–97. doi: 10.1177/10126902030381005

Harwood, C., Drew, A., & Knight, C. J. (2010). Parental stressors in professional youth football academies: A qualitative investigation of specializing stage parents. *Qualitative Research in Sport and Exercise, 2*(1), 39–55.

Harwood, C. G., Knight, C. J., Thrower, S. N., & Berrow, S. R. (2019). Advancing the study of parental involvement to optimize the psychosocial development and experiences of young athletes. *Psychology of Sport and Exercise, 42,* 66–73. doi: 10.1016/j.psychsport.2019.01.007

Hogg, M. A. (2001). A social identity theory of leadership. *Personality and Social Psychology Review, 5*(3), 184–200. doi: 10.1207/S15327957PSPR0503_1

Holt, N. L., Tamminen, K. A., Black, D. E., Sehn, Z. L., & Wall, M. P. (2008). Parental involvement in competitive youth sport settings. *Psychology of Sport and Exercise, 9*(5), 663–685. doi: 10.1016/j.psychsport.2007.08.001

Hughes, R., & Coakley, J. (1991). Positive deviance among athletes: The implications of overconformity to the sport ethic. *Sociology of Sport Journal, 8*(4), 307–325. doi: 10.1123/ssj.8.4.307

Kerr, G. A., & Stirling, A. E. (2012). Parents' reflections on their child's experiences of emotionally abusive coaching practices. *Journal of Applied Sport Psychology, 24*(2), 191–206. doi: 10.1080/10413200.2011.608413

Knight, C. J., Dorsch, T. E., Osai, K. V., Haderlie, K. L., & Sellars, P. A. (2016). Influences on parental involvement in youth sport. *Sport, Exercise, and Performance Psychology, 5*(2), 161–178. doi: 10.1037/spy0000053

Knight, C. J., & Harwood, C. G. (2009). Exploring parent-related coaching stressors in British tennis: A developmental investigation. *International Journal of Sports Science and Coaching*, 4(4), 545–565. doi: 10.1260/174795409790291448

Knight, C. J., & Holt, N. L. (2014). Parenting in youth tennis: Understanding and enhancing children's experiences. *Psychology of Sport and Exercise*, 15(2), 155–164. doi: 10.1016/j.psychsport.2013.10.010

Knight, C. J., & Newport, R. A. (2017). Understanding and working with parents of young athletes. In C. J. Knight, C. G. Harwood & D. Gould (Eds.), *Sport psychology for young athletes* (pp. 303–314). London: Routledge.

Lally, P., & Kerr, G. (2008). The effects of athlete retirement on parents. *Journal of Applied Sport Psychology*, 20(1), 42–56. doi: 10.1080/10413200701788172

Martinelli, L. A., Day, M. C., & Lowry, R. G. (2016). Sport coaches' experience of athlete injury: The development and regulation of guilt. *Sports Coaching Review*, 6(2), 162–178. doi: 10.1080/21640629.2016.1195550

McMahon, J. (2017). Creative analytical practices. In B. Smith & A. C. Sparkes (Eds.), *Routledge handbook of qualitative research in sport and exercise* (pp. 302–315) London: Routledge.

McMahon, J., Knight, C. J., & McGannon, K. R. (2018). Educating parents of children in sport about abuse using narrative pedagogy. *Sociology of Sport Journal*, 35(4), 314–323. doi: 10.1123/ssj.2017-0186

Mitchell, I., Evans, L., Rees, T., & Hardy, L. (2014). Stressors, social support, and tests of the buffering hypothesis: Effects on psychological responses of injured athletes. *British Journal of Health Psychology*, 19(3), 486–508. doi: 10.1111/bjhp.12046

National Society for the Prevention of Cruelty to Children (2017). *Physical abuse*. Retrieved from https://www.nspcc.org.uk/what-is-child-abuse/types-of-abuse/physical-abuse

Podlog, L., Kleinert, J., Dimmock, J., Miller, J., & Shipherd, A. M. (2012). A parental perspective on adolescent injury rehabilitation and return to sport experiences. *Journal of Applied Sport Psychology*, 24(2), 175–190. doi: 10.1080/10413200.2011.608102

Pynn, S. R., Neely, K. C., Ingstrup, M. S., Spence, J. C., Carson, V., Robinson, Z., & Holt, N. L. (2019). An intergenerational qualitative study of the good parenting ideal and active free play during middle childhood. *Children's Geographies*, 17(3), 266–277. doi: 10.1080/14733285.2018.1492702.

Richardson, L. (2000). New writing practices in qualitative research. *Sociology of Sport Journal*, 17(1), 5–20. doi: 10.1123/ssj.17.1.5

Scott, A. (2012). Making compromises in sports medicine: An examination of the health performance nexus in British Olympic sports. In D. Malcolm & P. Safai (Eds.), *The social organization of sports medicine: Critical sociocultural perspectives* (pp. 227–246). London: Routledge.

Smith, B., McGannon, K. R., & Williams, T. L. (2015). Ethnographic creative nonfiction: Exploring the whats, whys and hows. In G. Molnar & L. Purdy (Eds.), *Ethnographies in sport and exercise research* (pp. 73–88). New York: Routledge.

Smits, F., Jacobs, F., & Knoppers, A. (2017). 'Everything revolves around gymnastics': Athletes and parents make sense of elite youth sport. *Sport in Society*, 20(1), 66–83. doi: 10.1080/17430437.2015.1124564

Tofler, I. R., Knapp, P. K., & Lardon, M. T. (2005). Achievement by proxy distortion in sports: A distorted mentoring of high-achieving youth. Historical perspectives and clinical intervention with children, adolescents, and their families. *Clinics in Sports Medicine*, 24(4), 805–828. doi: 10.1016/j.csm.2005.06.007

Tourish, D., Collinson, D., & Barker, J. R. (2009). Manufacturing conformity: Leadership through coercive persuasion in business organizations. *Management*, 12(5), 360–383.

Tynan, R., & McEvilly, N. (2017). 'No pain, no gain': Former elite female gymnasts' engagements with pain and injury discourses. *Qualitative Research in Psychology*, *9*(4), 469–484. doi: 10.1080/2159676X.2017.1323778

Wadey, R., Day, M., Cavallerio, F., & Martinelli, L. (2018). Multilevel model of sport injury (MMSI): Can coaches impact and be impacted by injury? In R. Thelwell & M. Dicks (Eds.), *Professional advances in sports coaching* (pp. 336–357). London: Routledge.

Watchman, T., & Spencer-Cavaliere, N. (2017). Times have changed: Parent perspectives on children's free play and sport. *Psychology of Sport and Exercise*, *32*, 102–112. doi: 10.1016/j.psychsport.2017.06.008

Wiese-Bjornstal, D. M. (2019). Sociocultural aspects of sport injury and recovery. In E. O. Acevedo (Ed.), *Oxford research encyclopedia of sport, exercise and performance psychology*. Oxford, UK: Oxford University Press.

12 But We've Always Done It This Way

The Future of Qualitative Injury Research

Melissa Day and Kimberley Humphrey

Introduction

Over the past few decades numerous researchers have illustrated the steady growth of qualitative research in sport (e.g., Culver, Gilbert, & Sparkes, 2012; McGannon, Smith, Kendellen, & Gonsalves, 2019; Poucher, Tamminen, Caron, & Sweet, 2019). With this increase in published work comes the suggestion that qualitative research has not only gained in acceptance, but that qualitative researchers have become more innovative and more diverse in their approaches to research (Krane, 2017), as well as more cognizant of how to produce quality qualitive research (McGannon et al., 2019). The sport injury literature exemplifies this steady increase in the number of published studies. From 1990 to 1999 a total of 10 qualitative studies were published that focused on the acute injury process (from sustaining an injury to return to sport), while in comparison from 2000 to 2009 this number doubled to 20 published studies. In the following decade it has taken just six years (from 2010 to 2016) to reach and now exceed this number of publications, demonstrating the growing momentum of qualitative sport injury research (Humphrey, 2020).

This growing momentum of qualitative injury research should be celebrated given that it demonstrates the continual increase in the number of researchers who find value in using qualitative methods. Yet, caution must also be exercised, as, per Forscher's (1963) early warnings, an increased amount of research does not always create a useful foundation for building our understanding. Forscher's allegory of the decline of research provides us with a number of valuable considerations when surveying the current sport injury research landscape. Forscher depicted scientists as builders who aimed to build edifices (or bodies of knowledge) through the creation of bricks (or facts). As the story explains, the original pride shown in producing bricks of the highest quality to facilitate strong foundations for solid edifices gave way to an obsession with brick *making*. In order to make enough bricks in good time, brickmaking was rarely adventurous, difficult, or unusual. Forscher warned that without quality bricks then the edifice would crack; further, the land may become covered in bricks, making it difficult to construct an edifice.

The warnings gleaned from Forscher's story are evident in several contemporary reviews of qualitative research in sport. Specifically, such reviews have focused on the quality of methodology (e.g., the degree to which epistemology is linked to methodology, Culver et al., 2012; the danger of focusing on method over ontology, Giardina, 2017) and the breadth of research methodologies used (e.g., Culver et al., 2012; McHugh, 2017). Given that qualitative methodologies are now well recognized as a legitimate and valuable form of scholarship, the focus of contemporary review articles has shifted from needing to demonstrate the acceptance of qualitative methods to widening the horizons of qualitative researchers and ensuring methodological connoisseurship. As suggested by McGannon et al. (2019), connoisseurship is not simply about having more qualitative research, but encouraging a diversity of approaches grounded in appreciation, quality, and knowledge growth. Thus, just as Forscher suggested, efforts should be focused toward quality, ensuring strong foundations and encouraging research creativity. In line with contemporary perspectives, our aim in this chapter is not to jettison existing research but to explore the scope of possibility for future scholarship. To do this, we consider where there are opportunities in the research process to extend current practice. Our aim is not to provide an exhaustive list of future recommendations but to raise awareness of contemporary issues across the research process that may be curtailing qualitative sports injury research and to look to the future by envisaging how these issues may be overcome. Consequently, in this chapter we focus on three areas of the research process: (a) who are the "usual suspects" in injury research and how could alternative sampling strategies widen our understanding; (b) how can we expand upon traditional forms of data collection to include the use of place, objects, and the physical self; and (c) how can this knowledge be disseminated in more creative, user-friendly ways?

Current Quandaries and Curtailments

The Usual Suspects: Recruiting Beyond Severity and Time

In their seminal text on doing successful qualitative research, Braun and Clarke (2013) asked researchers to consider who the "usual suspects" are when sampling participants (p. 58). Within the sport injury literature, most often researchers have used purposeful sampling to focus on a particular subgroup or population of injured athletes. As Patton (2002) identified, this sampling strategy allows for the identification and selection of information-rich cases that will yield insights and in-depth understanding. In order to determine who might be "information-rich", sport injury researchers have frequently focused on the characteristics of the injury sustained, for example, participants are recruited based on injury severity (e.g., Mankad, Gordon, & Wallman, 2009), length of injury (e.g., Bianco, Malo, & Orlick, 1999; Gould, Udry, Bridges, & Beck, 1997), and/or type of injury sustained (e.g., Carson & Polman, 2012; Heijne, Axelsson, Werner, & Biguet, 2008). The aim of this strategy has often been to demonstrate the injury status of participants, verifying that the sample is representative of those who have sustained a sporting injury severe enough to incur a potential emotional response. Yet, such an approach is fraught with problems. First, it implies that there is a particular time point or severity after which an injury may impact on an individual. It does not account for individual factors such as injury history, how the injury was sustained, or the timing in the season for the athlete. Second, time points and terminology to describe the severity of injury vary across studies: for example, Bianco (2001) and Bianco et al. (1999) termed a 21-day time loss a "serious injury"; Ruddock-Hudson, O'Halloran, and Murphy (2014) suggested 8 weeks represented a "long-term" injury; whereas Gould et al. (1997) suggested 3 months of non-participation to be a season-ending injury. Rather than seeking global consensus on what constitutes severe injury, researchers might consider that the use of such terms for recruitment is devoid of meaning.

Finally, the use of such recruitment criteria operates at an intraindividual level of analysis, considering only how long the individual takes to resume play and does not take account of interpersonal (e.g., coach–athlete relationship), institutional (e.g., norms and values surrounding injury), cultural (e.g., media representations of injured athletes), and policy (e.g., National Governing Body policy surrounding injury) factors, all of which may influence when an athlete returns to sport. As Wadey, Day, Cavallerio, and Martinelli (2018) describe, there is currently an overemphasis at the intraindividual unit level of analysis in the sport injury literature. This emphasis is unsurprising when we consider that most recruitment strategies do not account for wider social-organizational-cultural influences that impact the sport injury process.

The key question here is how we might go beyond recruiting the usual suspects of injury research and consider the broader environment. First, we might reflect on the type of purposeful sampling used. Patton (2002) described 16 types of purposeful sampling yet predominantly injury research has used a criterion-i approach, which aims to identify and select all cases that meet some predetermined criteria of importance (e.g., severity, time). Rarely are the broader possibilities of purposeful sampling considered (Palinkas et al., 2015). Alternatives might include the use of criterion-e sampling (i.e., identifying and selecting all cases that exceed or fall outside a specified criterion), extreme or deviant cases (i.e., highlighting both the unusual and the typical), and confirming and disconfirming cases (i.e., once trends have been identified, deliberately seeking examples that counter this trend). Considering the wider possibilities of purposeful sampling may encourage researchers to compare and contrast, to identify similarities and differences, and to seek out hidden or deviant cases.

Second, when developing criteria for sampling, researchers might also consider how their research could account for wider social-organizational-cultural influences. Recruiting participants from within a specific club (e.g., Cavallerio, Wadey, & Wagstaff, 2016) or organization (e.g., Roderick, Waddington, & Parker, 2000) may allow for a broader understanding of injury. For example, Cavallerio et al.'s research described how the values of a rhythmic gymnastics club and the demands of the coach affected the occurrence and experience of overuse injuries in gymnasts. Through the use of ethnographic creative non-fiction Cavallerio's work illuminates how sociocultural values and norms of the club were learnt, accepted, and embodied by the gymnasts and ultimately led to overuse injuries. Such research opens the possibilities of exploring injury beyond an intraindividual level. Further research might consider how to recruit participants in order to explore relationships with significant others (e.g., injured-athlete–coach dyads or injured-athlete–coach–physiotherapist triads), wider cultural narratives (e.g., social media and the injured athlete), and policy (e.g., coach education and the development of policy regarding injury).

Recruiting beyond severity and time provides researchers with the opportunity to go beyond the usual suspects, to explore deviant cases, extreme cases, and disconfirming cases, thereby broadening our understanding of injury. Further, considering the wider social-organizational-cultural influences in our recruitment criteria moves us beyond focusing on individual responses to injury and consequently acknowledges the role that coaches, physiotherapists, sport cultures, and policies have on the injured athlete. Yet, in turn, such recruitment strategies also allow us to consider the reciprocal side of this relationship, exploring how injury impacts on those around the injured athlete, how it conforms to or challenges sport cultures, and how it may lead to policy change.

Describing the Indescribable: Moving Beyond Verbal Description

The experience of pain has long been recognized as a largely subjective experience, making it difficult to convey to others, particularly when pain sensations are not tangible or concrete (Strong et al., 2009). Further, as Linton (2005) suggested, our descriptions of our own pain and comprehension of others' pain will be influenced by a large variety of factors including our culture, family, nociceptive stimuli, environment, emotions, cognitions, and behaviors. Given this recognition of the difficulties associated with both describing and comprehending pain, the reliance on verbal qualitative methods (e.g., interviews, focus groups) to understand pain and injury is somewhat surprising. The sport injury literature exemplifies this reliance. Out of 51 acute sport injury papers published between 1990 and 2016, 43 studies used interviews to collect data, 33 of which were single one-off interviews and 10 of which used multiple interviews (Humphrey, 2020). Yet, verbalizing the injury process is not a discussion of pain *per se* as stories of injury are told through and about a body in pain. As Frank described, "the body is not mute, but it is inarticulate" (p. 27). Pain and the injured body are therefore central to understanding injury and consequently we must endeavor to provide more creative, nonverbal methods in order to not just hear the injury story but visualize it, read about it, feel it, and sense it. Such methods may help us to move away from taking cerebral approaches to injury research to, instead, considering the complex experiences of those who have undergone physical injury.

Outside of the sports domain, inspiration may be gained from researchers such as Kirkham, Smith, and Havsteen-Franklin (2015) whose study entitled "painting pain" asked participants to illustrate their experiences of living with chronic pain. Their analysis focused on how pain was represented as an object, the use of color to portray pain, and how pain changed over time. Participants described that using artwork was helpful and cathartic, allowing them to represent their experiences vividly and to challenge the perceptions of others by giving them a better insight into living with pain. As these participant statements indicate, using creative visual methods may provide participants with an alternative method of portraying their experiences, allowing the complex and indescribable to be seen rather than heard. Authors such as Phoenix (2010) provide support to such statements, suggesting that visual methods (e.g., painting, photography) can offer a different way of "knowing" physical culture which goes beyond the written and spoken word. Further, such methods have been shown to be well suited to a variety of populations including older adults (Baker & Wang, 2006) and children (Cope, Harvey, & Kirk, 2015) and for a variety of purposes including story creation (Busanich, McGannon, & Schinke, 2016) and recording events as they happen (Strachan & Davies, 2014). Yet, despite strong endorsements, qualitative injury research has been slow to move beyond verbal recollections and represents an exciting avenue for future research.

If the spoken word remains dominant in qualitative injury research, we might question whether the prevailing one-shot interview is enough to provide us with rich, comprehensive, in-depth detail about the injury process and the injured athlete. Authors such as Culver et al. (2012) have outlined the difficulties of gaining trust and rapport using one-off interviews, but do suggest that this type of interview may be useful for exploring events that follow a stage-by-stage temporal sequence, allowing the researcher to gain participants' views of each of these stages. The significance of Culver et al.'s (2012) suggestions to injury researchers will be dependent on the researcher's epistemology, with the potential to follow a stage-by-stage linear interview suiting the post-positivist researcher. Yet, as McGannon et al. (2019) highlight, the danger of using interviews as a "go to" or "default option" may risk "(unintentionally) missing opportunities to harness other methods that could contribute in different ways to understanding materiality and participant experiences, meaning making, and multisensory lives" (p. 12). Further, while Culver et al.'s suggestion may be appealing to some researchers, Day and Martinelli (2016) have warned that using linear interviews with injured participants means that during the early stages of interview, when rapport is likely to be at its weakest, participants could be asked to describe some of the most difficult aspects of their injury story.

Depending on the research question, sport injury researchers might consider the broader uses of interviews that go beyond one-to-one sedentary interviews. For example, interviews may be taken outside of the interview room environment using walking data collection (e.g., walking the training environment, completing a regular journey, or attempting a training session with someone in chronic pain). The walking interview provides the opportunity for the researcher to observe and not just hear an account (Jones et al., 2008), it may reduce power imbalances, particularly where the participant is familiar with the location and the participant and interviewer can walk side by side (Trell & Van Hoven, 2010), and can explore valuable connections between person and place (Holton & Riley, 2014). The use of this interview technique may be particularly poignant for injury researchers given that previous literature has described the centrality of place when recounting stories of injury. For example, as Martinelli, Day, and Lowry (2017) illustrated in their study on coach emotions following injury, place may be entangled in the decisions made both prior to and during injury and may prompt discussions on injury experiences. One coach described his critical decisions regarding the place of competition and state of the pitch prior to an injury occurring:

> The surface [football pitch] was tricky, wasn't dangerous but it was tricky … this game perhaps shouldn't be playable … should we have kept this game on today? … that was what was a bit more painful for me because I had, I had an influence on the surface. So I'd spoken to the groundsman, the officials and as a committee as such we decided to keep the match on.
>
> (Martinelli et al., 2017, p. 169)

Revisiting places critical to injury experiences may add to our knowledge, prompting further recollections and stories about injury. Further, players may associate place with successful (or unsuccessful) rehabilitation and return to sport:

> So then after some months I'm able to run down the side of the court. Just being able to jog along. I mean that was a GIGANTIC achievement, it meant SO much to me to be allowed to feel that you were running instead of walking. I mean that was a step that I can't, that I just can't explain. That people just don't understand unless they've tried that.
>
> (Thing, 2006, p. 368)

As the above examples demonstrate, place may be associated with particular emotions (e.g., guilt, excitement) and may be used to add detail and depth to injury stories. As Bairner suggests "memories bind us to particular places" (p. 18). The use of walking or place-based interviews may provide what de Leon and Cohen (2005) termed "walking probes", as elements of the surrounding environment can prompt more spontaneous discussions between researcher and participant. Although there may be a number of considerations to conducting these interviews, such as the physical restrictions of the injury and others (e.g., technical challenges of recording interviews, weather, who determines the route/location; Evans & Jones, 2011) injury researchers should consider the potential benefits of moving out of the interview room and engaging with participants "on the move".

In addition to place, sport injury researchers might also consider the use of objects in interviewing. As Woodward (2016) suggested, "the material properties of things are central to understanding the sensual, tactile, material and embodied ways in which social lives are lived and experienced" (p. 359). Objects may hold particular significance for injured athletes, representing who they were both before and after injury and might include clothing, sports equipment, medals/trophies, rehabilitation schedules, hospital scans or X-rays, and supports/bandages. Such objects frame everyday experiences of injury, emphasizing the tactile relationship between the injured body and the fabrics and materials that provide identity, healing, and physical support. For example, Allen-Collinson and Hockey wrote about the use of material to maintain their athletic identity after injury: "In wet weather we donned Gore-Tex jackets and waterproof running tights, clothing easily recognisable by fellow aficionados/as" (pp. 390–391). Laurendeau (2014) describes his experiences as an injured young athlete and his refusal of crutches, perceived to be a symbol of disability: "It's been four days, and you're sick and tired of lugging the crutches around school with you. Tossing the crutches into your locker, you drag yourself from class to class, angling your foot just so" (p. 14).

Further, objects may also hold powerful reminders of the moment that injury was sustained, not only for the injured athlete but also for teammates. Day and Schubert (2012) described how gymnasts witnessing injury avoided particular pieces of apparatus – "nobody went to bars that day after it happened" – as well as particular pieces of equipment: "They wanted us to get rid of the mat that she [injured gymnast] was using and that was something I was using as well" (p. 748). As these examples demonstrate, people, materials, and environments are entangled. Opening up dialogue about and around materials and environments that represent injury may therefore enhance participant storytelling during interview by conjuring emotions, memories, and providing a visual and tactile reminder of injury experiences. As Woodward (2016) suggests, the aim of research should not be to separate out the material and the social, but to keep these entanglements intact, thereby offering new insights and ways of thinking.

One final consideration for interviewing about sport injury is the centrality of the physical body. Exploring the stories that are told through, in, and out of the body may provide us with valuable understanding of how our social and psychological lives are fundamentally tied to and shaped by the body (Smith & Sparkes, 2009). Just as Frank (1995) suggests that illness calls attention to the body, sport injury provides a salient reminder of the fragility of the physical body and the potential transience of an athletic career. Understanding the injured body, the athlete's relationship with the body, how it is cared (or uncared) for, and how it is appreciated (or rejected) are fundamental to understanding injury experiences. As Hunt and Day (2018) describe in their study of chronic pain, all participant stories of pain were framed against a backdrop that described how it felt to play sport in a body without pain. For example:

> When I was younger and I could just do it, it was freeing, it was nice, you felt light and happy. When I became injured I felt almost trapped and confined by the limitations of my body so that whole limitless, weightless sort of bliss just disappeared.
>
> (p. 7)

The purpose of such description not only highlighted how the body felt different when in pain but fuelled future aspirations to achieve this bodily state again. Yet for many athletes, pain and injury are commonplace in training and competition. As Spencer described in his study of mixed martial arts, fighters learn how to react to the pain incurred when fighting, engaging in exercises that "callus" the body in order to withstand the rigors of the sport. As one participant described:

> The training sucks when you are training for a fight like that, it is painful, I had cauliflower ear, going into the fight every part of my body was injured, my body ached. So, I was super injured … I would I stop telling my coaches that I was injured because I was so embarrassed. I would go to physio, and I would not tell them everything because I thought they would think I was a hypochondriac.
>
> (Spencer, 2010, p. 128)

Spencer's work illustrates the marked physical changes that may occur to the body following sport injury. The occurrence of such changes after illness (e.g., cancer patients) and trauma (e.g., road accidents) have been suggested as fundamental to understanding identity and recovery (Hefferon, Grealy, & Mutrie, 2010). Yet, rarely do injury researchers ask about what it is like to live or continue to perform with visible reminders such as surgical scars or physical markers of injury. Finally, we might also consider asking about visible body modifications that may represent the injury experience. For example, Olympic double gold medal winner Kelly Holmes had the word "angel" tattooed on her shoulder, said to represent the feeling of running in her post-injury body at the Athens Olympics. Such modifications provide a powerful juxtaposition to her experiences of self-harm and bodily scars from cutting herself each day she was injured (Holmes, 2005). As authors such as Atkinson and Young (2001) have suggested, body modification may represent a "flesh journey", symbolically representing and physically chronicling changes in one's identity, relationships, thoughts, or emotions over time. Given the suggested emotional impact of injury, it is understandable that athletes who have battled injury may seek out such body modifications.

For us then, encouraging a diversity of approaches is not simply about moving away from one-to-one interviewing, but considering how we might better help participants to verbalize accounts of injury. For some, this may be through reconsidering the use of linear interview strategies and gaining a growing appreciation of the role of place, material objects, and the injured body. For others, or indeed in addition, this may be through the use of alternative mediums including the use of visual methods (e.g., photography, injury scrapbooks) or written mediums (e.g., letter writing, poetry). At the heart of these methods lie the research participant, and the consideration that injury experiences may be complex, fluid, and at times indescribable. Our choice of methodologies and methods needs to reflect the struggles some individuals may have with verbalizing all or part of their injury experience.

Disseminating Beyond Academia: Creative, Co-Constructed Dissemination

Our final point refers to a call made by Sparkes in 2002 which suggested that researchers should seek out alternative methods of dissemination in order to reach a wide range of audiences, not just our academic peers. As qualitative research in sport injury has continued to flourish there has been an emergence of more creative approaches, particularly in knowledge creation (see Chapter 15). As Smith and McGannon (2017) highlight, the emergence of journals such as *Qualitative Research in Sport, Exercise and Health* have supported the publication of different paradigms and theories, as well as encouraging innovative methods and methodologies. Similarly, conferences such as the International Conference for Qualitative Research in Sport, Exercise and Health have supported the dissemination of research through alternative forms of representation. Yet, dissemination can go far beyond academic publishing and conference presentations and more can still be done by injury researchers to ensure their research is relevant not only for other academics but sport therapists, physiotherapists, coaches, and other supporters of the injured athlete.

Creative analytical practices, as described by Richardson and St Pierre (2005), encompass a broad range of creative practices such as poetic representation, ethnodrama, and the use of video and performance-based mediums. These practices offer the opportunity to produce powerful and evocative representations of experiences, which, as Smith (2013, p. 135) suggests, helps researchers to "show rather then tell theory in and through story." Within the sport, exercise, and health literature there has been a growing increase in the range of creative methods being used to present research findings, including the use of poetry (e.g., Carless & Douglas, 2009), vignettes (e.g., Allen-Collinson, Owton, & Crust, 2016), creative nonfiction (e.g., Smith, Papathomas, Martin Ginis, & Latimer-Cheung, 2013), docudrama (McMahon, Zehntner, & McGannon, 2017), and infographics (Smith, Kirby Skinner, Wightman, Lucas, & Foster, 2019).

One of the key advantages to using these creative methods of dissemination is that information may be co-produced with individuals and organizations. For example, Smith et al. (2019) worked *with* over 350 disabled adults, 10 disability organizations, and 50 health professionals to test how evidence-based physical activity recommendations could be presented and to co-produce a resource. In using such co-production methods, problems can be identified and questions debated using many experts (of different kinds), to provide an evolving collective view (though rarely a consensus) on what the questions and challenges of the research are (Greenhalgh, Jackson, Shaw, & Janamian, 2016). As Smith et al.'s research demonstrates, co-producing may be used to ensure that information is disseminated in an affordable, user-friendly, understandable, and engaging way (Smith et al., 2019). Thus, sport injury researchers might consider who the stakeholders in their research are and how co-construction may help not only in moving beyond traditional academic publication pathways but also in creating valuable, impactful research.

Conclusion

So where does this leave the qualitative sport injury researcher? In this chapter we have encouraged injury researchers to "go beyond" usual practice, considering alternative sampling strategies, methodological creativity, and co-constructed dissemination. Such suggestions are not simply to encourage novelty, but provide the opportunity for different participants to tell or show their injury stories in a variety of different ways. Our hope is that such suggestions open alternative ways of understanding injury, allowing us to view the injury process through a different lens and inviting others to share in this new knowledge through more creative dissemination.

Critical Discussion Questions

1) In the first research quandary, we considered the "usual suspects" of injury research. Which populations are "left out" of injury research? You might consider factors such as age, class, gender, ethnicity, and type of injury.
2) In the second research quandary, we discuss the advantages of using painting as a method of understanding pain. What other alternatives are there to interviewing about pain and injury?
3) In the third research quandary, a number of suggestions are made for creative methods of disseminating information. What further methods of creative dissemination might be suitable for use in sport injury research and why?

References

Allen-Collinson, J., Owton, H., & Crust, L. (2016). Opening up dialogues and airways: Using vignettes to enrich asthma understandings in sport and exercise. *Qualitative Research in Sport, Exercise and Health*, *8*(4), 352–364. doi: 10.1080/2159676X.2016.1154097

Atkinson, M., & Young, K. (2001). Flesh journeys: Neo primitives and the contemporary rediscovery of radical body modification. *Deviant Behaviour*, *22*(2), 117–146. doi: 0163-9625/01

Baker, T. A., & Wang, C. C. (2006). Photovoice: Use of a participatory action research methods to explore the chronic pain experiences in older adults. *Qualitative Health Research*, *16*(10), 1405–1413. doi: 10.1177/104973206294118

Bianco, T. (2001). Social support and recovery from sport injury: elite skiers share their experiences. *Research Quarterly for Exercise and Sport*, *72*(4), 376–388.

Bianco, T., Malo, S., & Orlick, T. (1999). Sport injury and illness: Elite skiers describe their experiences. *Research Quarterly for Exercise and Sport*, *70*(2), 157–169. doi: 10.1080/02701367.1999.10608033

Braun, V., & Clarke, V. (2013). *Successful qualitative research*. London, UK: Sage.

Busanich, R., McGannon, K. R., & Schinke, R. J. (2016). Exploring disordered eating and embodiment in male distance runners through visual narrative methods. *Qualitative Research in Sport, Exercise and Health*, *8*(1), 95–112. doi: 10.1080/2159676X.2015.1028093

Carless, D., & Douglas, K. (2009). "We haven't got a seat on the bus for you" or "All the seats for mine": Narratives and career transition in professional golf. *Qualitative Research in Sport and Exercise*, 1, 51–66.

Carson, F., & Polman, R. C. J. (2012). Experiences of professional rugby union players returning to competition following anterior cruciate ligament reconstruction. *Physical Therapy in Sport*, *13*(1), 35–40. doi: 10.1016/j.ptsp.2010.10.007

Cavallerio, F., Wadey, R., & Wagstaff, C. (2016). Understanding overuse injuries in rhythmic gymnastics: A 12-month ethnographic study. *Psychology of Sport and Exercise, 25,* 100–109. doi: 10.1080/2159676X.2017.1335651

Cope, E., Harvey, S., & Kirk, D. (2015). Reflections on using visual methods in sports coaching. *Qualitative Research in Sport, Exercise and Health, 7*(1), 88–108. doi: 10.1080/2159676X.2013.877959

Culver, D. M., Gilbert, W., & Sparkes, A. (2012). Qualitative research in sport psychology journals: The next decade 2000–2009 and beyond. *The Sport Psychologist, 26*(2), 261–281. doi: 10.1123/tsp.26.2.261

Day, M., & Martinelli, L. (2016). The complexities of narrating athletic injuries. *Qualitative Methods in Psychology Bulletin, 22,* 14–21.

Day, M., & Schubert, N. (2012). The impact of witnessing athletic injury: A qualitative examination of vicarious trauma in artistic gymnastics. *Journal of Sport Sciences, 30*(8), 743–753. doi: 10.1080/02640414.2012.671530

Evans, J., & Jones, P. (2011). The walking interview: Methodology, mobility and place. *Applied Geography, 31*(2), 849–858. doi: 10.1016/j.apgeog.2010.09.005

Forscher, B. K. (1963). Chaos in the brickyard. *Science, 142*(3590), 339. doi: 10.1126/science.142.3590.339.

Frank, A. (1995). *The wounded storyteller.* London, UK: The University of Chicago Press.

Giardina, M. D. (2017). Challenges and opportunities for qualitative research: Future directions. In B. Smith & A. Sparkes (Eds.), *Routledge handbook of qualitative research in sport and exercise* (pp. 466–471). Oxon: Routledge.

Gould, D. R., Udry, E., Bridges, D., & Beck, L. (1997). Stress sources encountered when rehabilitating from season-ending ski injuries. *The Sport Psychologist, 11*(4), 361–378. doi: 10.1123/tsp.11.4.361

Greenhalgh, T., Jackson, C., Shaw, S., & Janamian, T. (2016). Achieving research impact through co-creation in community-based health services: Literature review and case study. *The Milbank Quarterly, 94*(2), 392–429. doi: 10.1111/1468-0009.12197

Hefferon, K., Grealy, M., & Mutrie, N. (2010). Transforming from cocoon to butterfly: The potential role of the body in the process of posttraumatic growth. *Journal of Humanistic Psychology, 50*(2), 224–247. doi: 10.1177/0022167809341996

Heijne, A., Axelsson, K., Werner, S., & Biguet, G. (2008). Rehabilitation and recovery after anterior cruciate ligament reconstruction: Patients' experiences. *Scandinavian Journal of Medicine and Science in Sports, 18*(3), 325–335. doi: 10.1111/j.1600-0838.2007.00700.x

Holmes, K. (2005). *Kelly Holmes: Black, white & gold. My autobiography.* Virgin Books.

Holton, M., & Riley, M. (2014). Talking on the move: Place based interviewing with undergraduate students. *Area, 46*(1), 59–65. doi: 10.1111/area.12070

Humphrey, K. (2020). *From knowledge to practice: Translating the psychosocial sports injury literature into a creative resource for sports injury rehabilitation professionals* (Unpublished Doctoral dissertation). University of Chichester, Chichester, United Kingdom.

Hunt, E., & Day, M. (2018). Narratives of chronic pain in sport. *Journal of Clinical Sport Psychology, 13*(1), 1–16. doi: 10.1123/jcsp.2017-0003

Jones, P., Bunce, G., Evans, J., Gibbs, H., & Ricketts Hein, J. (2008). Exploring space and place with walking interviews. *Journal of Research Practice, 4*(2), article D2. Retrieved from http://jrp.icaap.org/index.php/jrp/article/view/150

Kirkham, J., Smith, J., & Havsteen-Franklin, D. (2015). Painting pain: An interpretive phenomenological analysis of representations of living with chronic pain. *Health Psychology, 34*(4), 398–406. doi: 10.1037/hea0000139

Krane, V. (2017). Embracing the messiness of qualitative research: Challenges and opportunities for qualitative researchers in sport and exercise. In B. Smith & A. Sparkes (Eds.), *Routledge handbook of qualitative research in sport and exercise* (pp. 472–475). Oxon: Routledge.

Laurendeau, J. (2014). "Just tape it up for me, ok?": Masculinities, injury and embodied emotion. *Emotion, Space and Society, 12*, 11–17. doi: 10.1016/j.emospa.2013.03.010

Leon, J. P., & Cohen, J. H. (2005). Object and walking probes in ethnographic interviewing. Field Methods, 17, 200–204.

Linton, S. J. (2005). *Understanding pain for better clinical practice: A psychological perspective.* London: Elsevier.

Mankad, A., Gordon, S., & Wallman, K. (2009). Perceptions of emotional climate among injured athletes. *Journal of Clinical Sports Psychology, 3*(1), 1–14. doi: 10.1123/jcsp.3.1.1

Martinelli, L., Day, M., & Lowry, R. (2017). Sport coaches' experiences of athlete injury: The development and regulation of guilt. *Sports Coaching Review, 6*(2), 162–178. doi: 10.1080/21640629.2016.1195550

McGannon, K., Smith, B., Kendellen, K., & Gonsalves, C. A. (2019). Qualitative research in six sport and exercise psychology journals between 2010 and 2017: An updated and expanded review of trends and interpretations. *International Journal of Sport and Exercise Psychology.* doi: 10.1080/1612197X.2019.1655779

McHugh, T. (2017). Thinking about the future. In B. Smith & A. Sparkes (Eds.), *Routledge handbook of qualitative research in sport and exercise* (pp. 445–449). Oxon: Routledge.

McMahon, J., Zehntner, C., & McGannon, K. R. (2017). Fleshy, female and forty: A docudrama of a former elite swimmer who re-immersed herself into elite swimming culture. *Qualitative Research in Sport, Exercise and Health, 9*(5), 546–553. doi: 10.1080/2159676X.2017.1340328

Palinkas, L. A., Horwitz, S. M., Green, S. M., Wisdom, J. P., Duan, N., & Hoagwood, K. (2015). Purposeful sampling for qualitative data collection and analysis in mixed method implementation research. *Administration and Policy in Mental Health and Mental Health Services Research, 42*(5), 533–544. doi: 10.1007/s10488-013-0528-y

Patton, M. Q. (2002). *Qualitative research and evaluation methods* (3rd ed.). Thousand Oaks, CA: Sage Publications.

Phoenix, C. (2010). Seeing the world of physical culture: The potential of visual methods for qualitative research in sport and exercise. *Qualitative Research in Sport and Exercise, 2*(2), 93–108. doi: 10.1080/19398441.2010.488017

Poucher, Z. A., Tamminen, K. A., Caron, J., & Sweet, S. (2019). Thinking through and designing qualitative research studies: A focussed mapping review of 30 years of qualitative research in sport psychology. *International Review of Sport and Exercise Psychology, 13*, 163–186. doi: 10.1080/1750984X.2019.1656276

Richardson, L., & St. Pierre, E. (2005). Writing as a method of inquiry. In N. Denzin & Y. Lincoln (Eds.), *The sage handbook of qualitative research* (pp. 959–978). Thousand Oaks, CA: Sage Publications.

Roderick, M., Waddingdon, I., & Parker, G. (2000). Playing hurt: Managing injuries in English Professional Football. *International Review for the Sociology of Sport*, 35, 165–180.

Ruddock-Hudson, M., O'Halloran, P., & Murphy, G. (2014). The psychological impact of long-term injury on Australian Football League players. *Journal of Applied Sport Psychology, 26*(4), 377–394. doi: 10.1080/10413200.2014.897269

Smith, B. (2013). Sporting spinal cord injuries, social relations, and rehabilitation narratives: Aethnogrpaphic creative non-faction of becoming disabled through sport. *Social of Sport Journal*, 20, 132–152.

Smith, B., Kirby, N., Skinner, B., Wightman, L., Lucas, R., & Foster, C. (2019). Infographic. Physical activity for disabled adults. *British Journal of Sports Medicine, 53*(6), 335–336. doi: 10.1136/bjsports-2018-100158

Smith, B., & McGannon, K. R. (2017). Developmeing rigour in qualitative research: Problems and opportunities within sport and exercise psychology, 11, 101–121.

Smith, B., Papathomas, A., Martin Ginis, K. A., & Latimer-Cheung, A. E. (2013). Understanding physical activity in spinal cord injury rehabilitation: Translating and communicating research through stories. *Disability and Rehabilitation, 35*(24), 2046–2055. doi: 10.3109/09638288.2013.805821

Smith, B., & Sparkes, A. (2009). Narrative inquiry in sport and exercise psychology: What can it mean and why might we do it? *Psychology of Sport and Exercise, 10*(1), 1–11. doi: 10.1016/j.psychsport.2008.01.004

Spencer, D. C. (2010). Narratives of despair and loss: Pain, injury and masculinity in the sport of mixed martial arts. *Qualitative Research in Sport, Exercise and Health, 4*(1), 117–137. doi: 10.1080/2159676X.2011.653499

Strachan, L., & Davies, K. (2014). *Click!* Using photo elicitation to explore youth experiences and positive youth development in sport. *Qualitative Research in Sport, Exercise and Health, 7*(2), 170–191. doi: 10.1080/2159676X.2013.867410

Strong, J., Mathews, T., Sussex, R., New, F., Hoey, S., & Mitchell, G. (2009). Pain language and gender differences when describing a past pain event. *Pain, 145*(1–2), 86–95. doi: 10.1016/j.pain.2009.05.018

Thing, L. F. (2006). "Voices of the broken body." the resumption of non-professional female players' sports careers after anterior cruciate ligament injury. *The female player's dilemma: Is she willing to run the risk? Scandinavian Journal of Medicine and Science in Sports, 16*(5), 364–375. doi: 10.1111/j.1600-0838.2005.00452.x

Trell, E., & Van Hoven, B. (2010). Making sense of place: Exploring creative and (inter) active research methods with young people. *Fennia-International Journal of Geography, 188*(1), 91–104.

Wadey, R., Day, M., Cavallerio, F., & Martinelli, L. (2018). Multilevel model of sport injury (MMSI): Can coaches impact and be impacted by injury. In R. Thelwell & M. Dicks (Eds.,), *Professional advances in sports coaching: Research and practice* (pp. 408–440). London, UK: Routledge.

Woodward, S. (2016). Object interviews, material imaginings and 'unsettling' methods: Interdisciplinary approaches to understanding materials and material culture. *Qualitative Research, 16*(4), 359–374. doi: 10.1177/1468794115589647

13 Experimental Psychological Response to Injury Studies

Why So Few?

Kirsty Ledingham, Tom Williams, and Lynne Evans

Introduction

Over the last 20 years a growing body of research has examined the role of a number of psychological factors on athletes' responses to, and recovery from, sport injury (Brewer & Redmond, 2017). While this largely correlational and qualitative research has served to enhance our knowledge and understanding of a number of features of the injury process and athletes' injury experience, it has fallen short of providing an experimentally derived evidence base that can guide interventions with injured athletes. In this chapter we reflect upon why, since Cupal's (1998) seminal review, the proliferation of injury research has not extended to injury interventions and how this can be addressed. To this end, our intention here is to help inform the design of methodologically rigorous intervention studies that can extend the existing evidence base for the use of the different strategies to expedite athletes' recovery. The treatise is based on published injury intervention studies with injured athletic populations identified through a systematic literature search. Of the 14 experimental intervention studies we identified, 10 were randomized control trials (RCT) where participants were randomly allocated to groups, and 4 were non-randomized trial designs (n-RCT).

Critical Review of Experimental Intervention Research

From conception to completion, experimental studies provide researchers with a number of challenges. Based on the strengths and limitations of the existing research, we focus on five key areas that we believe have not only had a significant impact on the methodological quality of the studies conducted to date, but also represent the biggest barriers researchers conducting new research face; specifically, (a) recruiting large and homogenous samples, (b) ensuring baseline equivalence, (c) blinding, (d) standardized treatment protocol, and (e) validity and reliability of measures. Table 13.1 provides an overview of the studies considered as part of this review.

Table 13.1 Experimental (n = 14) and Non-Experimental (n = 8) Injury Response Intervention Studies

Authors	Intervention	Study Design	Participants	Injuries	Outcomes	Intervention Effects
Experimental						
Ross & Berger (1996)	Stress inoculation training	RCT – **Experimental group:** n = 30 received 2 × 1-hour stress inoculation training sessions. **Control group:** n = 30 no intervention.	60 male athletes aged 18–55 (M = 28.9).	Meniscus	Anxiety, pain, knee strength	Treatment group significantly less postsurgical pain and anxiety, and needed fewer days to return-to-recovery.
Theodorakis et al. (1996)	Goal-setting	Non-RCT – Quadricep strength training program for 4-sessions. **Experimental (injured):** n = 32 **Experimental (non-injured):** n = 29 **Control (non-injured):** n = 30 Both experimental groups set goals & received feedback between trails. **Control:** No intervention.	91 female athletes aged 18–24 (M = 22.0).	Knee Arthroscopic Surgery	Self-efficacy, self-satisfaction, knee extension	Significant effects in favour of both experimental groups compared to the control group for knee extension.

Theodorakis et al. (1997) Goal-setting	Non-RCT – Quadricep strength training program for 4 weeks × 3 sessions per week. **Experimental group:** $n = 20$ set performance and personal goals and received feedback. **Control group:** $n = 17$ no intervention.	37 student-athletes.	Knee Arthroscopic Surgery	Self-efficacy, self-satisfaction, anxiety, knee extension	Experimental group significantly greater knee extension self-satisfaction.
Theodorakis et al. (1998) Self-talk	RCT – Quadricep strength training program 6 training sessions × 3 per week. **Experimental group:** $n = 16$ received positive messages on a computer screen during sessions. **Control group:** $n = 14$ no intervention.	30 athletes aged 18–23 ($M = 19.2$).	Knee Arthroscopic Surgery	Anxiety, knee strength	Significant improvements in knee strength in favour of experimental group. No differences in anxiety.
Johnson (2000) Stress management, goal-setting, relaxation/ imagery	RCT – **Experimental group:** $n = 14$ received 3 intervention sessions (one per skill) lasting 15–25 minutes. **Control group:** $n = 44$ no intervention.	58 competitive athletes ($M = 23.7$).	Various	Psychosocial risk, mood, patient and physio self-rating of progress	Experimental group significantly higher overall mood and significantly less wishful thinking.

(Continued)

Table 13.1 Experimental (n = 14) and Non-Experimental (n = 8) Injury Response Intervention Studies (*Continued*)

Authors	Intervention	Study Design	Participants	Injuries	Outcomes	Intervention Effects
Cupal & Brewer (2001)	Relaxation & guided imagery	RCT – **Experimental group:** $n = 10$ received 10 intervention sessions every 2 weeks over 6 months. **Placebo group:** $n = 10$ received only SS from the same clinician. **Control group:** $n = 10$ no intervention.	30 competitive and recreational athletes aged 18–50 ($M = 28.2$).	ACL	Reinjury-anxiety, pain, knee strength	Significant differences in knee strength, reinjury anxiety, and pain in favor of experimental group compared to control and placebo.
Evans & Hardy (2002)	Goal-setting	RCT: **Experimental group:** $n = 13$ set goals with the sport psychologist every 7–10 days for 5 weeks. **SS control group:** $n = 13$ received only SS from the sport psychologist. **Control group:** $n = 13$ received a phone call every 10 days for 5–10 minutes from the sport psychologist.	77 injured athletes aged 17–39 ($M = 25.42$).	Various	Rehabilitation adherence, self/treatment efficacy, dispiritedness, reorganization	Significant differences in rehabilitation adherence and self-efficacy in favor of experimental group compared to SS control and control groups.
Maddison et al. (2006)	Modeling	RCT – **Experimental group:** $n = 30$ watched 2 coping videos (pre-surgery to 2 weeks post-surgery and 2–6 weeks post ACL surgery) **Control group:** $n = 28$ no intervention.	72 athletes aged 15–53 ($M = 30.0$).	ACL	Pain, anxiety, rehabilitation/ exercise self-efficacy, knee function	Significant differences in pre-operative pain, and efficacy in crutch use and rehabilitation exercises, and objective function at pre-discharge in favor of experimental group.

Study	Intervention	Design/Sample		Injury	Outcomes	Results
Christakou & Zervas (2007)	Relaxation and guided imagery	RCT – **Experimental group:** n = 9 received 12 individual relaxation/imagery sessions **Control group:** n = 9 no intervention.	18 male athletes aged 18–30 (M = 26.0).	Ankle sprains	Pain, edema, range of motion	No significant differences between groups.
Christakou et al. (2007)	Relaxation and guided imagery	RCT – **Experimental group:** n = 10 received 12 individual relaxation/imagery sessions **Control group:** n = 10 no intervention.	20 athletes aged 18–30 (M = 25.3).	Ankle sprains	Muscular endurance, dynamic balance, functional stability	Significant difference in favor of intervention for muscular endurance.
Beneka et al. (2013)	Self-talk	RCT – Participants attended laboratory 3 times within 7 days to complete a dynamic stability test. (n =15 in each group). **Experimental groups: (1)** instructional ST, **(2)** motivational ST **(3)** neutral ST. **Control group:** No intervention.	60 recreational athletes (M = 35.0).	Meniscus	Dynamic balance	Instructional and motivational experimental groups significantly better balance compared to control.
Mohammed et al. (2018)	Mindfulness	RCT – **Experimental group:** n = 10 received 8 weeks of mindfulness-based stress reduction (1 per week). **Control group:** n = 10 no intervention.	20 athletes aged 18–45 (M = 28.8).	Various	Mindfulness, pain, mood, anxiety, stress	No significant differences between groups.

(Continued)

Table 13.1 Experimental (n = 14) and Non-Experimental (n = 8) Injury Response Intervention Studies (*Continued*)

Authors	Intervention	Study Design	Participants	Injuries	Outcomes	Intervention Effects
Salim & Wadey (2018)	Emotional-disclosure	Non-RCT – **Experimental groups: Written-disclosure (WD)** – wrote about deepest thoughts and feelings **Verbal-disclosure (VD)** – talked about deepest thoughts and feelings **Control group:** wrote facts about daily events All participants completed 4 × 20-minute sessions 1 per week.	45 athletes formerly injured (*M* = 23.2).	Various	Growth, linguistic enquiry	VD group experienced more growth than WD and control between T2–T3. No significant difference between WD and control throughout.
Salim & Wadey (2019)	Gratitude visit	Non-RCT – **Experimental group:** *n* = 15 wrote & delivered a gratitude letter to a significant other. **Control group:** *n* = 15 no intervention.	30 formerly injured athletes (*M* = 21.8).	Various	Gratitude and growth	Experimental group greater relating (growth) to others between T1–T2, and T1–T3 than control – elaborated on in social validation.

Non-experimental

Gilbourne et al. (1996)	Goal-setting	Action research – 6-week goal-setting intervention within a specialist injury rehabilitation centre.	1 female athlete	ACL	Goal-setting diaries	Efficacy for the application of goal-setting intervention (specificity, identifiable phases, and reflections).
Evans et al. (2000)	Multimodal intervention	Action research – longitudinal multimodal intervention up to 12 months following injury.	3 rugby players aged between 23–26 ($M = 25$).	Various	Daily diaries, consultations with athlete/physio, case notes	Importance of emotional support (after setbacks), task support (mainly in the form of goal-setting), short- and long-term goals, flexible goals, confidence in limb.
Rock & Jones (2002)	Counseling skills	Case study – intervention sessions delivered at 3 days, 2, 4, 6, 8, and 10 weeks post-surgery. Sessions lasted 40–60 minutes.	3 athletes aged between 31–40 ($M = 35.3$)	ACL	Social support, adherence to rehabilitation, mood, perceived rehabilitation	Partial support (at a descriptive level) for counseling skills intervention.
Mankad et al. (2009a)	Written emotional-disclosure	Single-subject (repeated measures) – 5-week baseline; 3-consecutive-day intervention (expected to write for 20 minutes each day about injury experience); 4-week follow-up.	26-year-old male athlete.	ACL	Stress, mood disturbance, and self-esteem, linguistic analyses	Significant decreases in stress and mood disturbance and significant increase in self-esteem.

(Continued)

Table 13.1 Experimental (n = 14) and Non-Experimental (n = 8) Injury Response Intervention Studies (*Continued*)

Authors	Intervention	Study Design	Participants	Injuries	Outcomes	Intervention Effects
Mankad et al. (2009b)	Written emotional-disclosure	See Mankad et al. (2009a)	15 athletes aged 19–29 (M = 21.9).	Various	Stress, mood, immunological parameters	Significant main effects of time for intrusion, avoidance, mood, and CD4+.
Mankad & Gordon (2010)	Written emotional-disclosure	See Mankad et al. (2009a)	9 elite athletes, mean age 22.2 years.	Various	Psychological responses, rehabilitation beliefs, linguistic analyses	Significant changes in participants' psychological responses to injury and linguistic styles following intervention. No pre-post intervention effects for rehabilitation beliefs.
Mahoney & Hanrahan (2011)	Acceptance commitment therapy	Case study – standardized one-to-one sessions with trained therapist for 4 weeks	4 athletes aged 18–49 years (M = 27.3).	ACL	Acceptance, mindfulness, anxiety	Limited effectiveness of acceptance commitment therapy.
Shapiro & Etzel (2018)	Multimodal intervention (goal-setting, self-talk, relaxation/imagery)	Single subject (repeated measures) – 4-week multi-skill intervention	5 athletes mean age 19 years old.	Various	Use of mental skills, self-efficacy for rehabilitation and return-to-sport, adherence to rehabilitation, perceived recovery time	Limited change over course of study in self-efficacy for rehabilitation and return to sport, adherence, attitude, and speed of recovery.

Large and Homogenous Samples

One of the biggest challenges researchers face relates to sampling and the trade-offs that have to be made between sample size and composition; specifically whether heterogeneous samples (i.e., various injuries) to maximize sample size and expedite data collection are preferable to homogeneous samples. While the former have advantages over the latter, within experimental research heterogeneous samples can make it difficult to separate the intervention effects of the treatment from the result of the sequelae and functional progression of different injuries. However, a strength of the studies conducted to date has been that they have been homogenous with respect to injury type, for example, ankle sprains (Christakou & Zervas, 2007; Christakou, Zervas & Lavalle, 2007), anterior cruciate ligament tears (ACL; Cupal & Brewer, 2001; Maddison, Prapavessis & Clatworthy, 2006), and meniscus tears (Beneka et al., 2013; Ross & Berger, 1996). That said, the disproportionate number of studies examining knee injuries has arguably limited our ability to generalize the findings to other injured athletic populations.

In contrast to sample strengths, a common limitation of the RCT and n-RCT studies is their small sample sizes. To elaborate, only 3 out of the 14 studies included more than 15 participants in each condition. Large samples are usually required in order to provide sufficient power to detect statistically significant findings. However, the implications of small sample sizes and underpowered studies have not been an issue when detecting significant findings across studies, with only 1 of the 14 studies in this review (Christakou & Zervas, 2007) failing to demonstrate a statistically significant effect in favor of the treatment group on any outcomes.

Baseline Equivalence

In order to attribute the observed differences in outcomes between experimental and control groups to the intervention (as opposed to confounding variables such as injury severity), researchers must strive for pre-intervention baseline group equivalence. Typically, this is achieved through randomization to ensure each participant has an equal chance of being allocated to the various groups. A number of randomization procedures (with varying methodological rigor) have been adopted within the experimental injury research, including drawing lots (e.g., Christakou & Zervas, 2007), using computer software (e.g., Maddison et al., 2006), random block assignment (Cupal & Brewer, 2001), and alternative assignment (Ross & Berger, 1996). However, despite researchers' best attempts, imbalances between groups across potential confounding variables can still exist and are accentuated in studies with small sample sizes, such as those within the experimental sport injury intervention research, due to sampling error (i.e., unrepresentativeness of the samples).

To overcome these potential imbalances across known confounding variables, Evans and Hardy (2002) matched participants across groups according to their attending physiotherapist, the nature of the injury, stage of rehabilitation, sport, level of participation, and gender. When a match was obtained for a participant already assigned to a group, the new participant was randomly allocated to one of the other two groups. In doing so, the researchers not only strived to maintain baseline equivalence across a number of confounding variables, but also safeguarded equal numbers in each treatment condition (goal-setting, social support control, and control). This represents a far more rigorous, but time-intensive, approach to ensuring baseline equivalence compared to alternatively assigning participants to either the treatment or control condition based on who turned up first (Ross & Berger, 1996) or assigning every fourth participant to the intervention (Johnson, 2000). Suffice to say, the randomization procedure can have a profound effect on the inferences that can be drawn from the study's findings, and therefore it is essential that it be rigorous, explicit, and auditable.

Blinding

The third methodological challenge of conducting rigorous experimental research relates to the notion of "blinding"; specifically, to what extent are the participants aware of the nature of the study and to which group they have been assigned (blinded), and to what extent are the clinicians responsible for collecting the outcome measures aware of which group participants are allocated to (double-blinded)?

Perhaps surprisingly, in only 1 of the 14 experimental studies was the specific nature of the study masked from the participants. In Evans and Hardy (2002) participants were advised that the purpose of the study was to examine the psychological effects of injury in relation to athletes' psychological response and rehabilitation adherence, as opposed to the study being a goal-setting intervention involving experimental and control groups. That participants in other studies were not blind to the nature of the design and their specific involvement suggests they may have been subject to expectancy effects; these arise when the participants are aware that they are receiving a psychological intervention to facilitate their recovery. These risks are likely to be accentuated in studies such as Ross and Berger's (1996) in which participants in the stress inoculation treatment group were informed that they would likely experience anxiety and pain during rehabilitation, but that the interventions had been demonstrated to be effective in reducing distress and discomfort.

One way to overcome these expectancy effects is through the use of placebo groups. However, although commonly included within RCTs in other health domains, only two studies within the sport injury literature have included placebo-control groups (Cupal & Brewer, 2001; Evans & Hardy, 2002). In Cupal and Brewer's study participants in the placebo condition received the same amount of designated time for out-of-clinic rehabilitation activities and contact time with the clinician who delivered the imagery intervention to control for the non-specific effects of psychological treatments, such as hope, expectations of healing, and social support (Brewer & Redmond, 2017). In Evans and Hardy's study the need to control for expectancy effects was less of an issue because participants were blinded to the aims of the study. However, in order to control for the influential effects of social support, the authors included a social support control group, and in doing so, provided even stronger support for the efficacy of their goal-setting intervention.

In contrast, a methodological strength of four of the studies (Cupal & Brewer, 2001; Evans & Hardy, 2002; Johnson, 2000; Ross & Berger, 1996) was the blinding of the physiotherapist(s) responsible for measuring the outcomes to participants' group allocation. In the remaining ten studies, one study did not report who was responsible for assessing outcomes (Mohammed, Pappous, & Sharma, 2018), one did not say if the trained assessor was blinded (Maddison et al., 2006), three studies' outcomes were assessed by the researcher (Beneka et al., 2013; Christakou et al., 2007) or the researcher and the physiotherapist (Christakou & Zervas, 2007), and the remaining four studies included outcomes less susceptible to assessor bias, for example, questionnaires (e.g., Salim & Wadey, 2018) and functional measures (e.g., Theodorakis, Malliou, Papaioanna, Beneca, & Filactakidou, 1996).

Standardized Treatment Protocol

To develop effective intervention strategy guidelines for medical professionals and practitioners to employ with injured athletes, there needs to be far more procedural detail around the treatment (intervention) protocol within and across studies. Such detail should also relate to the checks conducted to ensure participants are complying with the treatment protocol, and that the treatment is being delivered in a consistent way across participants in the experimental condition(s).

Indeed, the essence of methodological intervention study rigor is that researchers provide sufficient procedural detail to allow other researchers to replicate the intervention. In some instances this is clearly more easily attainable than others. For example, brief interventions such as gratitude letters (Salim & Wadey, 2019), and modelling videos (Maddison et al., 2006) are more readily replicable than longitudinal interventions involving imagery, goal-setting, and mindfulness. In these cases, it is perhaps not surprising that the level of detail provided has been variable. For example, Mohammed et al. (2018) provide a detailed delineation of the eight-week mindfulness-based stress reduction intervention, whereas Johnson's (2000) multimodal (stress management/cognitive control, goal-setting, relaxation/guided imagery), and Evans and Hardy's (2002) goal-setting intervention provide insufficient detail around the content of the intervention to facilitate replication.

Furthermore, in order to ascertain the effectiveness of the intervention and participants compliance with it, researchers need to ensure that appropriate manipulation checks, and intervention compliance measures, have been employed to safeguard and delineate between their separate and potentially confounding effects. Again, this will be dependent upon the nature of the intervention. For example, there may be fewer issues associated with compliance to brief interventions such as Salim and Wadey's (2018) emotional-disclosure one. However, they become all the more important when there is an expectation and/or requirement for participants to engage in the intervention away from supervised sessions (e.g., Cupal & Brewer, 2001; Johnson, 2000).

In addition to ensuring participants comply with the intervention protocol, researchers should ensure consistency in the way the intervention protocol is delivered across experimental group participants. Unfortunately, these recommendations have only been adopted in one study. Cupal and Brewer (2001) not only provided a detailed account of each relaxation/imagery session, but also ensured the clinician administering the intervention adhered to the relaxation/imagery scripts by periodically video recording the sessions to ensure the intervention was delivered in a consistent manner across treatment condition participants.

Measures

A final methodological challenge for researchers looking to make appropriate inferences about intervention effects relates to the validity and reliability of outcome measures. Objective outcome assessments are desirable not least to overcome the potential effect of common method variance, which can arise when self-report questionnaires are used to measure both the predictor and outcome variables (Chang, van Witteloostuijn, & Eden, 2010). Fortunately, the majority of the studies conducted to date have incorporated objective recovery outcomes, including knee strength (e.g., Cupal & Brewer, 2001) and muscle endurance (Christakou et al., 2007) alongside more subjective indices of outcomes.

Furthermore, in order to assess the extent outcomes change as a result of the intervention *per se*, researchers must include repeated assessments of both the psychological factors and recovery outcomes. However, depending on the nature of the outcomes assessed, this can be more or less problematic. For example, following ACL reconstruction, knee strength measured on the isokinetic dynamometer is commonly assessed as a recovery outcome (e.g., Cupal & Brewer, 2001). However, patients are unable to undertake such testing due to the physical limitations imposed by surgery usually until approximately four weeks following surgery, limiting the ability to conduct pre-post assessments.

Alternate Intervention Study Approaches

Given the modest number of experimental intervention studies published to date, and the methodological challenges associated with them, we also reviewed intervention studies that employed single-subject (Mankad & Gordon, 2010; Mankad, Gordon, & Wallman, 2009a, b; Shapiro & Etzel, 2018), case study (Mahoney & Hanrahan, 2011; Rock & Jones, 2002), and action research designs (Evans, Hardy, & Fleming, 2000; Gilbourne, Taylor, Downie, & Newton, 1996) (see Table 13.1). We include these studies not only for the completeness of the treatise, but to elucidate how the strengths of these designs can help to overcome some of the limitations of the experimental ones.

Despite possessing less internal validity than RCT, single-subject designs offer an attractive quasi-experimental alternative not least because they require fewer participants, with each participant serving as their own control. Mankad and colleagues successfully adopted this approach in a series of studies that used an A-B-A withdrawal design, and included five weeks of baseline assessment, a three-day written emotional disclosure intervention, and a four-week follow-up. However, while such designs overcome issues associated with recruiting large and homogenous samples, their effectiveness is dependent upon stable baseline assessments in the dependent variable (e.g., mood) so that post-intervention changes can be attributed to the intervention. Unfortunately, given that athletes' emotional responses fluctuate throughout rehabilitation, with emotions becoming less intense and more positive as time progresses (e.g., Brewer et al., 2007), it can be difficult to separate the intervention effects from naturally occurring change as a result of the athletes' progression through rehabilitation.

Case study designs, such as those reported by Mahoney and Hanrahan (2011) and Rock and Jones (2002), done well can provide an in-depth and idiographic approach that demonstrates (at a descriptive level) the effectiveness of an intervention on outcome variables, as well as possible mechanisms that explain its effects. For example, using pluralist methodologies (qualitative follow-ups to complement initial quantitative findings) and triangulation to maximize the reliability and validity of their findings, Rock and Jones provided tentative support for the effectiveness of a 12-week counselling-skills intervention on three athletes' perceptions of mood, pain, and rehabilitation following ACL surgery.

Impactful intervention research requires evidence of more than just the effectiveness of the "treatment"; practitioners require evidence about processes, social context, participant engagement, collaboration, and flexibility. However, such factors are typically removed from (quasi)experimental designs in an attempt to reduce confounding factors and bias. Designs such as action research offer opportunities to learn about factors excluded from positivist RCT and single-subject designs. This notion of theoretical pluralism (i.e., what is weak in one is strong in the other) is particularly important when evaluating (and indeed designing) complex sport injury interventions.

Two action research studies that embrace the complexity of the cyclic research process and in which researchers and participants collaboratively plan, act, reflect, and modify the intervention, have been conducted in an injury context (Evans et al., 2000; Gilbourne et al., 1996). Whereas Gilbourne et al.'s study comprised a six-week goal-setting intervention, Evans et al.'s evolved to be a multi-modal (including goal-setting, imagery, simulation training, social support, verbal persuasion) to respond to the multifaceted needs of the athletes. Results evidenced a number of notable findings that reflected the changing context, which would not have been possible without the longitudinal engagement, and a flexible, evolving, and collaborative intervention approach. For example, emotional support emerged as particularly salient when participants were faced with additional demands and setbacks; intervention effectiveness was inextricably linked to goal flexibility; the use of short- and long-term performance and process goals, and task support created a climate of increased motivation and facilitated athletes' adherence to the rehabilitation. Notwithstanding the limitations of these, and other studies, researchers should not dismiss the contribution that alternative approaches such as those considered here can make to evidence-based practice.

Future Research Implications

To build on our discussion of the intervention research conducted to date we move on to what we consider some of the key recommendations for researchers to foster evidence-based intervention practice. To this end, given the significant challenges associated with it, sampling seems a fitting place to start. The integrity of the sample is key to researchers' ability to confidently infer that the intended effects on outcome variables can be attributed to the intervention itself. In order to safeguard this, a priori decisions about sample attributes need to be supplemented by more pragmatic decisions around access, feasibility, and timing (e.g., relative to injury onset and duration, and time of season). Networks of influence, particularly where researchers have established, or can foster, collaborative relationships with medical professionals, physiotherapists, athletic trainers, coaches, and conditioning staff can help facilitate access to injured athletes, and ensure access to samples of appropriate size and composition (e.g., homogenous or heterogeneous samples). Arguably the greatest benefits will be derived from such networks when conducting experimental studies that require matching participants on key attributes across experimental and control groups – in these instances physicians, physiotherapists, and athletic trainers can play an instrumental role in helping with the matching of participants, providing feedback on their clinical progress and any setbacks they might encounter; and, where applicable, an independent assessment of recovery outcomes of interest (e.g., rehabilitation adherence and functional outcomes). In terms of group assignment in RCT designs, in our opinion, the stratified randomization procedures employed by Evans and Hardy (2002) and Salim and Wadey (2019) represent the most appropriate approach to ensuring baseline equivalence, equal group size, and integrity across treatments and negating potential confounding effects.

With regard to the logistics of implementing the intervention itself, adherence to the intervention is likely to be maximized when the burden on participants is minimized – albeit without compromising engagement in, and compliance with, the intervention itself. Typically, intervention studies require participant engagement of between one and two months for experimental studies and up to season-long for mixed methods and qualitative approaches. Given the importance of participant adherence to the integrity and rigor of intervention studies, as well as the meaningfulness of the findings, there is an onus on researchers to reduce the burden on participants involved in interventions studies. One approach to this was that adopted by Christakou et al. (2007) in which the relaxation and imagery treatment group completed each intervention session immediately after their physical rehabilitation session. Not only did this make it logistically easier for participants to attend the intervention sessions, but, given the intervention was designed to mirror physical components of rehabilitation, this approach most likely optimized the effectiveness of the intervention. Unfortunately this approach may not be as suitable for intervention approaches that require, or would benefit from, being introduced or practiced away the formal physical rehabilitation environment. In these instances the researcher may have to make some pragmatic decisions around fostering the effectiveness of strategy use vis-à-vis intervention effects, optimizing adherence, and minimizing potential confounds.

As part of quality assuring and safeguarding the integrity of intervention study design and the meaningfulness of intervention effects, we also recommend researchers try to account for the patient–practitioner interaction and control for any potential confounding effects. In an injury context, social support is arguably the most influential confounding variable, and as such should be controlled for, ideally by including a social support control group alongside a traditional one. Ensuring participants receive the same contact and contact time, with the same person across experimental and control groups, would allow researchers to separate the effects of social support from the intervention itself. However, the feature that has arguably detracted from the quality of intervention studies most is the lack of procedural and intervention content detail. Not only does this lack of detail preclude replication, it makes quality assurance problematic and leaves intervention effects uncertain. To overcome this, researchers should ensure they provide sufficient detail when reporting intervention studies, particularly with regard to treatment/experimental conditions. In interventions involving strategies such as goal-setting, this might include designing workbooks or goal-setting sheets for recording purposes that provide a broad template for others to follow, for example, in relation to the number, type, and nature of the goals and goal-setting process engaged in.

Intervention strategies that involve a significant cognitive component (e.g., imagery) and use away from formalized intervention sessions may require pre-intervention checks to assess individuals' baseline ability and pre-intervention use (Christakou & Zervas, 2007). Measures of adherence, which might include weekly logs or diaries and the use of peer debriefing to record the number of times and nature of participants' engagement with the treatment, could further facilitate replicability. Where feasible and acceptable it may also be worth filming intervention sessions (e.g., Cupal & Brewer, 2001). Finally, wherever possible researchers should consider integrating social validation or "exit" interviews post-intervention, similar to those employed by Salim and Wadey (2019). These qualitative methods offer numerous advantages in relation to contextualizing intervention effectiveness and interpreting quantitative findings, as well as helping participants' assimilate post-intervention appraisals and injury and intervention experience.

Conclusion

Our intention in this chapter has been to reflect on and elucidate what we consider to be some of the barriers to conducting experimental intervention research as a basis for propagating the need for an experimentally derived evidence base that can guide interventions with injured athletes. To this end we have drawn on the existing research to help illustrate some of the strengths and limitations of study designs, prior to suggesting how the strengths might be harnessed and the limitations alleviated. In the interests of completeness, as well as methodological and conceptual rigor, we included non-experimental designs in the current treatise. We hope that this inclusive approach will help inform the design of methodologically rigorous intervention studies in the future.

Critical Discussion Questions

1) How would you go about designing and implementing the optimal intervention study to examine the effectiveness of your strategy(ies) of choice?
2) Discuss the challenges associated with experimental as opposed to non-experimental intervention study designs?
3) What challenges does delivering longitudinal as opposed to brief-duration interventions present researchers with?

References

Beneka, A., Malliou, P., Gioftsidou, A., Kofotolis, N., Rokka, S., Mavromoustakos, S., & Godolias, G. (2013). Effects of instructional and motivational self-talk on balance performance in knee injured. *European Journal of Physiotherapy*, *15*(2), 56–63. doi: 10.3109/21679169.2013.776109

Brewer, B. W., Cornelius, A. E., Sklar, J. H., Van Raalte, J. L., Tennen, H., Armeli, S., & Brickner, J. C. (2007). Pain and negative mood during rehabilitation after anterior cruciate ligament reconstruction: A daily process analysis. *Scandinavian Journal of Medicine and Science in Sports*, *17*(5), 520–529. doi: 10.1111/j.1600-0838.2006.00601.x

Brewer, B. W., & Redmond, C. J. (2017). *Psychology of sport injury*. Champaign, IL: Human Kinetics.

Chang, S. J., van Wittleloostuijn, A., & Eden, L. (2010). From the editors: Common method variance in international business research. *Journal of International Business Studies*, *41*(2), 178–184. doi: 10.1057/jibs.2009.88

Christakou, A., & Zervas, Y. (2007). The effectiveness of imagery on pain, edema, and range of motion in athletes with a grade II ankle sprain. *Physical Therapy in Sport*, *8*(3), 130–140. doi: 10.1016/j.ptsp.2007.03.005

Christakou, A., Zervas, Y., & Lavallee, D. (2007). The adjunctive role of imagery on the functional rehabilitation of a grade II ankle sprain. *Human Movement Science*, *26*(1), 141–154. doi: 10.1016/j.humov.2006.07.010

Cupal, D. D. (1998). Psychological interventions in sport injury prevention and rehabilitation. *Journal of Applied Sport Psychology*, *10*(1), 103–123. doi: 10.1080/10413209808406380

Cupal, D. D., & Brewer, B. W. (2001). Effects of relaxation and guided imagery on knee strength, reinjury anxiety, and pain following anterior cruciate ligament reconstruction. *Rehabilitation Psychology*, *46*(1), 28–43. doi: 10.1037/0090-5550.46.1.28

Evans, L., & Hardy, L. (2002). Injury rehabilitation: A goal-setting intervention study. *Research Quarterly for Exercise and Sport*, *73*(3), 310–319. doi: 10.1080/02701367.2002.10609025

Evans, L., Hardy, L., & Fleming, S. (2000). Intervention strategies with injured athletes: An action research study. *The Sport Psychologist*, *14*(2), 188–206. doi: 10.1123/tsp.14.2.188

Gilbourne, D., Taylor, A., Downie, G., & Newton, P. (1996). Goal-setting during sports injury rehabilitation: A presentation of underlying theory, administration procedure, and an athlete case study. *Sport Exercise and Injury*, *2*, 1–10.

Johnson, U. (2000). Short-term psychological intervention: A study of long-term-injured competitive athletes. *Journal of Sport Rehabilitation, 9*(3), 207–218. doi: 10.1123/jsr.9.3.207

Maddison, R., Prapavessis, H., & Clatworthy, M. (2006). Modeling and rehabilitation following anterior cruciate ligament reconstruction. *Annals of Behavioral Medicine, 31*(1), 89–98. doi: 10.1207/s15324796abm3101_13

Mahoney, J., & Hanrahan, S. J. (2011). A brief educational intervention using acceptance and commitment therapy: Four injured athletes' experiences. *Journal of Clinical Sport Psychology, 5*(3), 252–273. doi: 10.1123/jcsp.5.3.252

Mankad, A., & Gordon, S. (2010). Psycholinguistic changes in athletes' grief response to injury after written emotional disclosure. *Journal of Sport Rehabilitation, 19*(3), 328–342. doi: 10.1123/jsr.19.3.328

Mankad, A., Gordon, S., & Wallman, K. (2009a). Psycholinguistic analysis of emotional disclosure: A case study in sport injury. *Journal of Clinical Sport Psychology, 3*(2), 182–196. doi: 10.1123/jcsp.3.2.182

Mankad, A., Gordon, S., & Wallman, K. (2009b). Psycho-immunological effects of written emotional disclosure during long-term injury rehabilitation. *Journal of Clinical Sport Psychology, 3*(3), 205–217. doi: 10.1123/jcsp.3.3.205

Mohammed, W. A., Pappous, A., & Sharma, D. (2018). Effect of mindfulness based stress reduction (MBSR) in increasing pain tolerance and improving the mental health of injured athletes. *Frontiers in Psychology, 9*, 722–732. doi: 10.3389/fpsyg.2018.00722

Rock, J. A., & Jones, M. V. (2002). A preliminary investigation into the use of counseling skills in support of rehabilitation from sport injury. *Journal of Sport Rehabilitation, 11*(4), 284–304. doi: 10.1123/jsr.11.4.284

Ross, M. J., & Berger, R. S. (1996). Effects of stress inoculation training on athletes' postsurgical pain and rehabilitation after orthopedic injury. *Journal of Consulting and Clinical Psychology, 64*(2), 406–410. doi: 10.1037/0022-006X.64.2.406

Salim, J., & Wadey, R. (2018). Can emotional disclosure promote sport injury-related growth? *Journal of Applied Sport Psychology, 30*(4), 367–387. doi: 10.1080/10413200.2017.1417338

Salim, J., & Wadey, R. (2019). Using gratitude to promote sport injury–related growth. *Journal of Applied Sport Psychology*, 1–20. doi: 10.1080/10413200.2019.1626515

Shapiro, J., & Etzel, E. (2018). An individualized multimodal mental skills intervention for injured college athletes. *Journal of Contemporary Athletics, 12*, 237–252.

Theodorakis, Y., Beneca, A., Goudas, M., Antoniou, P., & Malliou, P. (1998). The effect of self-talk on injury rehabilitation. *European Yearbook of Sport Psychology, 2*, 124–135.

Theodorakis, Y., Beneca, A., Malliou, P., & Goudas, M. (1997). Examining psychological factors during injury rehabilitation. *Journal of Sport Rehabilitation, 6*(4), 355–363. doi: 10.1123/jsr.6.4.355

Theodorakis, Y., Malliou, P., Papaioannou, A., Beneca, A., & Filactakidou, A. (1996). The effect of personal goals, self-efficacy, and self-satisfaction on injury rehabilitation. *Journal of Sport Rehabilitation, 5*(3), 214–223. doi: 10.1123/jsr.5.3.214

14 Introducing Knowledge Translation Into the Field of Sport Injury Psychology

The Art of Improving Research Uptake in Practice

Fiona J. Leggat

Introduction

Sport injury psychology is a flourishing field of research. The increased research attention it is receiving, and the overall maturity of the field, can be evidenced in recent books (e.g., Brewer & Redmond, 2016) and systematic reviews (e.g., Ivarsson, Tranaeus, Johnson, & Stenling, 2017). However, despite the critical importance of these empirical developments for our theoretical knowledge and professional practice, it is surprising to note that recent researchers have argued that the models and theories driving sport injury psychology research are not "fit for purpose" when it comes to applied practice, perpetuating a research–practice gap (Hess, Gnacinski, & Meyer, 2019; Wadey et al., 2019). A critical pursual of the sport injury psychology literature, as well as consideration of theoretical advancements in other fields of research (e.g., healthcare research), soon reveals one potential reason for the evidence–practice gap, which concerns *how* researchers are currently doing their research. To expand, up until now, the common methodological approach by injury researchers who have published research in sport psychology has been to construct their own research question, devise their own methodologies and methods, collect data on participants (e.g., injured athletes), interpret datasets themselves, write up their results, and disseminate the findings through conferences and peer-reviewed journals. While this approach has its merits (e.g., theoretical advancement), I would argue that this methodological approach restricts the uptake of empirical research in practice. In this chapter I propose another way of doing research, which focuses on working "with" rather than "on" participants. As Verhagen (2012) suggests, "if Mohammed will not come to the mountain, then the mountain must come to Mohammed" (p. 8), to help bridge the evidence–practice or "know–do" gap.

In this chapter, I introduce one methodological approach that has been shown to help bridge the evidence–practice or "know–do" gap in healthcare and exercise psychology (e.g. Smith, Tomasone, Latimer-Cheung, & Martin Ginis, 2015), that has not yet been considered in the sport injury psychology literature: that is, knowledge translation (KT). This chapter presents an introduction to KT with a specific focus on integrated knowledge translation (iKT), and how it can be utilized to help bridge the "know–do" gap. The chapter closes with future research directions and critical discussion questions.

What is Knowledge Translation?

It is important to firstly to understand what KT is (and is not). Terms including knowledge exchange, research utilization, dissemination, diffusion, and implementation research (McKibbon et al., 2010) have all been used to describe KT, resulting in conceptual confusion (Bowen & Graham, 2013a). Yet, it could be argued few of these truly reflect KT. Defined originally by the Canadian Institute of Health Research (CIHR), KT is a dynamic and iterative process. This process includes the synthesis, dissemination, exchange, and ethically sound application of knowledge to improve health, provide more effective health services and products, and strengthen the health care system. This process takes place within a complex system of interactions between researchers and knowledge users which may vary in intensity, complexity, and level of engagement depending on the nature of the research and the findings as well as the needs of the particular knowledge user (CIHR, 2016). This refers to KT as a process, comprised of multiple phases, and thus as a noun. In contrast, other terminology used, including dissemination and implementation, describe verbs, which, instead, represent actions and parts of the KT process (Graham et al., 2006). These terms do not resemble KT in its entirety, and thus, Straus, Tetroe, and Graham (2013b) suggest such individual phases "are not usually sufficient on their own to ensure appropriate knowledge use" (p. 4). Like geographical preferences, some nations have instead taken a preference to these action-based terms over that of the KT term. For example, in Canada, KT as a term is prolific, while in the United Kingdom and Europe "implementation research" has gained greater momentum, and given rise to the journal of *Implementation Science* (Graham et al., 2006; Straus et al., 2013b). However, as an action, implementation is only one phase of the iterative KT process. Adding further complexity to the terminology phenomena, KT is not simply comprised of one paradigm.

Different Types of Knowledge Translation

Two contrasting paradigms or types of KT exist: the knowledge transfer paradigm and the engagement paradigm. These are better known as end-of-project KT and integrated KT (iKT), respectively (Straus et al., 2013b). To outline, end-of-project KT views the reason for the evidence–practice gap as a problem in knowledge transfer (Bowen & Graham, 2013b); for example, the intended audience is not ready to hear the knowledge, or the implementation or dissemination of knowledge is inadequately reaching the audience. Given that coaches and applied practitioners in the sport sciences show a lack of preference for knowledge from journal articles and conference presentations (Fullagar, McCall, Impellizzeri, Favero, & Coutts, 2019), research being dispersed in this format may, in part, also explain the gap in sport injury psychology; the knowledge dissemination is not practical for users.

In contrast, iKT views the gap as a problem in knowledge production, whereby audiences are failing to draw upon knowledge because it does not address the real-world priorities and practice problems they face (Bowen & Graham, 2013b). Accordingly, iKT is rooted in participatory research with the integration of knowledge users, decision makers, and researchers to co-produce research as equals (Bowen & Graham, 2013a). Knowledge users are individuals (e.g., coaches, physiotherapists, psychologists, injured athletes) who are likely to use the knowledge generated, whereas decision makers (e.g. managers, policymakers, governing bodies) are those who have the authority to evoke change to policies, programs, or practices, and authorize iKT activities. Put simply, iKT is conducted *with* and not *on* users; co-production is the vital component. Co-production promotes a two-way system of communication, whereby all co-producers (knowledge users, decision makers and researchers) should be actively involved in the whole KT process (Gagliardi, Kothari, & Graham, 2017) in recognition that each community can bring unique and valuable expertise of the practice problem and the needs of the setting (Kothari & Wathen, 2017). In iKT, such expertise and practical knowledge from co-producers is often regarded as knowledge (see Box 14.1). This is known as tacit knowledge (Kothari, Bickford, Edwards, Dobbins, & Meyer, 2011), which can provide researchers with otherwise unattainable knowledge regarding how iKT activities and interventions may be viewed and experienced by users (Williams & Glasby, 2010).

BOX 14.1: WHAT IS CONSIDERED "KNOWLEDGE"?

The distinction of the word "knowledge" in the title of KT outlines that knowledge should be regarded as more than just research, and include all forms of knowing (e.g., grey literature, administrative data, organizational context); otherwise KT would be research translation (Straus et al., 2013b). Despite this, knowledge has largely been interpreted and distinguished by many as research evidence (Kothari et al., 2011). This may, in part, be explained by the biomedical roots of healthcare, where KT originates, comprised traditionally of those with biomedical (e.g., positivist) epistemologies (Bowen & Graham, 2013b). In contrast, for those with epistemologies rooted in the social sciences (e.g. constructivist), non-research sources of evidence (e.g. tacit knowledge, grey literature) are additionally recognized. For those considering using iKT for sport injury psychology projects, a holistic view of knowledge, encompassing all ways of knowing, is recommended given the need to understand the practice environment and contextual influences (Wadey et al., 2019). However, individuals should also seek to reflect upon their own epistemologies.

At present, it could be argued that much of the sport injury psychology knowledge translation efforts fall into the end-of-project KT paradigm. For example, research is conducted by researchers, and then attempted to be disseminated to knowledge users. Although researchers may consult knowledge users during dissemination (e.g., Ollivier, Aston, & Price, 2018), this is not regarded as iKT due to the paradigms underpinning view of the "know–do" gap. Given the remarks that sport injury psychology research may not be "fit for purpose" (e.g., Hess et al., 2019), iKT and co-producing research to meet the specific needs of those in practice settings may be a solution. Thus, less in accordance with the notion, "build it and they will come", but rather, "build it with them, and they are already there" (Greenhalgh, Jackson, Shaw, & Janamian, 2016, p. 414), co-production may not only create more relevant knowledge, but also increase the uptake in practice. Although a great number of strengths of iKT have been illustrated, the co-production process can also be challenging, with costs that individuals should weigh up prior to initiating iKT (see Table 14.1). If iKT is deemed advantageous, it then begs the question, how can we "do" it?

Table 14.1 Summary of Strengths, Challenges, and Costs of iKT

Strengths	*Challenges and Costs*
Improved research quality due to…	Six categorizations of cost:
• More user-relevant research questions.[a] • Greater suitability of methodologies chosen.[b] • Enhanced intepretation of findings.[b]	• Practical cost, personal researcher cost, professional researcher cost, research cost, knowledge user/decision maker cost, and cost to science as a profession.[c]
Improved research uptake due to…	Managing time and resources.[a b d]
	Communication with all co-producers.[b]
• A greater value seen in the use of research by knowledge users.[a] • Feelings of ownership in what is produced.[b]	Overcoming previous poor experiences of research collaboration.[b]
Formation of new relationships and connections with those in practice settings.[b]	Aligning roles and expectations of co-producers in the process.[a b]
Improved knowledge on the research process in knowledge users.[b]	Managing differing needs and priorities of all co-producers.[a b]
Prompt future collaborative research projects.[a]	Coping with co-producer lack of skill or understanding in iKT.[a d]

[a] Gagliardi, Berta, Kothari, Boyko, and Urquhart (2016)
[b] Bowen, Botting, Graham, and Huebner (2017)
[c] Olivier, Kothari, and Mays (2019)
[d] Gagliardi and Dobrow (2016)

How Can We "Do" Knowledge Translation?

Theoretical Underpinning

Before "jumping straight into the waters" of iKT, sport injury psychology researchers would do well to first consider their theoretical underpinnings of the iKT process. Within the broader KT literature, 159 different theoretical underpinnings have been drawn upon (see Strifler et al., 2018). One of these includes the Knowledge to Action (KTA) Cycle (see Figure 14.1), which was developed by Graham and colleagues in 2006. The KTA Cycle, categorized as a full-spectrum process model (Esmail et al., 2020; Nilsen, 2015), aims to describe and guide the whole process of conducing KT. The model is comprised of two concepts: a knowledge creation funnel and an action cycle. Derived from a concept analysis of 31 planned action theories (Graham et al., 2006; Straus et al., 2013b), the KTA Cycle is a highly cited theoretical approach to KT. Although healthcare dominant, its use spans many domains (see Field, Booth, Ilott, & Gerrish, 2014) including physical activity promotion (Smith et al., 2015), and exercise adherence (Babatunde, MacDermid, & MacIntyre, 2017). In part, this may be due to its capacity to elicit change at individual, community, organization, and system levels, in conjunction with its practicality for both end-of-project KT and iKT (Straus et al., 2013b). Given the recent attention on taking a system-level approach in sport injury psychology (Wadey, Day, Cavallerio, & Martinelli, 2018) this provides another justification for this methodology. For the purposes of the

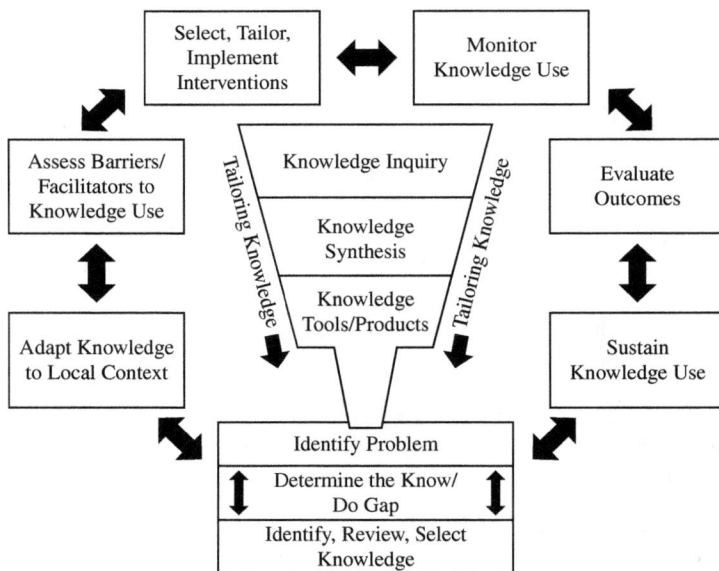

Figure 14.1 The Knowledge to Action (KTA) Cycle (Graham et al., 2006).

present chapter, the process of iKT will be outlined using the KTA Cycle. The next paragraph gives a practical outlook on the process of conducting iKT based upon the KTA Cycle, while also outlining key considerations for sport injury psychology researchers to reflect upon and debate.

The Process of iKT

To illustrate both the KTA Cycle and the process of iKT, each phase of the cycle will be outlined with key considerations presented. These considerations are derived from those acknowledged in the literature and my own personal experiences. It should be noted that although seemingly cyclical, the authors of the KTA Cycle describe the concepts as dynamic and interchangeable with fluid boundaries, whereby phases in the knowledge funnel may occur simultaneously or in conjunction with those in the action cycle (Graham et al., 2006). Therefore, this outline is not prescriptive, but acts simply a guide to researchers. Both the knowledge funnel and the action cycle are described below.

Knowledge Funnel

This component, designed to filter and tailor knowledge, is divided into three phases to tailor knowledge to the practice problem: *knowledge inquiry*, *knowledge synthesis*, and *knowledge tools/products* (Graham et al., 2006; Straus et al., 2013b). Before initiating the funnel, co-production teams may wish to align their views on what they constitute as "knowledge" (see Box 14.1). *Knowledge inquiry* is that where knowledge, such as primary empirical studies, is searched for and gathered to gain a broad knowledge base (Graham et al., 2006). Such a phase may parallel that of a literature search; however, all co-producers should be involved to ensure knowledge is gathered from all appropriate sources (e.g., grey literature). If existing knowledge of the practice problem is insufficient – which is likely the case for adopting iKT over end-of-project KT – co-producers should gather additional knowledge (e.g., conduct empirical research).

Knowledge synthesis refers to the synergy of such knowledge to form a more specialized knowledge base on the practice problem. Co-producers may take advantage of recent systematic reviews in the field at this point to aid with synthesis (e.g., Ivarsson et al., 2017). However, if such a specific synthesis is absent from the sport injury psychology literature, or if the knowledge did not previously exist to conduct a synthesis, co-producers may seek to conduct such a synthesis or review themselves.

Finally, the creation of *knowledge tools/products* refers to the development of educational modules, decision aids, practice guidelines, or other materials whose purpose it is to present the synthesized and useful knowledge to the practice problem, in a user-friendly and easily accessible format (Straus et al., 2013b). Through this process, co-production with all communities is integral to understand what knowledge is most useful and how it should be delivered. The development of tools to measure the use of the knowledge may also be developed here (e.g., Babatunde et al., 2017). This represents an exciting and influential phase for sport injury psychology practice.

Action Cycle

In comparison to the knowledge funnel, the action cycle aims to guide the application of the knowledge to those who need it (e.g., applied practitioners/injured athletes). The cycle consists of seven phases, each influenced by one another, and of phases in the knowledge funnel (Graham et al., 2006; Straus et al., 2013b).

The first phase of the action cycle is divided into three parts. First, *identification of the problem*, whereby the need for specific knowledge production to address a practice problem is recognized (Graham et al., 2006). Arguably, this phase may be actioned before that of the *knowledge inquiry* phase; without identification of the problem, the broader knowledge to "solve" it cannot be gathered. Specifically, with iKT, such a practice problem may be raised by those in the setting (e.g., applied practitioners/coaches) and brought to the attention of researchers (Kothari & Wathen, 2017) and not vice versa. Once a problem is addressed and knowledge explored to "solve" it, co-producers should aim to *determine the know–do gap*; in short, to establish how much additional knowledge is required. Subsequent to the gathering and synthesizing of knowledge, the final action is to *select and review knowledge* pertinent to the problem (Graham et al., 2006). At this point, knowledge is chosen for use based upon its specificity and usefulness to users. While all co-producers may provide valuable insight into such knowledge selection, knowledge appraisal skills should also be considered.

The second phase refers to the "*adaptation of knowledge to local context*" and within this phase, knowledge selected is tailored to the demands of the setting (e.g., sport) and circumstances (e.g., injury) while considering its value, usefulness, and appropriateness (Graham et al., 2006). This phase may be conducted in conjunction with the creation of knowledge tools/products with all co-producers. For example, existing tools may be modified for applicability in different sports. Although few guidelines exist for how to conduct this phase, qualitative co-production activities (e.g., Laur & Keller, 2015) alongside more systematic approaches for guideline adaptations (see Fervers et al., 2011) are advocated.

Next is the "*assessment of barrier and facilitators to knowledge use*". Barriers and facilitators include factors related to the knowledge itself, to the knowledge users (e.g. coaches/applied practitioners/injured athletes), and to the setting where the knowledge may be used (Graham et al., 2006). For example, contextual demands, such as stressors of applied practitioners may influence the use of knowledge in practice (e.g., Kerai, Wadey, & Salim, 2019). To fully understand these factors, additional theoretical approaches and data collection may be required. Drawing upon a determinant framework may help to understand and explore factors influencing knowledge implementation and use (see Nilsen, 2015 for a review), while additional data collection methods, such as observation, focus groups, setting, and questionnaires, may identify more contextually specific influences. The findings from this phase will likely inform the selection of knowledge products and interventions to ensure barriers and facilitators are minimized or maximized respectively.

Phase four, "*select, tailor and implement interventions*", outlines the process of planning and executing interventions to facilitate the uptake of knowledge tools/products in practice (Graham et al., 2006), often referred to as dissemination or implementation. Described as an "art" (Wensing, Bosch, & Grol, 2013), selecting and tailoring an intervention to a setting can require many different considerations (see Box 14.2). Involvement from all co-producer parties at this point is paramount to ensure intervention components are both feasible and applicable to knowledge users. Additional literature, from fields including behavior change, may be drawn upon to maximize chances of effectiveness in acknowledgment of barriers and facilitators identified. The phase should conclude with the implementation or the piloting of the intervention in the practice setting.

BOX 14.2: SELECTING INTERVENTIONS IN IKT

Ideally, the choice of an intervention should be guided by research evidence on the effectiveness of various interventions. However, given the specificity of knowledge and uniqueness of contextual settings, it is important to creatively construct tailored interventions in order to promote and sustain knowledge use (Wensing et al., 2013). It is beyond the scope of this chapter to discuss the variety of KT interventions used, but co-producers should seek to consider these factors when selecting their intervention:

- The purpose of the intervention (e.g., behavior change, education).
- The target of the intervention (e.g., trainees, experienced psychologists, coaches).
- The overcoming of barriers, and maximization of facilitators to knowledge use (e.g., intervention mapping using theory or common-sense (Verhagen, 2012; Wensing et al., 2013)).
- The components used in the intervention (e.g., single vs. multi-component). There is little research to suggest "better is more"; however, interventions targeting different barriers/facilitators may lead to a more successful uptake (Wensing et al., 2013).
- The type of the intervention components (e.g., passive, such as written guidelines and dyadic lectures or/and active, such as outreach visits, interactive talks).
- The method to measure the intervention effectiveness (e.g., research design).

Once implemented, the next phase is to *monitor knowledge use*. Such a step is necessary to determine how and to what extent the knowledge products from the intervention have been used in practice (Graham et al., 2006). Different knowledge users (i.e., coaches/injured athletes) and types of knowledge (i.e., conceptual/instrumental) may require different measurement methods, as one method may not be suitable for all users (Graham et al., 2006; Straus, Tetroe, Bhattacharyya, Zwarenstein, & Graham, 2013a). Should co-producers recognize any initial issues with the intervention, or deem that it has brought about a less-than-desired uptake of knowledge in practice, previous phases may be revisited (e.g., reassessing barriers to knowledge use). If a desired uptake is reached, the penultimate phase may be conducted.

The aim of the phase *evaluating outcomes* is to determine the outcomes of the knowledge uptake in practice, both intended and unintended (Graham et al., 2006). Although the evaluation takes place at this point, planning of the evaluation may have taken place when designing the intervention. Typically, mixed method designs are advocated here to gather both robust evidence on effectiveness and greater detail regarding how the intervention was received and experienced by users (Straus et al., 2013a). As in the monitoring phase, evaluation methods used may be population, outcome, and setting dependent. Evaluations of the iKT process and co-production experience with co-producers may additionally be carried out here.

Should outcomes of the knowledge uptake be desirable, iKT projects should proceed to the final phase of the KTA Cycle, *sustain knowledge use*. This refers to efforts to support the continued use of knowledge products (Graham et al. 2006). Barriers to knowledge use and the initial problem itself may alter and adapt over time, but the process for managing the change is suggested to be the same; an individual in a practice setting (e.g., coach) may recognize a practice problem and seek to initiate a co-production effort, restarting the KTA Cycle loop. When planning for sustainable knowledge use, other elements to consider include the scalability and spread of the knowledge products. For example, a knowledge product may be disseminated online for use in other practice settings (e.g., Babatunde et al., 2017).

Challenges Ahead for Sport Injury Psychology Researchers Doing iKT

Navigating the iKT Literature

The first challenge becomes evident when delving into the iKT literature for the first time. As in KT, the terminology used to describe iKT is often labeled with different terminology, with collaborative research, engaged scholarship, and mode-two knowledge production, to name a few (Gagliardi et al., 2017). This makes true iKT hard to unmask. Similarly, iKT is often confused with community-based participatory research (CBPR; Jull, Giles & Graham, 2017). To aid with the identification of iKT literature from CBPR, two key differences can be observed. First, in iKT, knowledge users or decision makers should identify the practice problem in their setting (Jull et al., 2017). This is unlike CBPR, which is largely researcher-driven. Second, in iKT, a co-producer should also possess the authority to evoke change in the practice setting using the knowledge produced (Kothari & Wathen,

2017). In CBPR, such authority may not be possessed. Due to such mislabeling, research using both CBPR and iKT terms should be interpreted with caution. Future iKT researchers should be encouraged to use search terms from past iKT reviews (see Gagliardi, Berta, Kothari, Boyko, & Urquhart, 2016) when searching for literature; although experienced researchers have also noted difficulties in unearthing iKT studies (Gagliardi et al., 2017).

Selecting Co-Production Activities

The second challenge is concerned with selecting the most effective co-production activities. These are consistently poorly described (Gagliardi et al., 2016, 2017) with the type, intensity, and frequency of activities for the most effective co-production and positive outcomes still unknown (Banner et al., 2019; Gagliardi et al., 2016, 2017; Kothari & Wathen, 2017). There is also little consensus as to what components within the activities are most effective. It has been illustrated that meetings are most frequently used (Gagliardi et al., 2016), but effectiveness of this is relatively unknown. Based upon their scoping review, Gagliardi et al. (2016) have urged researchers "to capture and report the full extent of iKT activities" (p. 10), acknowledging that the reporting of these must improve for the field to advance. The authors suggest the use of the WIDER checklist to do this. The checklist recommends describing the activity, mode of delivery (intensity, duration, timing), content, co-producers and their role, the setting, and adherence (see Albrecht, Archibald, Arseneau, & Scott, 2013). As the activity reporting quality is weak, and it is relatively unknown which activities are most effective for co-production, communication with all co-producers to ascertain what activities might be most appropriate is recommended. It is hoped the relative "experts" can provide greater guidance on what activities work best for them given the knowledge they want to contribute, their environment, and contextual demands.

Co-Producer Involvement

A third challenge regards the level of involvement for each party of co-producers. The level of engagement in iKT activities are infrequently reported, and therefore it is relatively unknown how much co-producer involvement is needed to create positive outcomes (Banner et al., 2019). Gagliardi et al. (2016) identified that co-producer involvement most frequently occurred in phases identifying the practice problem and developing the intervention, with minimal involvement elsewhere. Additionally, researchers have neglected to go beyond merely stating co-producer involvement, and illustrate "how and when" different co-producers are involved. Researchers have suggested the "how" is especially pertinent, and should be obtained from the perspective of the co-producer (Kothari & Wathen, 2017); researchers may perceive they are giving responsibility and voice to co-producers, when they may not always be drawing from that voice. Given the underlying assumption, and reports that co-producer involvement positively influences outcomes in iKT, sport injury psychology researchers are encouraged to measure, evaluate, and report co-production in iKT activities to assess this connotation further (Gagliardi et al., 2016; Kothari & Wathen, 2017). Researchers should also aim to involve co-producers in all phases of the iKT process to identify how these individuals' influence at different phases can affect the outcomes. To measure co-producer engagement, the IAP2 spectrum of patient engagement (IAP, n.d.) has been proposed (Banner et al., 2019), yet encouraging reflexive practice among all co-producers may also provide insight, and thus should be encouraged.

Creating and Maintaining Relationships with Co-Producers

Finally, developing rapport and relationships with co-producers can be the largest challenge in iKT, particularly given that relationships are perhaps the most vital component to the success of iKT (Kothari & Wathen, 2017). With the practicality of continual engagement, geographical location, time, differing priorities and attitudes, and lack of iKT understanding noted as barriers to the iKT process, many of these barriers also inhibit the formation of relationships (Gagliardi et al., 2016). For example, identifying and aligning the needs, expectations, and priorities of all co-producers can take large amounts of time and effort, yet these are necessary to prompt positive outcomes (Bowen, Botting, Graham, & Huebner, 2017). While some barriers can be overcome in a simple fashion (e.g., geographical location through the use of technology), others are more challenging. For example, bad past experiences with researchers may severely inhibit knowledge users' trust and sharing of knowledge with researchers in iKT (Bowen et al., 2017). Thus, at the onset of a project Gagliardi et al. (2017) suggest great investment is required by co-producers to grapple with and understand the collaborative nature of an iKT project. In the same way as a practitioner may seek to build up rapport with an injured athlete, all co-producers should establish relationships and thus, an allocation of time for this "getting to know you" process is paramount.

Future sport injury psychology researchers using iKT are therefore encouraged to maintain and develop relationships with practice settings, given the potential of iKT as an avenue of research. Drawing from qualitative traditions, immersive methods, such as ethnography, may provide an opportunity for researchers wishing to forge relationships and better understand practice settings (Baumbusch et al., 2018). For example, immersion can facilitate communication with, and promote an enhanced understanding of, users and their setting. Reflexive methods are also recommended during the development of relationships, encouraging researchers to remain aware of their motivations and biases, while working with the agendas and priorities of others.

Future Research Implications

In this chapter, I have introduced iKT by describing what it is (and is not) and how it can be done. Thus, my main future research direction is that iKT is taken up by researchers in the field of sport injury psychology to reduce the research–practice gap. However, within this broader suggestion, I offer two additional directions for future research. First, researchers in sport injury psychology need to begin to start conducting research "with" and not just "on" others, which, among other things, includes co-constructing research questions, methodologies, findings, and practice/policy. By working with applied practitioners, coaches, managers, and athletes, and drawing from their experiential knowledge, gaps in knowledge production may become apparent and more specific research needs may arise. This change in the way we do research will allow more relevant co-produced research to be created and utilized in the practice setting. Second, sport injury psychology researchers would do well to write reflective diaries, perhaps confessional tales of the iKT process, so others can benefit from their experiences. Indeed, tales of the entire process and how it evolves from conception to sustaining knowledge use would not only be beneficial to the sport injury psychology literature but also help to extend and lead the way in the broader iKT research, given that little is known about the outcomes of iKT outside of health care.

Conclusion

The process of KT, and specifically iKT, is an underutilized methodological approach in sport injury psychology. It allows real-world practice needs to dictate research, resulting in the production of meaningful work with positive practice outcomes. The multiple considerations in each phase and its lack of a "one-size-fits-all" approach makes iKT appealing to both quantitative and qualitative researchers alike, with projects that can aid small case study settings and large-scale organizational operations. Through iKT, a bridge can be built between researchers and the practice world, enabling the field of research to advance and ultimately provide a better service for injured athletes and those who work with them. If you, the reader, are interested in providing more impactful research, iKT provides an exciting solution!

Critical Discussion Questions

1) Reflect on your current research interests in sport injury psychology. Who might benefit from your type of research in your local geographical area (e.g., governing body, local sporting team)? How might you start to build a working relationship with them?
2) Consider the phase of knowledge product development. What creative and innovative ways could sport injury psychology researchers better disseminate their research beyond academic conferences and journals to maximize the uptake of research findings?
3) Moving beyond the status quo of doing research *on* injured athletes, what iKT activities/methods could future researchers use to work *with* injured athletes?

References

Albrecht, L., Archibald, M., Arseneau, D., & Scott, S. D. (2013). Development of a checklist to assess the quality of reporting of knowledge translation interventions using the Workgroup for Intervention Development and Evaluation Research (WIDER) recommendations. *Implementation Science 8*, 52. doi: 10.1186/1748-5908-8-52

Babatunde, F. O., MacDermid, J. C., & MacIntyre, N. (2017). A therapist-focused knowledge translation intervention for improving patient adherence in musculoskeletal physiotherapy practice. *Archives of Physiotherapy 7*, 1 doi: 10.1186/s40945-016-0029-x

Banner, D., Bains, M., Carroll, S., Kandola, D. K., Rolfe, D. E., Wong, C., & Graham, I. D. (2019). Patient and public engagement in integrated knowledge translation research: Are we there yet? *Research Involvement and Engagement 5, 8*. doi: 10.1186/s40900-019-0139-1

Baumbusch, J., Wu, S., Lauck, S. B., Banner, D., O'Shea, T., & Achtem, L. (2018). Exploring the synergies between focused ethnography and integrated knowledge translation. *Health Research Policy and Systems 16, 103*. doi: 10.1186/s12961-018-0376-z

Bowen, S., Botting, I., Graham, I. D., & Huebner, L. (2017). *Beyond* "two cultures": Guidance for establishing effective researcher/health system partnerships. *International Journal of Health Policy and Management, 6*(1), 27–42. doi: 10.15171/ijhpm.2016.71

Bowen, S., & Graham, I. D. (2013a). From knowledge translation to engaged scholarship: Promoting research relevance and utilization. *Archives of Physical Medicine and Rehabilitation, 94*(1) (Suppl.1), S3–S8. doi: 10.1016/j.apmr.2012.04.037

Bowen, S., & Graham, I. D. (2013b). Integrated knowledge translation. In S. Straus, J. Tetroe, & I. Graham (Eds.), *Knowledge translation in healthcare: Moving evidence to practice* (pp. 14–23). Chichester, UK: Wiley-Blackwell.

Brewer, B. W., & Redmond, C. J. (2016). *Psychology of sport injury*. Champaign, IL: Human Kinetics.

Canadian Institute of Health Research (CIHR). (2016). Knowledge translation. Retrieved April 16, 2020 from http://www.cihr-irsc.gc.ca/e/29418.html

Esmail, R., Hanson, H. M., Holroyd-Leduc, J., Brown, S., Strifler, L., Straus, S. E., Niven, D.J., & Clement, F. M. (2020). A scoping review of full-spectrum knowledge translation theories, models, and frameworks. *Implementation Science, 15*, 11. doi: 10.1186/s13012-020-0964-5

Fervers, B., Burgers, J. S., Voellinger, R., Brouwers, M., Browman, G. P., Graham, I. D., Harrison, M. B., … Burnand, B. (2011). Guideline adaptation: An approach to enhance efficiency in guideline development and improve utilisation. *BMJ Quality and Safety, 20*(3), 228–236. doi: 10.1136/bmjqs.2010.043257

Field, B., Booth, A., Ilott, I., & Gerrish, K. (2014). Using the knowledge to action framework in practice: A citation analysis and systematic review. *Implementation Science, 9, 172*. doi: 10.1186/s13012-014-0172-2

Fullagar, H. K., McCall, A., Impellizzeri, F. M., Favero, T., & Coutts, A. J. (2019). The translation of sport science research to the field: A current opinion and overview on the perceptions of practitioners, researchers and coaches. *Sports Medicine, 49*(12), 1817–1824. doi: 10.1007/s40279-019-01139-0

Gagliardi, A. R., Berta, W., Kothari, A., Boyko, J., & Urquhart, R. (2016). Integrated knowledge translation (IKT) in health care: A scoping review. *Implementation Science, 11, 38*. doi: 10.1186/s13012-016-0399-1

Gagliardi, A. R., & Dobrow, M. (2016). Identifying the conditions needed for integrated knowledge translation (IKT) in health care organizations: Qualitative interviews with researchers and research users. *BMC Health Services Research, 16*, 256 doi: 10.1186/s12913-016-1533-0

Gagliardi, A. R., Kothari, A., & Graham, I. D. (2017). Research agenda for integrated knowledge translation (IKT) in healthcare: What we know and do not yet know. *Journal of Epidemiology and Community Health, 71*(2), 105–106. doi: 10.1136/jech-2016-207743

Graham, I. D., Logan, J., Harrison, M. B., Straus, S. E., Tetroe, J., Caswell, W., & Robinson, N. (2006). Lost in knowledge translation: Time for a map? *Journal of Continuing Education in the Health Professions, 26*(1), 13–24. doi: 10.1002/chp.47

Greenhalgh, T., Jackson, C., Shaw, S., & Janamian, T. (2016). Achieving research impact through co-creation in community-based health services: Literature review and case study. *The Milbank Quarterly, 94*(2), 392–429. doi: 10.1111/1468-0009.12197

Hess, C. W., Gnacinski, S. L., & Meyer, B. B. (2019). A review of the sport-injury and -rehabilitation literature: From abstraction to application. *The Sport Psychologist, 33*(3), 232–243. doi: 10.1123/tsp.2018-0043

International Association for Public Participation. (n.d.). IAP2 spectrum of patient engagement. Retrieved on April 16, 2020 from https://www.iap2.org/page/pillars

Ivarsson, A., Tranaeus, U., Johnson, U., & Stenling, A. (2017). Negative psychological responses of injury and rehabilitation adherence effects on return to play in competitive athletes: A systematic review and meta-analysis. *Open Access Journal of Sports Medicine, 8*, 27–32. doi: 10.2147/OAJSM.S112688

Jull, J., Giles, A., & Graham, I. D. (2017). Community-based participatory research and integrated knowledge translation: Advancing the co-creation of knowledge. *Implementation Science, 12*, 150. doi: 10.1186/s13012-017-0696-3

Kerai, S., Wadey, R., & Salim, J. (2019). Stressors experienced in elite sport by physiotherapists. *Sport, Exercise, and Performance Psychology, 8*(3), 255–272. doi: 10.1037/spy0000154

Kothari, A. R., Bickford, J. J., Edwards, N., Dobbins, M. J., & Meyer, M. (2011). Uncovering tacit knowledge: A pilot study to broaden the concept of knowledge in knowledge translation. *BMC Health Services Research, 11, 198*. doi: 10.1186/1472-6963-11-198

Kothari, A., & Wathen, C. N. (2017). Integrated knowledge translation: Digging deeper, moving forward. *Journal of Epidemiology and Community Health, 71*(6), 619–623. doi: 10.1136/jech-2016-208490

Laur, C., & Keller, H. H. (2015). Implementing best practice in hospital multidisciplinary nutritional care: An example of using the knowledge-to action process for a research program. *Journal of Multidisciplinary Healthcare, 8*, 463–472. doi: 10.2147/JMDH.S93103

McKibbon, K. A., Lokker, C., Wilczynski, N. L., Ciliska, D., Dobbins, M., Davis, D. A., Haynes, R.B., & Straus, S. E. (2010). A cross-sectional study of the number and frequency of terms used to refer to knowledge translation in a body of health literature in 2006: A Tower of Babel? *Implementation Science, 5, 16*. doi: 10.1186/1748-5908-5-16

Nilsen, P. (2015). Making sense of implementation theories, models and frameworks. *Implementation Science, 10*, 53 doi: 10.1186/s13012-015-0242-0

Oliver, K., Kothari, A., & Mays, N. (2019). The dark side of coproduction: Do the costs outweigh the benefits for Health Research? *Health Research Policy and Systems, 17*, 33. doi: 10.1186/s12961-019-0432-3

Ollivier, R., Aston, M., & Price, S. (2018). From research participants to video stars: Engaging families in end-of-grant knowledge translation. *Journal of Family Nursing, 24*(4), 612–620. doi: 10.1177/1074840718809414

Smith, B., Tomasone, J. R., Latimer-Cheung, A. E., & Martin Ginis, K. A. (2015). Narrative as a knowledge translation tool for facilitating impact: Translating physical activity knowledge to disabled people and health professionals. *Health Psychology, 34*(4), 303–313. doi: 10.1037/hea0000113

Straus, S. E., Tetroe, J., Bhattacharyya, O., Zwarenstein, M., & Graham, I. D. (2013a). Monitoring knowledge use and evaluating outcomes. In S. E. Straus, J. Tetroe & I. D.

Graham (Eds.), *Knowledge translation in healthcare: Moving evidence to practice* (pp. 227–236). Chichester, UK: Wiley-Blackwell.

Straus, S. E., Tetroe, J., & Graham, I. D. (2013b). Knowledge translation: What it is and what it isn't. In S. E. Straus, J. Tetroe & I. D. Graham (Eds.), *Knowledge translation in healthcare: Moving evidence to practice* (pp. 3–13). Chichester, UK: Wiley.

Strifler, L., Cardoso, R., McGowan, J., Cogo, E., Nincic, V., Khan, P. A., Scott, A... Straus, S. (2018). Scoping review identifies number of knowledge translation theories, models and frameworks with limited use. *Journal of Clinical Epidemiology, 100*, 92–102. doi: 10.1016/j.jclinepi.2018.04.008

Verhagen, E. (2012). If athletes will not adopt preventative measures, effective measures must adopt athletes. *Current Sports Medicine Reports, 11*(1), 7–8. doi: 10.1249/JSR.0b013e318240dabd

Wadey, R., Day, M., Cavallerio, F., & Martinelli, L. (2018). The multilevel model of sport injury: Can coaches impact and be impacted by injury? In R. Thelwell & M. Dicks (Eds.), *Professional advances in sports coaching: Research and practice* (pp. 336–357). New York: Routledge.

Wadey, R., Roy, K., Evans, L., Howells, K., Salim, J., & Diss, C. (2019). Sport psychology consultants' perspectives on facilitating sport injury-related growth. *The Sport Psychologist, 33*(3), 244–255. doi: 10.1123/tsp.2018-0110

Wensing, M., Bosch, M., & Grol, R. (2013). Developing and selecting knowledge translation interventions. In S. Straus, J. Tetroe & I. Graham (Eds.), *Knowledge translation in healthcare: Moving evidence to practice* (pp. 227–236). Chichester, UK: Wiley-Blackwell.

Williams, I., & Glasby, J. (2010). Making "what works" work: The use of knowledge in UK health and social care decision-making. *Policy and Society, 29*(2), 95–102. doi: 10.1016/j.polsoc.2010.03.002

15 "But It Is Bad!" "Yes, But Is It Really as Bad as You Have Indicated on Here?" "Absolutely!"

Challenging Injured Athletes' Irrational Beliefs: Not a Straightforward Exercise

Robert Morris

Introduction

In this chapter, I present the case of "Joanne", an international canoe slalom athlete in her late twenties going through a protracted period of injury, to contextualize the challenges that there may be when trying to challenge athletes' irrational beliefs about their injury and rehabilitation process. I will draw upon rational emotive behavioral therapy (REBT), humanistic counseling, and multidisciplinary meetings as underpinning approaches to the work carried out. In doing so, I will highlight the need to fully understand the context within which you are working (see Brown, Gould, & Foster 2005) and to be flexible in the approach administered. Following this, I will engage in critical reflection of the work carried out, highlighting the key learnings and future research avenues that surface on the back of the case presented.

Context and Presenting Issue

Joanne was an international athlete who had previously attended the Olympic Games as an athlete competing in canoe slalom. She was in the middle of a second Olympic cycle, where she had expectations of medaling, when she ruptured ligaments in her shoulder during a training run. The injury would result in her having several months out of training and competing. This injury was one that required surgery and a protracted period of rehabilitation before Joanne would be able to compete again.

I was approached by "Colin", the physiotherapist of Joanne, to work with Joanne one month after she had had an operation on her shoulder to try and repair the damage she had sustained. Colin informed me that Joanne was really struggling to cope with her injury, she was experiencing extremely low mood, and was viewing the injury as catastrophic. Because of her psychological state, she was struggling to adhere to the physical recovery and the exercises she needed to complete. Colin also informed me that, realistically, her chances of competing at the Olympic Games were in serious doubt and that Joanne viewed this as devastating because this Olympic Games was one where she had high expectations and was in an excellent position to achieve success. Joanne had put all her efforts toward this success, sacrificing time with friends and family, and delaying or postponing outside interests, including family holidays, for sporting success (cf. Douglas & Carless, 2009).

Following my initial conversations with Colin, I met with Joanne to get further context around her current feelings and situation. Joanne informed me that she had never experienced any situations like the one she was currently in; she had never had any long-term injuries and she had not been in a situation where she was at risk of missing any major competitions. For Joanne, this was both demoralizing and upsetting (see Chapter 8), and she was struggling to cope with the shock of what had happened. Equally, Joanne was feeling physical pain (see Chapter 5) due to the operation she had and was feeling low as a result. It was, in Joanne's words

> the worst period in my life; I'm constantly in pain and just feel down all the time. I am going to miss the Olympics where I had a really good chance of winning at least a medal and all my hard work over the last few years has been wasted. It is devastating. I'm devastated.

Needs Analysis and Intervention

From my initial evaluation of the conversations I had been having with Joanne and Colin, it was clear to me that Joanne was having several irrational beliefs about her injury; particularly that it was devastating and that it was the worst period in her life. Upon reflection of this situation, I immediately considered that REBT may be an approach I could use to work with Joanne – it is an approach that has garnered significant research evidence in sport in recent years (e.g., Turner & Barker, 2013, 2014) and was an approach I had successfully used before with a client who had a long-term injury (e.g., Morris, Tod, & Eubank, 2017). The current situation had echoes of what the literature highlighted as irrational beliefs (e.g., "the worst period in my life; all my hard work over the last few years has been wasted; it is devastating; I'm devastated"), and of the previous situations I had worked in where REBT was an effective intervention for supporting injured athletes (e.g., long-term injured, experiencing reduced functioning and mood as a consequence of the injury rehabilitation process).

As a result of this needs analysis, I decided that using REBT would be the best approach to take in this instance, drawing on the framework of Turner and Barker (2014), as I had done previously. Using an REBT framework would involve a period of education around what REBT is and how thinking more rationally can help with delineating what is *actually* a crisis period from *perceptions* of what is a crisis period, followed by a period of disputation, an effective rational belief phrase, and a reinforcement phrase.

Education Phase

For the first few weeks of the intervention, Joanne and I engaged in an education phase, with the intention that at the end of this phase Joanne would be better informed about the fact that during the injury it was not the adversity (injury; A) itself that was causing the difficulties she was experiencing. Rather, it was her belief (B) about the adversity (injury) and how catastrophic it was that determined her emotional and behavioral responses (C; see Turner & Barker, 2013, 2014). To do this, I engaged in a period of information dissemination with Joanne, where we discussed the diverse ways that she could react to her injury and the benefits (and negatives) of each. In doing this, Joanne and I were able to conceptualize more clearly what is controllable (e.g., her thoughts and feelings around the injury) and uncontrollable (e.g., the pain she was feeling) in the injury rehabilitation process. From this phrase of education, Joanne indicated that she had become more aware of the fact it was not the injury itself that was causing her to experience negative emotions and behavioral responses but actually her beliefs about the injury (i.e., "the worst period in my life; all my hard work over the last few years has been wasted; it is devastating; I'm devastated") and suggested that the education phase was valuable in getting a clearer perspective on what she can and cannot control in her rehabilitation process.

Disputation (D)

The second phase of the intervention was a period of disputation, with the aim of questioning Joanne's beliefs around how catastrophic the situation she was in was. Having used the approach of the "badness scale" previously (see Ellis, Gordon, Neenan, & Palmer, 1997), I decided that this approach may be suitable in the current context as it would mean that I was able to challenge Joanne's beliefs around how bad the current situation was in relation to other – (what I would consider) more serious – situations that may occur in everyday life. To do this, I first got Joanne to rate on a scale of 0% (not bad at all) to 100% (the worst thing that could ever happen) where she would rate her current injury situation. At the point at which we engaged in this work, Joanne rated her injury situation as 80% bad. Subsequently, to try and challenge Joanne's beliefs around how bad her injury truly was, I gave her a range of adversities that she may encounter throughout her life, including stubbing her toe, being paralyzed, contracting an incurable disease, never playing sport again, losing a loved one, and losing an important match, and asked her to rate these on the same scale of 0% (not bad at all) to 100% (the worst thing that could ever happen). Joanne rated stubbing her toe at 5% bad, being paralyzed at 100% bad, contracting an incurable disease at 90% bad, never playing sport again at 85% bad, losing a loved one at 100% bad, and losing an important match at 50% bad.

After rating the elements I gave her on the badness scale, I asked Joanne if she would like to reconsider any of her ratings, in particular her injury situation. Joanne looked at me confused – "What do you mean?" I explained that the idea behind the badness scale was to get someone to reflect on truly how bad a certain situation (i.e., the injury in this context) was. "But it is bad!" came the reply. "Yes, but is it really as bad as you have indicated on here?" I responded. "Absolutely!" was Joanne's response. Joanne went on to explain that she truly believed her injury and the chances of missing out on the Olympics was 80% bad – this was something she had spent the majority of her life working toward, it was something she spent a significant amount of time in her day preparing for, and it was, at this moment in time, the most important factor in her life. Joanne explained that she felt I was patronizing her and that I did not understand her or her sport. "This is the one thing I have worked on for so long – right now it is my life! It may actually be my only chance of going to the Olympics and it could be gone. You won't change my mind on this …".

As a practitioner, I came out of this session deflated – the athlete I had spent a period of time building up a relationship with and felt I had started to do some effective work with felt I was patronizing her – ultimately harming our relationship and the work I was doing. I questioned whether or not I would be able to recover the consultancy and if I did, what I would need to do to do this. I questioned if I should change the consultancy approach I took, ditching the REBT approach for an alternative, or continue the disputation period through to its conclusion. Ultimately, I concluded, after a protracted period of reflection, that if I continued my current approach with REBT I may risk further harming a relationship which I had spent a period of time developing, especially when the client had already suggested she felt patronized by my challenging of her beliefs. Upon further reflection of the situation, I started to consider that the situation Joanne was in was, in her opinion, catastrophic. I reflected that, as a practitioner, my role is not necessarily to judge how someone is feeling, but to help and support them through their own development. This situation truly made me reflect on the value of sport to some people; even if, from the outside, something feels irrational and that it should be challenged, for some people this *is* the case.

Humanistic Counseling

After reflecting upon the approach I had previously taken when working with Joanne, both by myself and with colleagues, I decided that it may be best for me to engage in a period of humanistic counseling (see Rogers, 1959), drawing upon my natural philosophy, as a way of supporting the recovery process. In doing so, I was trying to allow the conversation to evolve from the context, allowing Joanne to discuss what was important to her at that moment in time, and then, subsequently, support her with determining her own way forward to manage these important issues. Working in this way was done with the aim of achieving self-actualization and fulfilment (see Rogers, 1951). Issues that Joanne wanted to discuss included: how she could overcome the emotional challenges she was experiencing as a result of her injury; how she could cope with the idea of missing out on the Olympic Games – something she had worked for intensely for a significant period of time and with a significant effort; why she was taking part in canoe and the importance of it for her as an individual; and how she could prepare for the possibility of not returning from her injury and having to retire (and the emotional consequences of this).

Through protracted humanistic consultancy sessions focused around these elements, Joanne was able to start to work through the challenges she was experiencing and start to make her own decisions about what was the best way forward. Decisions Joanne made included focusing on acceptance of the current situation (and the possibility of missing the Olympics) and developing a broader identity to ensure that during periods of difficulty she had other elements to her life that she could focus on. Through conversations, Joanne also discussed having a better understanding of the injury and expected recovery pathway to appease the unknowns of the process and give a realistic understanding of the outcomes. It was through these conversations that Joanne decided that she would like to have more multidisciplinary meetings about her injury rehabilitation (cf. Hess, Gnacinski, & Meyer, 2019), where all staff involved in the process would be able to give their perspectives on how the recovery was progressing.

Multidisciplinary Team Support

In addition to the humanistic support that I was providing on a one-to-one basis, therefore, it was decided that, as a group, we would make the conscious decision to meet bi-monthly, to discuss the rehabilitation and how all aspects of this process were going. Meetings included Joanne, me as the psychologist, and the physiotherapist, surgeon, and strength and conditioning coaches working with Joanne. Specifically, I discussed the emotional and psychological support being provided and how Joanne was progressing in these areas; the physiotherapist discussed the physical support around the management of the injury they were providing; the surgeon discussed the expert support they were providing on the recovery process, including stage of rehabilitation and expected recover points; and the strength and conditioning coach discussed the training program Joanne had been working to, aimed at improving and maintain physical conditioning throughout the rehabilitation process. The conversations we had as a multidisciplinary team were aimed at facilitating Joanne's understanding of where she was up to in her rehabilitation, allowing her to understand what was realistic and unrealistic at that stage, and identifying more clearly the approach she would like to take moving forward. Essentially, these meetings gave Joanne scope to make necessary decisions about her rehabilitation process and gave her an overall understanding of the process from multiple perspectives – something she did not have previously when people were working more in silos. It was also during these meetings that challenges around the rehabilitation were discussed. These included, for example, the fact that Joanne was recovering well physically, but, at times, was unwilling to push herself due to psychological fear of her injury reoccurring. This information meant that Joanne and I could work on aspects like her fear of reinjury through our humanistic support sessions.

Outcome Analysis

Joanne and I met bi-monthly for our counseling sessions throughout her 12-month injury layoff and, during alternative weeks, met with the rest of the multidisciplinary team to discuss her injury recovery. Throughout this period there were several physical and psychological challenges; there was the need to change rehabilitation program at one stage due to continued shoulder pain which was expected to subside but did not. Such changes were difficult for Joanne – she wanted to be back competing as soon as possible, but there were several delays during her rehabilitation, such as these, which hindered this. These delays meant that Joanne missed the Olympic Games and the possibility of competing for a medal, something which she had been working toward for several years. However, because of the work we were able to do with Joanne, she was able to cope effectively with these challenges, and all others that she was presented with during the rehabilitation process. Joanne reflected:

> The support provided was great because it allowed me to understand more about who I am, the injury I had, and what I could and could not do during the recovery process. I think the start was a real struggle for me because I was devastated that what I had planned for was not going to happen – I had worked half my life to get in a position to win an Olympic medal and that was just gone. I just wanted to chat about it – being "rational" was not in my thoughts. So, I struggled with that initially. But I get it now – it's not the worst thing that can happen. However, I just needed to chat about the injury and understand the process to realize that. That was the important bit. I don't think that [the REBT] was needed.

Practitioner feedback from Joanne's physiotherapist, strength and conditioning coach, and surgeon also suggested that the work that had been conducted was effective in supporting the recovery process. These staff reflected that Joanne had showed a more positive outlook on her recovery process and had been more rational in her thinking as the process moved on, dealing with challenges that cropped up throughout the rehabilitation process well. Colin (Joanne's physiotherapist) reflected:

> The process of giving Joanne more knowledge of her rehabilitation process definitely worked. Joanne went from someone who was being unrealistic and irrational in her thinking, to someone who was understanding and more accepting of what needed to be done. Keeping athletes involved can help them stay motivated, rather than them thinking that something is being done to them.

My own reflections also highlight the apparent changes that took place, which I observed when working with Joanne through her rehabilitation. One reflection, taken from my case notes, said:

> The work which has been conducted with Joanne has resulted in her appearing to be more relaxed and confident about her rehabilitation process. She

appears to be more comfortable with being injured and what is required to overcome the challenges she is facing – she also appears to have dealt with the fact she is not going to the Olympics – as devastating as it is – well.

Collectively, these reflections highlight that Joanne did experience changes in her way of thinking about the injury rehabilitation process. She appeared to become more rational, as is evidenced by both her own reflections and those of the practitioners she was working with. But it did not appear to be the REBT that was effective in this regard; rather, it seemed it was taking an alternative approach with Joanne, focused around the development of a caring and nurturing environment where she was able to self-explore that allowed this to happen. Equally, Joanne appeared to become more confident about how her rehabilitation process would progress; having a knowledge and understanding of the physical and psychological factors influencing recovery was crucial in this regard.

Critical Reflections

Sport Psychology (in Injury) Is Context Specific

As can be seen in the case of Joanne, REBT is not for everyone. The challenges outlined earlier, including the time and context within which Joanne was competing, meant that, although Joanne's beliefs were not considered "rational" to me as a psychologist, this did not matter. For Joanne at that moment in time and in that context, this truly was the worst thing that could happen. To Joanne, the injury came at a period where she was building up to the Olympic Games, a competition she had been preparing to compete at for the past decade. Competing at the Olympic Games (and potentially winning an Olympic Medal) was everything Joanne had wanted and put her effort into; it was everything those around her had been preparing for as well, doing everything they could do to help. Joanne almost felt that, in our initial conversations, I was being patronizing and did not truly understand her and her context. By behaving in this way, I did not supply the best support I could for Joanne. This situation and reflection on the case allowed me to deliberate the balance between client and practitioner and whose interests are being served and by which techniques we should support clients. In the current context, by using a previous example to drive the work I carried out with the current client, I missed the context, the pain, the suffering, and, ultimately, the challenges this athlete was going through. To this athlete, at this moment in time, it *was* the worst thing she had gone through and it *was* the hardest thing to recover from.

Importance of Broader Philosophical Understanding for Injury Support

The case of Joanne also highlights the value of understanding and drawing upon broader philosophical positions and techniques when working with athletes, depending upon their specific needs. In working with Joanne, I originally called upon REBT, derived from cognitive therapy. Over time, however, it was clear that a broader counseling-based approach was needed. In the current context, the counseling approach was used to support Joanne with the emotional challenges of the injury she had suffered. Although REBT may be useful in some contexts in disputing irrational beliefs, as was the case with Joanne, the beliefs and challenges were much deeper rooted. Sport – in particular, canoe – was Joanne's main focus in her life; she had sacrificed a lot to be in the position she was in. Although in some cases disputing the beliefs she had around canoe would provide an element of relief, as her beliefs were so engrained in her identity as an individual, it would not provide long-term relief. Only broader conversations around the purpose of what she was doing and her identity would likely provide relief, as it did in the current context. These differing approaches do require diverse ways of working and different understandings of broader philosophical approaches to sport psychology.

Use of the Multidisciplinary Team for Injury Recovery

In some instances, sport psychology can exist in silos. It is common during an injury rehabilitation process for support staff to have their own specific role and purpose. In the case of Joanne, for example, I was tasked with providing emotional and psychological support; the physiotherapist was tasked with providing physical support around the management of the injury; the surgeon provided expert support on the recovery process, including stages of rehabilitation and expected recover points; and the strength and conditioning coach was tasked with improving and maintaining physical conditioning throughout the rehabilitation process. Although existing in silos with specific purposes, the case of Joanne highlights the value of the multidisciplinary team working collectively as part of a broader support program. The bi-monthly meetings that took place were a valuable opportunity for me, as the psychologist, to gain a greater understanding of the psychological factors influencing recovery. It was only through these meetings, for example, that I was able to understand that Joanne was recovering well physically, but was unwilling to push her rehabilitation because her beliefs about the injury had made her feel so despondent and dejected about not going to the Olympic Games that she had reacted by using avoidance-focused coping, wanting to avoid anything that reminded her about the injury. This information only became apparent to me through gathering information at multidisciplinary meetings – Joanne was not as open about these feelings as she might have been in meetings we had, but the broader multidisciplinary team knew that the operation had been successful and that there were no physical concerns, but that Joanne was still not pushing herself to her full potential.

Future Research Implications

The case outlined in the current chapter raises several questions that can inform future research. First, the current case raises the need for more research to be conducted on when and why techniques such as REBT can and should be used. As is shown in the current case, REBT may be inappropriate and counterproductive to the development of an appropriate practitioner–client allegiance, making consultancy ineffective. Future research, therefore, which focuses on understanding the use of REBT in injury recovery, may help to identify when such an approach may be effective and at which time point in injury recovery this approach may be suitable. Additional practice-based evidence of "unsuccessful" consultancy will also help to generate a more nuanced and well-considered evidence-base to inform sport psychology practice.

The case of Joanne also highlights the need to understand, more broadly, the approaches that can be taken when working in injury rehabilitation, and the value of these approaches. In this case, there was a need for me, as the practitioner, to flex my approach. Research that explores, first, how, why, and when practitioners should or could flex, and, second, the skills required in this regard can help ensure that practitioners are not left unprepared should the need arise. This type of research could be supplemented by a series of case studies, where practitioners working with athletes through injury rehabilitations outline and discuss the approaches they have taken, the rationale for their approaches, and the outcomes of the work. These case studies could include, for example, a variety of philosophical underpinnings including cognitive behavioral, humanistic, narrative therapy, existential, and psychodynamic approaches. Practitioners may then be able to extrapolate from the case studies to their own contexts, identifying potential interventions that may work with clients they are working with.

Finally, the case of Joanne also outlines the need to understand more broadly the value of multidisciplinary teams in injury rehabilitation. As is outlined, the use of multidisciplinary meetings was crucial to determine what stage of recovery Joanne was at, both physically and psychologically, and identify any gaps in support or areas that needed to be changed. Research that explores the value of having multidisciplinary teams working collectively, as in this case, to support injured athletes (or explores the most effective ways of working collectively in a multidisciplinary team in this regard) can help ensure that appropriate support is being provided throughout the recovery process, maybe reducing the challenges that athletes may experience, such as irrational beliefs about their injury (cf. Hess et al., 2019).

Conclusion

In this chapter, I presented the case of "Joanne", an international canoe slalom athlete in her late twenties going through a protracted period of injury, to contextualize the challenges that there may be when trying to challenge athletes' irrational beliefs about their injury and rehabilitation process. In drawing upon (and failing) with an REBT approach, I outline the value of understanding and using, where appropriate, alternative approaches to sport psychology practice, in this case humanistic counseling as an underpinning approach with integrative multidisciplinary meetings as supplementary. In doing this, I also highlight the need to fully understand the context within which you are working. The chapter concludes with a series of critical reflections and future research considerations that emerge from the case, including the need to research when and where certain psychological interventions may be appropriate in injury rehabilitation, when the use of alternative approaches may be appropriate, and what value working in a multidisciplinary team may have to reduce negative emotional reactions to injury.

Critical Discussion Questions

1) How does the context you are working in and the background of the client influence the types of interventions you are able to use in sport psychology practice, with particular focus on the values and beliefs of the client?
2) What might be the advantages and disadvantages of being eclectic and flexible in your approach to working with athletes during injury rehabilitation and what are the ways that sport psychology practitioners (e.g., their histories, history of intervention, needs, desires, perceptions) influence service delivery processes and outcomes when working with injured athletes?
3) What advantages and disadvantages might there be to be working within a multidisciplinary team when working with injured athletes, especially when developing effective multidisciplinary interventions to support the process?

References

Brown, C. H., Gould, D., & Foster, S. (2005). A framework for developing contextual intelligence (CI). *The Sport Psychologist, 19*(1), 51–62. doi: 10.1123/tsp.19.1.51

Douglas, K., & Carless, D. (2009). Abandoning the performance narrative: Two women's stories of transition from professional sport. *Journal of Applied Sport Psychology, 21*(2), 213–230. doi: 10.1080/10413200902795109

Ellis, A., Gordon, J., Neenan, M., & Palmer, S. (1997). *Stress counselling: A rational emotive behavior approach*. London: Cassell.

Hess, C. W., Gnacinski, S. L., & Meyer, B. B. (2019). A review of the sport-injury and -rehabilitation literature: From abstraction to application. *The Sport Psychologist, 33*(3), 232–243. doi: 10.1123/tsp.2018-0043

Morris, R., Tod, D., & Eubank, M. (2017). "It's the end of the world as we know it (and I feel fine)": the use of Rational Emotive Behavioral Therapy (REBT) to increase function and reduce irrational beliefs of an injured athlete. In M. Turner & R. Bennett (Eds.), *Rational emotive behavioral therapy in sport and exercise* (pp. 220–230). London: Routledge

Rogers, C. (1951). *Client-centered therapy: Its current practice, implications and theory*. London: Constable.

Rogers, C. R. (1959). A theory of therapy, personality, and interpersonal relationships, as developed in the client-centered framework. In S. Koch (Ed.), *Psychology, A study of a science, Vol. III: Formulations of the person and the social context* (pp. 198–256). New York: McGraw-Hill.

Turner, M. J., & Barker, J. B. (2013). Examining the efficacy of rational-emotive behavior therapy (REBT) on irrational beliefs and anxiety in elite youth cricketers. *Journal of Applied Sport Psychology, 25*(1), 131–147. doi: 10.1080/10413200.2011.574311

Turner, M. J., & Barker, J. B. (2014). Using rational-emotive behaviour therapy with athletes. *The Sport Psychologist, 28*(1), 75–90. doi: 10.1123/tsp.2013-0012

16 Less Control, More Flexibility

Using Acceptance and Commitment Therapy With Injured Athletes

Sarah Cecil

Introduction

When we write stories, they should be a good read. As an applied psychologist I would back myself to "tell" good stories, whether they be fireside chats, corridor conversations, or meaningful consultancies. Writing a good story on the other hand is a whole different proposition. As a lifelong admirer of authors who sculpt a beautiful story, I hold the not uncommon dream that I have a book in me; in the meantime, please let me share my story of working with injured athletes in an intensive rehabilitation unit in Great Britain. It does have a beginning, a middle, and an end, so Mr Graham, my most memorable English teacher, will be pleased.

At the beginning of my career I worked predominantly from a cognitive behavioural therapy perspective. Currently, in the middle of my career, I predominantly use acceptance and commitment therapy (ACT). The first person to introduce me to some of the concepts behind ACT was an injured British Lion[1] (i.e., John[2]) whom I conducted my MSc dissertation on. This was back in 1997 and consisted of a "goal setting" intervention based on Vallerand's (1997) model of hierarchical motivation over an 18-week period. John not only provided me with rich data for my dissertation but more importantly provided me invaluable insight into his high-performance mindset and how to embrace the challenges of professional sport and injury. This was very early on in my professional career. Over 20 years later it still feels memorable and, like all athletes and coaches, has influenced my practice. Rereading the interview transcript it emerges that John displayed strong value-based goal setting, a willingness to experience uncomfortable thoughts and feelings, including uncertainty, pain, and fear, as well as self-awareness, a capacity to notice his thoughts, and a strong ability to be present focused. On reflection, he displayed the concept of psychological flexibility, described by Bond et al. (2011) as the willingness to remain in contact with undesirable internal experiences in the service of your values and important goals. Given the recent call for more practice-based evidence in the sport injury literature to help reduce the gap between theory and practice (Wadey et al., 2019), and considering the small evidence base of using ACT with injured athletes (e.g., Bennett & Lindsay, 2016; Mahnoney & Hanrahan, 2011), the aim of this chapter is to reflect on my experiences of utilizing ACT, and by doing so I hope to contribute to practice-based evidence.

Acceptance and Commitment Therapy: A Brief Review

ACT is recommended as a therapy for chronic pain, anxiety, and depression (Society of Clinical Psychology, 2016) and is emerging as a therapy for sport injury rehabilitation (Bennett & Lindsay, 2016; Mahnoney & Hanrahan, 2011). The basic premise for ACT is that it is not thoughts, emotions, and feelings *per se* that cause suffering, but the struggle *not* to have them. At the heart of ACT is the notion of psychological flexibility, which is described as the ability to adapt to a situation with awareness, openness, and focus and to take effective action, guided by your values (Hayes, Srosahl, & Wilson, 2011). Russ Harris (2019) in his book, *The Confidence Gap*, follows on from Phil Knight (2019) by beautifully describing ACT and psychological flexibility in a nutshell as: "be present, open up and do what matters". This is supported by Degaetano, Wolanin, Marks, and Eastin (2016) who suggest that psychological inflexibility (i.e., the act of attempting to control or eliminate uncomfortable thoughts, feelings, and sensations) may hinder the rehabilitation process. Indeed, active avoidance of negative internal experiences may be more influential on adherence to rehabilitation than the content of the internal experiences. When working with athletes, coaches, and sport science staff I would quote Russ Harris in terms of psychological flexibility and also share that the aim of ACT is to accept uncomfortable thoughts and feelings and take them along for the ride as you move forward toward what is important to you.

Starting in 2003, ACT is part of the third wave of psychotherapies, which focus more on the relationship a person has with their thoughts as opposed to the content (Hayes & Hoffman, 2017). The second wave came in the 1970s with the emergence of cognitive behavioral therapy (CBT) and the focus on changing thoughts which had followed on from the first wave of behavioral therapy that focused on the application of learning theories. A key skill/behavior when working with ACT is the acceptance of unwanted thoughts and feeling as opposed to the active avoidance or alterations of these thoughts. This acceptance is obviously easier said than done, especially in a sporting world where skill development is often focused around a deficit model in which the aim is to change incorrect movement. Thus, when trying to "land" or "sell" the concept of ACT in sport it is important to illustrate the impact of this type of therapy, which can be challenging given the limited evidence-base in sport injury psychology; more about this later, but know that the evidence of impact will always lie with the athlete, as unpicking their sporting successes will provide you with clues to their existing psychological flexibility skills. My formal introduction to ACT was in 2005 when I attended a 2-day course which helped to develop my practice, just as John had done back in 1997.

Psychological Flexibility

Time for a little more about psychological flexibility. The best paper I have read on psychological flexibility is by Kashdan and Rottenberg (2010). I highly recommend that you take a look. They view psychological flexibility as a fluid concept which unfolds over time and is dynamic in nature. They reinforce the notion that it entails being open, aware, and committed to behaviors that are congruent with personal values in a similar vein to Hayes et al. (2011). This is linked to the ability to adapt your behavior and mindset in different situations in order to not compromise social or personal functioning and encapsulates the very human skill of balancing competing desires and needs. Indeed, they fix the concept within the context that people experience: "Thus, rather than focusing on specific content (within a person), definitions of psychological flexibility have to incorporate repeated transactions between people and their environmental contexts" (p. 2). This quote for me demonstrates two things: first, that psychological flexibility is a skill which can be honed; and second, that I would view it as a verb not a noun – something we do, rather than something we are.

With regard to injury and rehabilitation, two areas of research discussed by Kashdan and Rottenberg (2010) are of particular interest to me. First, the research demonstrating correlational relationships between cardiac vagal control (CVC) and psychological flexibility. CVC is identified through beat-to-beat variability in heart rate and is linked to the parasympathetic nervous system functioning. Steven Porges's (1995) book, *Polyvagal Theory*, is a key textbook in this area. High CVC is linked to greater resiliency when faced with daily life stressors (Fabes & Eisenberg, 1997) and also to a number of constructs such as attentional flexibility (Suess, Porges, & Plude, 1994), executive functioning (Hansen, Johnsen, & Thayer, 2003), and self-regulation (Segerstrom & Solberg Nes, 2007). This collective research may suggest that we can use psychological flexibility to increase our parasympathetic activity, which may well facilitate rehabilitation both physically and mentally. Second, the description of the work done by Creswell et al. (2007) on using functional neuroimaging to observe limbic system activation when rapidly labeling thoughts as negative or positive coinciding with less openness and receptivity to ongoing thoughts and feelings. In contrast, prefrontal cortex activity is observed when there is openness, curiosity, and a shift away from judging thoughts and feelings, which coincides with a reduction in limbic activity. This links to the work done on the triune brain (Maclean, 1990) and human functioning, which has been utilized widely by applied practitioners in sport psychology predominantly for performance but also for injury in terms of understanding and managing perceptions of threat.

In summary, psychological flexibility is at the heart of ACT and at the heart of both the ACT Hexaflex and the ACT matrix. Another key element of both of these is experiential avoidance. Experiential avoidance relates to utilizing strategies to evade or escape from undesirable internal events or their antecedents. In my work I have utilized the Hexaflex more frequently within an injury context, so that is what I will focus on in this chapter. That said, I would encourage you to read the ACT matrix nonetheless as an equally usable concept. There are six key principles in the ACT Hexaflex (see Figure 16.1): Values, Acceptance, Self as Context, Cognitive Defusion, Committed Action, and Be Present. In this chapter I focus on how I utilized the ACT Hexaflex at the Team Great Britain Intensive Rehabilitation Unit (IRU). I worked at the unit for over five years from 2012 to

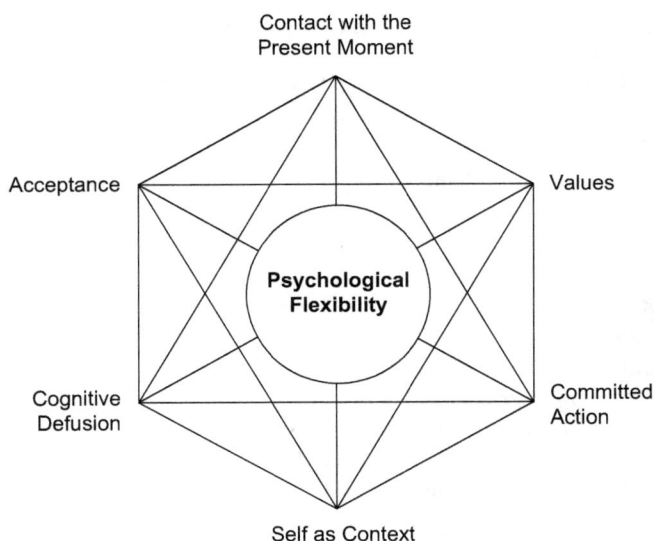

Figure 16.1 The ACT Hexaflex Model. © Steven C. Hayes. Used by permission.

2017. During this time, I did further training on ACT following on from the initial training I had done in 2005. The aim of this chapter is to give the reader an insight into applied practice and also to be open about the work I do in the field in order to provide an opportunity for athletes, practitioners, and academics to see "behind the closed doors" of professional practice and get "under the skin" of practitioners' lived experiences.

Using ACT With Injured Athletes: My Reflections

Before I reflect on my experiences, it is first important to provide some context. The IRU is based at Bisham Abbey (England) and is a residential rehabilitation unit with a full multidisciplinary team (MDT). My role there as a sport psychologist was twofold. First, to do a brief psychology assessment with the athletes on the Monday and use this to inform the subsequent work during the week. Second, to provide a psychology formulation and messaging strategy to the rest of the MDT team during the weekly case conferencing and planning for each athlete. Following the Monday screening I would then have a second consultation with the athletes on Wednesday morning in which further formulation and work would be done predominantly from an ACT perspective. The minimum contact time I had with the injured athletes was two sessions during a week. The athletes usually stayed at the IRU for between one and two weeks; some would return after a week or two back in their sports. Most of the athletes who came to the IRU would have an individual sport psychologist who they would be working with in their sport and I would make contact with the sport psychologist prior to their arrival at the IRU. I utilized the six key principles from the Hexaflex in the assessment and interventions with the athletes. The brief psychological assessment was a 45-minute case formulation process in which a series of 6 questions were asked to "unpick" the presenting state of athletes with regard to psychological flexibility and experiential avoidance (see Table 16.1). These two roles will be discussed in more depth in the following sections.

Brief Psychological Assessment With Injured Athlete

The discussion around Questions 1, 4, 5, and 6 during the brief psychological assessment would start to unearth what is important to the athlete from a wider perspective and would lead into initial conversations about values and why the athlete is choosing their sporting journey. This would build on existing information that had been fed in by their team from their sport and usually their own sport psychologist. Insights Discovery profiles were widely used across Olympic and Paralympic sports at this time and this would be an additional source of information. Using this approach I would start to gain clarity around an athlete's "why". This type of conversation was facilitated by the focus of work by Simon Sinek (2011), which was relatively commonplace across elite sport at that time.

Questions 2–6 helped to uncover acceptance/experiential avoidance and committed action. Often athletes would be focusing their actions on moving away (not always gently) from unwanted thoughts and feelings. Some athletes were fused with their thoughts, feelings, or an actual experience. Degaetano et al. (2016) suggest that psychological inflexibility may hinder the rehabilitation process. Active avoidance of negative internal experiences may be more influential on adherence to rehabilitation than the content of the internal experiences. If the athletes displayed experiential avoidance I would spend more time in the Wednesday session exploring the usefulness of this approach. Questions 2–6 further provided insight into acceptance of internal experiences. It gave insight into how well the athletes have processed key events in their injury history and rehabilitation process to date.

Table 16.1 Bespoke IRU Psychological Screening Tool

1. What one thing could we know about you that would really help you get the most out of your time at the IRU?
2. In the last two weeks do you feel that your thoughts and feelings are getting in the way of your rehabilitation?
3. Do you think it is ok to experience pain?
4. In comparison to others you know, how do you feel you are managing your rehabilitation/life?
5. Has anything changed since you knew you were coming into the IRU?
6. If you woke up tomorrow, and one thing had changed to show that you're progressing well in your rehab, what would that one thing be?

Experience has highlighted to me that this lack of processing, making sense, and acceptance of experiences to date are a key part of rehabilitation.

In terms of self as context, the ability to notice oneself and to understand what is constant about you over time and what changes is another key element of ACT. Question 1 would give an initial insight into this through the self-awareness of the athlete as well as how they spoke about themselves and their injury. In terms of being present, again, at this time, a lot of athletes were familiar with the concepts inherent in mindfulness and also would most likely have a good ability to be present when training and competing in their sports. With regard to cognitive defusion, and especially cognitive defusion exercises, these would be explored, when useful, on the Wednesday. At the end of the screening on Monday I would then create an initial formulation based on the ACT Hexaflex to share with the rest of the team and to also ask for their support in gathering more data. The intervention work would begin during the screening as the purpose of the 45 minutes was to assess where athletes were in their processing journey and to initiate the next steps, which would be further explored in the next session.

The next steps with an athlete in the IRU would be to incorporate the information gathered by the rest of the MDT on my next touchpoint with the team on the Wednesday morning briefing. This may lead to adjustment to the Hexaflex formulation and also inform the focus of my work during the next 45-minute session with the athlete. Most of the athletes had a sport psychologist working with them back in their sport, thus any work I would do would be incorporated into their existing work and I would provide guidance to their sport psychologist on any additional work that could be done post departure from the IRU.

Further Formulation and Interventions With Injured Athletes

At heart, ACT is a pragmatic therapy and thus it is always useful to explore how well the current strategies are working for the athlete. In my experience, it was also important to start with values when utilizing the ACT Hexaflex. During the Wednesday session I would frequently do a values card exercise to help unearth and highlight the values that were important to the athlete. This work also included gaining clarity on the difference between values and goals, and the importance in rehabilitation of making value-based decisions. For example, an athlete may have the goal of going to the Olympics and have a value of persistence. Goal-based decisions focused purely around the Olympics could lead to an athlete not adhering as the goal now seemed impossible because they were injured or overdoing rehabilitation exercises in order to get there. Focusing instead on the value of persistence leads an athlete to persist during rehabilitation. Obviously athletes have more than one value and the identification of these help the athlete gain clarity on how to make good decisions with the bigger picture in mind. Goals continue to be important but it is important to ensure that goals and values are congruent and alligned. This work helps uncover what the individual focus of committed actions are. From my perspective, the committed actions to emerge would be the goals which were congruent with the values of the athlete. Often further work needed to be done on self as context and acceptance to enable this.

In terms of self as context I would tend to use either the "mirror exercise" or utilize a mindfulness self as context script. The mirror exercise, which can often produce strong emotions (as much ACT work can), involves the athlete looking at themselves in the mirror as you talk through their awareness and perception of themselves over time. In general, I would ask them if they could remember what it felt like to be their age minus five years and also imagine what it might feel like to be their age plus five years. Most athletes are in the age range 18–25 so experience taught me that thinking much beyond 30 was at times hard to imagine. As well as exploring changes and consistency over time I would also ask them to share the different roles they played (e.g., as an athlete, child, sibling, friend, partner). The aim of the session is to give them insight into what is constant and also to notice how they can notice themselves and have a distance between their thoughts, feelings, and perceptions and their constant self. This is not always the "gentlest" of exercise so it was important to recognize the readiness of the athlete and their pe, rception of safety and trust in me and the team at the IRU. For neophyte practitioners these are important issues to consider when using experiential exercises and thus, as always, the therapeutic alliance needs to be built, contracting needs to be continual, and rapport has to be established. This "readiness" is hard to quantify but signs I would look out for are good eye contact, a feeling of openness and vulnerability from the athlete, a desire for change from the athlete, and signs from their body language.

The mindfulness self as context exercise is "gentler" and requires the athlete simply to follow your voice as you guide them. The script contains a mixture of a generic mindfulness exercise combined with questions about the athlete other time, context, and situation. Again, the aim is to increase the athlete's awareness of the different roles they play and to be able to notice themselves and their thoughts and emotions. Occasionally athletes who liked my voice would record the sessions and were able to play them back to continue this exercise; all would be guided to mindfulness resources that had elements of self as context.

The main aim of my interventions is to enable athletes to process thoughts, feelings, and experiences for them to move forward in their rehabilitation in a valued direction. Through experience I have found that athletes can be "stuck" in their rehabilitation process as they have not processed and/or challenged thoughts, beliefs, emotions, and experiences. In addition, many athletes arrive at the IRU in a state of threat due to their injury and other life experiences and moving them through this state of threat and into a perceived state of safety is a key component of the work done in the IRU. Once values and self as context had been explored, the next step was to do further work on the notion of acceptance in contrast to avoidance. This would emerge from further explorations of uncomfortable thoughts and feelings that the athletes were experiencing and their current strategies they were using. It was always important to tread carefully at this stage as it would be easy to start to label existing strategies as bad and new ones as the answer. It is more useful to explore whether existing strategies are still working or being of use and to discuss how these may have worked in the past but may no longer be useful. This helps to shift toward flexibility of thinking and also highlights that different strategies may serve different purposes and also that things may shift over time. Labeling strategies as good or bad can maintain avoidance as well as cognitive fusion. It was not uncommon at this time to utilize a cognitive defusion experiential exercise to explore both the notion of acceptance and also of finding a gap in fused cognitions. The two I utilized most frequently were the often-used metaphor and the monster (tug-of-war) exercise. My offer to the reader is to play around with different experiential exercises till you land on ones that make sense, work for you, and which you can deliver with conviction (and a twist of humor).

The benefits of the Hexaflex are that athletes report feeling and thinking differently quite quickly. It seems to help those who are aware of their avoidance to shift their mindset and thus be in a position to start to process their experience, thoughts, and emotions. A caveat to this is that occasionally I would unpick a sporting success as a starting point for athletes who were understandably resistant to exploring thoughts and feelings around their injury. When debriefing a successful performance, elements of the Hexaflex would often emerge, notably around acceptance, noticing without judgment, and a commitment to the bigger picture and values.

The final piece of work was around committed action, ensuring this was aligned to values and not in the pursuit of avoidance of uncomfortable thoughts and feelings. This would align with the focus of the work that the MDT team had begun formulating during the case conferencing as well as the changes that the athlete highlighted in response to Question 6 in the screening. Each session would end with gaining consent from the athlete on what they wanted to share with the rest of the IRU MDT team and then what would be written in the discharge summary, which would be sent back to the sport (including the sport psychologist). Most commonly the athletes would give consent for a more detailed debrief with their sport psychologist and this would be done verbally to support the discharge summary. The bulk of the work was brief intervention work sandwiched between the existing work of a sport psychology colleague. Some athletes were longer term and thus the focus of the work was necessarily slower in pace but with the same aim of increasing psychological flexibility.

The evidence-base for ACT and the Hexaflex is predominantly outside of sport. There is experiential practice-based evidence in my work, but future research is needed to further understand its validity and veracity. The athletes in my care were often at a vulnerable time in their journey. At times it was the first long stop on their journey; often ACT was a catalyst for the emergence of an altered story, leading to a narrative entrenched in their values and a choice to approach uncomfortable thoughts and feelings. Increasing an athlete's ability to notice their thoughts and feeling without judgment, to notice their consistent self over time, and to focus on performance-based value decision leads to a positive shift for the athletes. This was reported from various sources; never described as psychological flexibility *per se* but often as a shift in perspective, adherence, and ownership. During the week itself what was often visible to staff was the reduction in reactive behaviors and instead there was a gap between stimulus and response in which athletes were able to make conscious value-based decisions.

Future Research Implications

I am conscious that this is a single story set in a unique rehabilitation environment. As a profession it may be time to get into the consulting space in order to explore the interplay between therapeutic approach, practitioner, and athlete with regard to injury. The story above is full of potentially idiosyncratic pitfalls and further understanding is needed of real-time sport psychology with injured athletes. As a profession, the lack of observations, peer supervision, and team therapy mean that applied practice guidelines are often through the eyes of the individual practitioner. There is also often a gap between researchers and practitioners. Performance-analyzed individual case studies of sport psychologists in practice may be part of the next frontier in applied sport psychology.

Conclusion

Starting a sentence with "personally" probably breaks all types of rules, and especially in a book on critical perspectives. Nevertheless, *personally*, I have found ACT and the Hexaflex to be a consistent impacting framework in my work in rehabilitation. Promoting psychological flexibility gently facilitates the processing of experiences, thoughts, and emotions, enabling athletes to tell a different story about their injury experience and to move forward in a committed direction aligned to their values. Psychological flexibility promotes the skill of responding rather than reacting and helps athlete with injuries be best prepared for the reality they choose.

Critical Discussion Questions

1) What is the difference between values and goal setting?
2) Why is self-as-context an important concept in the psychology of rehabilitation?
3) What is the relationship between avoidance, processing of an experience, and rehabilitation adherence?

Notes

1 The British & Irish Lions is a rugby union team.
2 Pseudonym.

References

Bennett, J., & Lindsay, P. (2016). An acceptance commitment and mindfulness-based intervention for a female hockey player experiencing post injury performance anxiety. *Sport and Exercise Psychology Review*, *12*, 36–45. doi: 10.1080/16506073.2015.1098724

Bond, F. W., Hayes, S. C., Baer, R. A., Carpenter, K. M., Guenole, N., Orcutt, H. K. (2011). Preliminary psychometric properties of the Acceptance and Action Questionnaire–II: A revised measure of psychological inflexibility and experiential avoidance. *Behavior Therapy, 42*(4), 676–688. doi: 10.1016/j.beth.2011.03.007

Creswell, J. D., Way, B. M., Eisenberger, N. I., & Lieberman, M. D. (2007). Neural correlates of dispositional mindfulness during affect labeling. *Psychosomatic Medicine, 69*(6), 560–565. doi: 10.1097/PSY.0b013e3180f6171f

Degaetano, J. J., Wolanin, A. T., Marks, D. R., & Eastin, S. M. (2016). The role of psychological flexibility in injury rehabilitation. *Journal of Clinical Psychology, 10*(3), 192–205. doi: 10.1123/jcsp.2014-0023

Fabes, R. A., & Eisenberg, N. (1997). Regulatory control and adults' stress-related responses to daily life events. *Journal of Personality and Social Psychology, 73*(5), 1107–1117. doi: 10.1037//0022-3514.73.5.1107

Hansen, A. L., Johnsen, B. H., & Thayer, J. F. (2003). Vagal influence in the regulation of attention and working memory. *International Journal of Psychophysiology, 48*(3), 263–274. doi: 10.1016/S0167-8760(03)00073-4

Harris, R. (2019). *The confidence gap.* London: Robinson.

Hayes, S. C., & Hofmann, S. G. (2017). The third wave of cognitive behavioural therapy and the rise of process-based care. *World Psychiatry, 16*(3), 245–246. doi: 10.1002/wps.20442

Hayes, S. C., Strosahl, K. D., & Wilson, K. G. (2011). *Acceptance and commitment therapy: The process and pratice of mindful change.* New York: Guildford Press.

Kashdan, T. B., & Rottenberg, J. (2010). Psychological flexibility as a fundamental aspect of health. *Clinical Psychology Review, 30*(7), 865–878. doi: 10.1016/j.cpr.2010.03.001

Knight, P. (2019). *Shoe dog: A memoir by the creator of Nike.* London: Simon & Schuster.

Maclean, P. D. (1990). *The triune brain in evolution: Role in Paleocereral functions.* New York: Plenum Press.

Mahoney, J., & Hanrahan, S. J. (2011). A brief educational intervention using acceptance and commitment therapy: Faour injured athletes' experiences. *Journal of Clinical Sport Psychology, 5*, 252–273. doi: 10.1123/jcsp.5.3.252

Porges, S. W. (1995). Orienting in a defensive world: Mammalian modifications of our evolutionary heritage. A polyvagal theory. *Psychophysiology, 32*(4), 301–318. doi: 10.1111/j.1469-8986.1995.tb01213.x

Segerstrom, S. C., & Nes, L. S. (2007). Heart rate variability reflects self-regulatory strength, effort, and fatigue. *Psychological Science, 18*(3), 275–281. doi: 10.1111/j.1469-8986.1995.tb01213.x

Sinek, S. (2011). *Start with why: How great leaders inspire everyone to take Action.* London: Penguin.

Society of Clinical Psychology, American Psychological Association. Division 12.(2016)*Psychological treatments.* Retrieved from http://www.div12.org/

Suess, P. E., Porges, S. W., & Plude, D. J. (1994). Cardiac vagal tone and sustained attention in school-aged children. *Psychophysiology, 31*(1), 17–22. doi: 10.1111/j.1469-8986.1994.tb01020.x

Vallerand, R. J. (1997). Towards a hierarchical model of intrinsic and extrinsic motivation. In M. P. Zanna (Ed.), *Advances in experimental social psychology* (pp. 271–360). New York, NY: Academic Press.

Wadey, R., Roy, K., Evans, L., Howells, K., Salim, J., & Diss, C. (2019). Sport psychology consultants' perspectives on facilitating sport injury-related growth. *The Sport Psychologist, 33*(3), 244–255. doi: 10.1123/tsp.2018-0110

17 "This Is the Final Jump," I Respond. Why, Why Do I Utter Those Words?

Using Storytelling in Sport Injury Rehabilitation

Monna Arvinen-Barrow, Damien Clement, and Brian Hemmings

Introduction

The filming crew wanted to leave, and it was all down to me. Pete has been sitting bored by the ski lifts for the past two hours, AJ is too tired, and my jumps are almost impossible to get a good shot of. "Is this it," Pete asks? "Yes, this is it. This is the final jump," I respond. Why, why do I utter those words? This is the final jump of the shoot. What's more tragic is that this jump would also be the last of my career. At the top, I radio the others: "Ready?" "Yeah, go!" "3-2-1 DROP."

I drop in, speed, and approach the jump backwards. This is normal. I was born to do this! I think dying is the reason I was born. But I don't die. I survive. A fast wind catches me just as I reach the take-off. I am moving fast, so I can't feel it. I take off, start spinning. 180 degrees, ok. 360 degrees, ok. 540 degrees, ok? No. Not even close. I continue to go higher, even though the landing had already started. This is going far. Too far. Way too far. I continue spinning, and overshoot the landing. I can't stop. 1080 degrees – check, 1170 degrees – check, 1240 degrees, PAM.

Silence. Darkness. The end.

(Hyysalo, 2016, pp. 36–37)

Pekka Hyysalo was only 19 years old when he encountered a freestyle skiing accident that resulted in a life-threatening traumatic brain injury. As part of his healing, Hyysalo wrote an autobiography (Hyysalo, 2016) of his injury, subsequent rehabilitation, and journey back to life without freestyle skiing. In the book, Hyysalo explains how telling his story has helped him better cope with his injury and transition process: "I nearly drowned, but then came FightBack" (Hyysalo, 2016, p. 7).

Although Hyysalo's injury was unique in its severity and recovery, his story is one of many stories of sport injury that reflect challenge, triumph, survival, and, in his case, personal growth. By telling his story in a book, Hyysalo also contributes to the long history of storytelling. Throughout the history of humankind, stories and narratives have been used to communicate knowledge and experience between people in a variety of contexts (Burns, 2001). Dobrin (2013) argues that stories can provide a way of structuring our understanding of events in addition to helping "root us in an on-going stream of history", consequently enhancing our sense of belonging, personal growth, and identity development. Furthermore, storytelling has been used as a technique to bring about cognitive and behavioral change and to facilitate problem-solving in the therapeutic, business, education, and personal development settings (Berman & Brown, 2000; Watkins, 2001). This chapter will apply the concept of storytelling within applied sport psychology practice; specifically, in the context of sport injury rehabilitation.

Critical Reflections

Sport injuries are a worldwide phenomenon among sport participants of all ages (Conn, Annest, & Gilchrist, 2003; Konttinen et al., 2011; Maffulli et al., 2010; Uitenbroek, 1996). Since the late 1960s, researchers and applied practitioners have focused on understanding how psychological factors may contribute to sport injury occurrence, rehabilitation, and return to participation (e.g., Jackson et al., 1978; Ogilvie, 1966; Valiant, 1981). Typical psychological responses to sport injury include a range of cognitive appraisals, emotional and behavioral responses interacting in a bidirectional, cyclical manner (Wiese-Bjornstal, 2010; Wiese-Bjornstal, Smith, Shaffer, & Morrey, 1998). Consistent with the stress and coping theory (Lazarus & Folkman, 1984), these psychological responses are initiated by the athlete's injury-related cognitive appraisals (e.g., "what does this injury mean to me"). These appraisals arise from a conjoining of personal and situational factors and typically fall under one of three categories. Appraisals related to injury's impact on one's life is perceived as: (a) irrelevant (e.g., "this will not impact me in any way"); (b) benign-positive (e.g., "I needed this break from sport"); or (c) stressful ("I cannot believe this happened to me at this moment in time"; Brewer & Redmond, 2017).

Theoretically, much of the psychology of sport injury literature has been dominated by stress and coping theory, and a cognitive-behavioral perspective in general (e.g., Brewer, 1994; Wiese-Bjornstal et al., 1998; Williams & Andersen, 1998). Thus, it is not surprising that much of intervention research has also focused on testing the efficacy of cognitive-affective-behavioral techniques in sport injury rehabilitation (Hess, Gnacinski, & Meyer, 2019; Ievleva & Orlick, 1991). Interventions such as goal-setting, imagery, and cognitive restructuring have been implemented with a goal of addressing and/or modifying potentially maladaptive and harmful thought patterns, emotional and/or behavioral responses (e.g., Evans & Hardy, 2002; Evans, Hardy, & Fleming, 2000; Evans, Jones, & Mullen, 2004; Flint, 2007).

More recently, researchers have called for adopting an interprofessional and person-centered approach to sport injury rehabilitation (e.g., Arvinen-Barrow

& Clement, 2019; Hess et al., 2019; Wadey, Day, Cavallerio, & Martinelli, 2018). Such an approach calls for a humanistic, person-centered perspective to working with injured athletes, and focuses on the following fundamental factors: establishing a client–practitioner relationship, consultant genuineness, nonjudgmental caring, empathy, and the lived human experience (Hill, 2001). One way to facilitate humanistic, person-centered perspective to sport psychology consultancy is through storytelling. Considered as an established concept in a range of academic disciplines and applied practice (Laurell & Söderman, 2018), storytelling as a strategy has also become popular across different healthcare domains. However, storytelling has received limited research attention in applied sport psychology practice. This chapter, therefore, is novel in that it aims to discuss the intricacies of storytelling as applied to the context of sport injury rehabilitation.

It Is All Storytelling: In Life, in Sport, in Injury

In this chapter, storytelling is loosely defined as an interactive act of using written, oral, electronic, or visual means of communication to tell a story in an effort to enable understanding of self or a situation. In life, storytelling has formed a significant part of human history. Since the dawn of time, we as humans have used stories as a form of self-expression and as a strategy to make sense of life (Scaletti & Hocking, 2010; Ward, 2007). Stories, as told by all of us, "are an integral part of our social lives and the way in which we communicate ourselves, and indeed our identity, to the world" (Czarniawska, 2004, cited in Tompkins, 2009, p. 125).

Sport also has a long tradition of incorporating historical events, successful athlete stories, and setbacks into their communities (Davis, 2012). Take Michael Jordan, one of the greatest basketball players of all time, who, as a sophomore in high school was not selected for the varsity basketball team due to being too short (5'11") and not skilled enough. Jordan's story of how "he grew 4 inches and worked out constantly" (Poppel, 2015, 17 October), is a popular sport story told worldwide on the value of hard work, determination, and motivation.

One of the most memorable injury stories is that of a British sprinter Derek Redmond. His resilience through last minute withdrawal, due to injury, from the 1988 Olympic Games, subsequent multiple surgeries, and then the infamous hamstring injury during the 1992 Olympic Games semi-final, is a story told to highlight the importance of never stopping in the face of hardship, and even referenced in a presidential speech by President Barack Obama: "Derek Redmond bravely making it through with little help, moments of euphoria after years of hard work. Moments when the human spirit triumphs over injury that should have been impossible to overcome."

Stories Come in Different Forms, and All Shapes and Sizes

Consistent with the definition of storytelling used in this chapter, storytelling in sport injury rehabilitation can take different forms. *Written* stories can refer to injured-athlete self-narratives, diaries, journals. They can also take the form of published (auto)biographies and memoirs of athletes (e.g., Hyysalo, 2016; Newman, Howells, & Fletcher, 2016; Roy & Swift, 1998; Sparkes, 2004), educational case-studies and success stories (e.g., Arvinen-Barrow & Clement, 2019; Sachs, Tashman, & Razon, 2020), relevant religious scriptures (Waumsley, 2015), and other written texts such as letters, poems, and/or inspirational quotes.

Oral stories on the other hand can be those told verbally by the injured athlete, the applied sport psychology consultant, the sport medicine professional, teammates, peer-support group members, coaches, and significant others. Oral stories can also be *electronic*, and thus take the form of a podcast, Ted Talk, audiobook, and songs with relevant lyrics, to name a few.

> My daily treatments were awful. It was a daily reminder of being injured. Every day. For ninety solid days in a row. On day two, my athletic trainer asked me if I wanted to have music while she did manual massage on my back. I said yes. That day, I randomly chose *Feel no Pain* by Sade. Somehow it made me feel better. The next day, I was not in the mood for rehab so I said I wanted to listen to a song by The Theme Song that described my mood at the time (I can't really say the name of the song here, it is so explicit, lol). Selecting a song of the day became a game – every day I would want to listen to a different song and even educate my AT about music she had never hear of. There were Justin Timberlake days, Pink days, and at times, explicit 2Pac kind of days. And finally, *I'm Outta Here* day.

Electronic stories also overlap with *visual* stories. Sport-related movies, such as *A League of Their Own*, *Million Dollar Baby*, and *Cinderella Man*, each bring a sport injury story to life beyond the written word (e.g., Boyle, Millington, & Vertinsky, 2006). Similarly, documentaries of injury stories (e.g., Andy Murray, *Resurfacing*), and other media formats (e.g., interviews) can all become stories of education, inspiration, support, and hope for injured athletes. It is also important to recognize that visual stories can also take the form of drawings, paintings, pictures, and different forms graphic art in a range of visual platforms. Encouraging injured athletes to create different types of visual stories to make sense of their injury experience can be a powerful way to communicate and make sense of a lived experience (Bartolli, 2019).

> One of my clients loves taking pictures and uses his Instagram account to capture his days. While he was injured, we purposefully used this to summarize his injury journey each day, capturing his progress, mood, and thoughts. He named his injury Mr. Blake, the torn shoulder labrum. #MrBlake and #MrBlakeToRecovery were born. The photographic story of the injury process was very inspiring, and each day a new photo would appear on his Instagram feed to represent his injury process. In our meetings, we would then discuss and unpack these photos, and the meanings behind the images.

There Is a Power in Every Story It Provokes Thoughts, Feelings, and Actions

Storytelling serves both a biological and psychosocial function (McCann, Barto, & Goldman, 2019). Experienced and regulated by the amygdala, the part of the brain that plays a central role in social interaction, communication, and emotion recognition, stories are rooted deeply in our neural pathways. The human brain prefers a story over scientific data, and through the process of storytelling, the brain develops a connection between the storyteller and the listener (McCann et al., 2019).

From the storyteller's perspective, creating and telling a story can help organize thoughts, providing the individual with an opportunity to organize and structure the information in a meaningful way. Rutledge (2011, 16 January) argues that stories are how we as humans think and make sense of the meaning of life. Stories can help the injured athlete make sense of their injury experience, and gain an understanding of what happened, and what steps to take next in the process of healing and recovery. Storytelling also engenders a range of emotions associated with the story – ranging from anger, sadness, and anxiety to feelings of joy, excitement, and relief. Depending on how the story is listened to, this emotional process can also result in feelings of validation, understanding, and empathy, for both the storyteller (self-compassion) and the listener. Rutledge (2011, January 16) also argues that stories can provide order. Having structure and familiarity can be comforting and enables the process of systematic exploration of practical behavioral solutions to the problem at hand – in this case – the sport injury rehabilitation and recovery.

I, You, We, They: We All Have a Story to Tell

When it comes to storytelling in sport injury rehabilitation, every member of the rehabilitation team enters the rehabilitation with a myriad of personal stories that have the potential to be relevant to the injury experience. It is therefore important to recognize that the role of storyteller in the injury rehabilitation may vary, and at times the most impactful or relevant stories may come from an unexpected source.

The most obvious one, is of course, the injured athlete. Just like Hyysalo, the injured athlete holds a powerful position as the storyteller of their own narrative. The injury experience is theirs to own, and to recount, should they so choose. At the time when many athletes perceive lack of control over their bodies, knowing that their lived experience of the injury, and the story that emerges from it, is something only they can tell, can be a powerful way to regain control over their situation. Through telling their stories, injured athletes can process what has happened in a personal and meaningful way, hopefully enabling injury acceptance, and ultimately, better recovery outcomes:

> I am like, six months post-surgery now. At times I cannot believe this happened to me. I tore my ACL. I TORE my ACL. There was a time, I did not think I would make it to six months post-op. But here I am. Almost ready to go back. So close, but so far. And now I am ready to talk about it.

The applied sport psychology consultant or the sport medicine professional (e.g., athletic trainer, physiotherapist, orthopedic surgeon) working with the injured athlete can also be an impactful storyteller during sport injury rehabilitation. The personalized lived experiences from the field can be compelling (Sachs et al., 2020), particularly as a means to make a connection with the injured athlete. Using metaphors (Lindsay, Thomas, & Douglas, 2010) from other sports and past experiences to demonstrate the significance of an injury to a young patient can go a long way in changing their cognitive appraisals of the injury, and thus impacting patients' emotional and behavioral responses:

> "I would be worried if you were an Irish dancer and you had that broken toe" – says the surgeon to an anxious swimmer two weeks before state championships. "But you are not an Irish dancer, so you can train as much as your pain allows. I have seen many of these toes, and each and every one of them, have eventually healed as normal."

The Art of Storytelling

Effective stories in sport injury rehabilitation do not necessarily need to come from sport, or be injury-related. They can come from personal experiences in life and the lives of others (Gallo, 2019; Waumsley, 2015). What matters is that the story told is constructed and told in a way that allows the listener to take away meaning (Waumsley, 2015). That, in a nutshell is the art of storytelling.

Putnam (2019) outlines three specific steps for effective storytelling: Build Your Storybank, Incorporate Your Stories, and Deliver Your Stories. *Build Your Storybank* refers to the process of finding the content and sources of your stories, and outlining them in terms of the message, the source of the story, and the name of the story. *Incorporate Your Stories* refers to the process of determining whether the story will serve as (a) an illustration to follow a key message or (b) create an experience to precede a key message (Putnam, 2019). This step also asks the storyteller to determine whether the story fits within a didactic or experiential learning framework.

In *Deliver Your Stories*, Putnam (2019) highlights the intricacies of storytelling for maximum impact. Putnam highlights three main components for effective art of storytelling; keep it short, use pauses, and the importance of showing, not telling. When reviewing a masterclass on storytelling, Waumsley (2015) also emphasizes the importance of *how* stories are told – the tone, the pitch, the speed, the emotion:

> We were treated to a brief history of storytelling by Brian, who regaled stories from Freud, to modern day hairdressers; from his own youth, to the rich and famous of today, from The Bible and from sport. All were told with warmth, humour, passion, tenderness, emotion and a congruence that allowed us all to take from them whatever felt meaningful to us. This is the art – to tell a story that gets a message across; one within which there holds a powerful

metaphor to which the listener can draw a parallel between the action in it and their own lives.

(Berman & Brown, 2000; cited in Waumsley, 2015, p. 100)

Future Research Implications

In this chapter, we have highlighted the potential for using storytelling in sport injury rehabilitation in myriad ways. In doing so, we have also demonstrated that thus far, much of the evidence in support is anecdotal, or drawn from other health-care domains. Just like other active ingredients (Tod, Hardy, Lavallee, Eubank, & Ronkainen, 2019) of effective sport psychology consulting, the role for, and the use of, storytelling in sport injury rehabilitation needs to be empirically tested. Are stories used in sport injury rehabilitation? If so, what kind of stories are used? How and for what purpose are these stories used? It would also be imperative to establish the *be, know*, and *do* (Tod, Hutter, & Eubank, 2017) of effective storytelling practice from the consultants and the injured athlete perspective. What personal characteristics are viewed as effective for storytelling in sport injury rehabilitation? How effective are stories in helping the injured athletes achieve their goals and resolve their psychological concerns related to sport injury rehabilitation? How are stories and storytelling enhancing the applied sport psychology consultant's ability to provide interprofessional and athlete-centered care?

Conclusion

This chapter aimed to apply the concept of storytelling within applied sport psychology practice; specifically, in the context of sport injury rehabilitation. Traditionally used in various cultural contexts throughout history, stories and storytelling are an integral part of life, sport, and sport injury. Stories can come from numerous sources and be told by a range of individuals involved in the sport injury process. Stories can be powerful ingredients for applied sport psychology consultants, as they can connect and unite individuals to shared reality, and they "play an important role in "bringing an understanding presence that assists with the telling of the story" (Brown & de Jong, 2018, p. 41). In short, the purpose of stories, and the storyteller, is "not to tell you how to think, but to give you questions to think upon" (Brandon Sanderson, fantasy and science fiction writer; personal communicaation).

Critical Discussion Questions

1) Stories are inherently personal, cultural, and relational and often consist of individuals close to the storyteller. What, if any, ethical implications are there to consider when using storytelling in sport injury rehabilitation?
2) Since stories are predicated on individual experiences, is there a need for the applied sport psychology consultant to evaluate the truthfulness of the

content, particularly if the story relates to the injury in question and the story is used to foster acceptance of injury and its resulting outcome?

3) How can stories and storytelling fit into the medical and rehabilitation process? Can stories be used to challenge and change the intended medical and/or rehabilitation protocol?

References

Arvinen-Barrow, M., & Clement, D. (Eds.). (2019). *The psychology of sport and performance injury: An interprofessional case-based approach*. Abington, UK: Routledge.

Bartolli, A. (2019). Every picture tells a story: Combining interpretative phenomenological analysis with visual research. *Qualitative Social Work*. doi: 10.1177/1473325019858664

Berman, M., & Brown, D. (2000). *The power of metaphor: Story telling & guided journeys for teachers, trainers & therapists*. Carmarthen: Crown House Publishing Company.

Boyle, E., Millington, B., & Vertinsky, P. (2006). Representing the female pugilist: Narratives of race, gender, and disability in Million Dollar Baby. *Sociology of Sport Journal, 23*(2), 99–116. doi: 10.1123/ssj.23.2.99

Brewer, B. W. (1994). Review and critique of models of psychological adjustment to athletic injury. *Journal of Applied Sport Psychology, 6*(1), 87–100. doi: 10.1080/10413209408406467

Brewer, B. W., & Redmond, C. J. (2017). *Psychology of sport injury*. Champaign, IL: Human Kinetics.

Brown, G., & de Jong, J. J. W. (2018). Cancer storytelling: A study of well-being expressions made by patients. *Journal of Pastoral Care and Counseling, 72*(1), 37–44. doi: 10.1177%2F1542305018754796

Burns, G. W. (2001). *101 healing stories: Using metaphors in therapy*. New York: John Wiley & Sons Inc.

Conn, J. M., Annest, J. L., & Gilchrist, J. (2003). Sports and recreation related injury episodes in the US population, 1997–99. *Injury Prevention, 9*(2), 117–123. doi: 10.1016/j.jsams.2006.03.004

Davis, J. A. (2012). *The Olympic Games effect: How sports marketing builds strong brands*. New York: John Wiley & Sons.

Dobrin, A. (2013). Story-telling is necessary for human survival: We need to be part of a story no matter how shallow or manipulative it may be. *Psychology Today*. Retrieved from https://www.psychologytoday.com/us/blog/am-i-right/201308/story-telling-is-necessary-human-survival

Evans, L., & Hardy, L. (2002). Injury rehabilitation: A goal-setting intervention study. *Research Quarterly for Exercise and Sport, 73*(3), 310–319. doi: 10.1080/02701367.2002.10609025

Evans, L., Hardy, L., & Fleming, S. (2000). Intervention strategies with injured athletes: An action research study. *The Sport Psychologist, 14*(2), 188–206. doi: 10.1123/tsp.14.2.188

Evans, L., Jones, L., & Mullen, R. (2004). An imagery intervention during the competitive season with an elite rugby union player. *The Sport Psychologist, 18*(3), 252–271. doi: 10.1123/tsp.18.3.252

Flint, F. A. (2007). Modeling in injury rehabilitation: Seeing helps believing. In D. Pargman (Ed.), *Psychological bases of sport injuries* (3rd ed., pp. 95–108). Morgantown, WV: Fitness Information Technology.

Gallo, C. (2019). Storytelling to inspire, educate, and engage. *American Journal of Health Promotion, 33*(3), 469–472. doi: 10.1177/0890117119825525b

Hess, C. W., Gnacinski, S. L., & Meyer, B. B. (2019). A review of the sport injury and rehabilitation literature: From abstraction to application. *Journal of Applied Sport Psychology, 33*(3), 232–243. doi: 10.1123/tsp.2018-0043

Hill, K. L. (2001). *Frameworks for sport psychologists.* Champaign, IL: Human Kinetics.

Hyysalo, P. (2016). *FightBack: Toinen mahdollisuus [FightBack: Second chance).* Helsinki: Tammi Publishers.

Ievleva, L., & Orlick, T. (1991). Mental links to enhanced healing: An exploratory study. *The Sport Psychologist, 5*(1), 25–40. doi: 10.1123/tsp.5.1.25

Jackson, D. W., Jarrett, H., Barley, D., Kausch, J., Swanson, J. J., & Powell, J. W. (1978). Injury prediction in the young athlete. *American Journal of Sports Medicine, 6*(1), 6–14. doi: 10.1177/036354657800600103

Konttinen, N., Mononen, K., Pihlaja, T., Sipari, T., Arvinen-Barrow, M., & Selanne, H. (2011). Urheiluvammojen esiintyminen ja niiden hoito nuorisourheilussa – Kohderyhmänä 1995 syntyneet urheilijat [Sport injury occurence and treatment in youth sports – Athletes born in 1995 as a target population]. *KIHUn julkaisusarja nro, 25 (PDF-julkaisu),* 1–16. Retrieved from http://www.kihu.jyu.fi/tuotokset/haku/index.php?hae=Tee+haku#TOC2011

Laurell, C., & Söderman, S. (2018). Sports, storytelling and social media: A review and conceptualization. *International Journal of Sports Marketing and Sponsorship, 19*(3), 338–349. doi: 10.1108/IJSMS-11-2016-0084

Lazarus, R. S., & Folkman, S. (1984). *Stress, appraisal, and coping.* New York, NY: Springer Publishing Company.

Lindsay, P., Thomas, O., & Douglas, G. (2010). A framework to explore and transform client-generated metaphors in applied sport psychology. *The Sport Psychologist, 24*(1), 97–112. doi: 10.1123/tsp.24.1.97

Maffulli, N., Giuseppe Longo, U., Gougoulias, N., Caine, D., & Denaro, V. (2010). Sport injuries: A review of outcomes. *British Medical Bulletin, 97,* 47–80. doi: 10.1093/bmb/ldq026

McCann, S., Barto, J., & Goldman, N. (2019). Learning through story listening. *American Journal of Health Promotion, 33*(3), 477–481. doi: 10.1177/0890117119825525e

Newman, H. J. H., Howells, K. L., & Fletcher, D. (2016). The dark side of top level sport: An autobiographic study of depressive experiences in elite sport performers. *Frontiers in Psychology, 7*(868). doi: 10.3389/fpsyg.2016.00868

Ogilvie, B. C. (1966). *Problem athletes and how to handle them.* London, UK: Pelham.

Poppel, S. (2015, 17 October). Michael Jordan didn't make varsity – At first. *Newsweek.* Retrieved from https://www.newsweek.com/missing-cut-382954

Putnam, L. (2019). How to be a storyteller (even if you think you're not). *American Journal of Health Promotion, 33*(3), 472–475. doi: 10.1177/0890117119825525c

Roy, T., & Swift, E. M. (1998). *Eleven seconds: A story of tragedy, courage, & triumph.* New York: Grand Central Publishing.

Rutledge, P. B. (2011, 16 January). The psychological power of storytelling: Stories leap frog technology, taking us to authentic experience. *Psychology Today.* Retrieved from https://www.psychologytoday.com/us/blog/positively-media/201101/the-psychological-power-storytelling

Sachs, M., Tashman, L. S., & Razon, S. (Eds.). (2020). *Performance excellence: Stories of success from the real world of sport and exercise psychology.* Lanham, MD: Rowman & Littlefield.

Scaletti, R., & Hocking, C. (2010). Healing through story telling: An integrated approach for children experiencing grief. *New Zealand Journal of Occupational Therapy, 57*(2), 66–71.

Sparkes, A. C. (2004). Bodies, narratives, selves, and autobiography: The example of Lance Armstrong. *Journal of Sport and Social Issues, 28*(4), 397–428. doi: 10.1177/0193723504269907

Tod, D., Hardy, J., Lavallee, D., Eubank, M., & Ronkainen, N. (2019). Practitioners' narratives regarding active ingredients in service delivery: Collaboration-based problem solving. *Psychology of Sport and Exercise, 43*, 350–358. doi: 10.1016/j.psychsport.2019.04.009

Tod, D., Hutter, R. I. V., & Eubank, M. (2017). Professional development for sport psychology practice. *Current Opinion in Psychology, 16*, 134–137. doi: 10.1016/j.copsyc.2017.05.007.

Tompkins, A. (2009). "It was a great day when…": An exploratory case study of reflective learning through storytelling. *Journal of Hospitality, Leisure, Sport and Tourism Education, 8*(2), 123–131. doi: 10.3794/johlste.82.198

Uitenbroek, D. G. (1996). Sports, exercise, and other causes of injuries: Results of a population survey. *Research Quarterly for Exercise and Sport, 67*(4), 380–385. doi: 10.1080/02701367.1996.10607969

Valiant, P. M. (1981). Personality and injury in competitive runners. *Perceptual and Motor Skills, 53*(1), 251–253. doi: 10.2466/pms.1981.53.1.251

Wadey, R., Day, M., Cavallerio, F., & Martinelli, L. (2018). The multi-level model of sport injury: Can coaches impact and be impacted by injury? In R. Thelwell & M. Dicks (Eds.), *Professional advances in sports coaching: Research and practice* (pp. 408–440). Abingdon, UK: Routledge.

Ward, R. S. (2007). Physical therapy: Stories that must be told. *Physical Therapy, 87*(11), 1555–1557. doi: 10.2522/ptj.2007.presidential.address

Watkins, J. (2001). *Adventures in human understanding: Stories for exploring the self.* Carmarthen: Crown House Publishing Company.

Waumsley, J. A. (2015). Masterclass in applied sport psychology – 'Being creative in your practice: using storytelling with athletes'. *Sport and Exercise Psychology Review, 11*(1), 100–101.

Wiese-Bjornstal, D. M. (2010). Psychology and socioculture affect injury risk, response, and recovery in high-intensity athletes: A consensus statement. *Scandinavian Journal of Medicine and Science in Sports, 20*, 103–111. doi: 10.1111/j.1600-0838.2010.01195.x

Wiese-Bjornstal, D. M., Smith, A. M., Shaffer, S. M., & Morrey, M. A. (1998). An integrated model of response to sport injury: Psychological and dociological dynamics. *Journal of Applied Sport Psychology, 10*(1), 46–69. doi: 10.1080/10413209808406377

Williams, J. M., & Andersen, M. B. (1998). Psychosocial antecedents of sport injury: Review and critique of the stress and injury model. *Journal of Applied Sport Psychology, 10*(1), 5–25. doi: 10.1080/10413209808406375

18 Textbooks Don't Tell It Like It Is

Tales From Working in the Field With Injured Athletes

Renee Newcomer Appaneal

Introduction

The reality of applied work, particularly that which occurs in elite sport and within a multidisciplinary support team environment, is complex and dynamic. Most of the time this work is wonderfully rewarding, yet it can also be a complicated, uncomfortable, and unsustainable situation from which one needs to escape! Textbooks provide information on basic elements of professional practice, or what consulting involves. These resources are generally aimed at enhancing declarative knowledge, or awareness and understanding of factual information; though applying one's expertise in any situation requires contextual intelligence, or knowing how to practice (Brown, Gould, & Foster, 2005). And how to "do" sport psychology, especially at the pointy end of elite sport, reflects a craft that is purposefully developed. This does not simply accumulate over time or with mere exposure, rather it requires active intentional reflection to promote learning and growth. A few adverse experiences along the way do a great deal to remind (and at times force) us to pause and reflect, and perhaps reconsider how we work.

I have worked with athletes dealing with injury and illness for nearly 25 years within a multidisciplinary rehabilitation setting, but also while on tour with teams competing at international events. As I reflect upon these roles, there is a complex mix of emotions. Overall, I believe my work with athletes and their support teams has been effective, but there are experiences that I am not sure about. It would be easier (and preferable) to share only the "success" stories. Instead, I will describe some of the more uncomfortable experiences I've had providing support to athletes with injuries, which is an area I consider to be lacking in the applied sport psychology literature. In this chapter, I present three vignettes: "In Staging Camp with Tonya", "Getting Steve Back to the Snow", and "Educating Eloise". For ethical reasons, I use pseudonyms and have employed certain safeguards to preserve the anonymity of the athletes concerned. Following these vignettes, I share my reflections and my "survival pack" to help me navigate difficult situations like these. The chapter closes with future research directions and critical discussion questions.

Setting the Scene

Before jumping into the vignettes, I provide a quick snapshot of my background, professional philosophy, and most frequently used frameworks – all of which inform my practice. My hybrid background includes graduate and post-graduate training in exercise and sport science, counseling, clinical and health psychology, and behavioral medicine. I work from an integrated sport science perspective, which, among other areas, considers psychosocial and behavioral aspects in addition to medical, nutritional, physiological, biomechanical, motor development, and learning and skill acquisition.

My professional philosophy involves a foundational belief that people are generally doing the best they can in whatever circumstances they are dealing with at the time. I aim to work collaboratively with an athlete, as equal partners, toward mutually agreed-upon objectives. I view psychology as integral to both health and performance, and seek to provide a service that enhances well-being, promotes mental health, and strives toward excellence. I do not consider health and performance as dichotomous goals; however, I respect others' preferences to separate them and appreciate the situations that create tension between them. For example, when faced with a career- or life-threatening health condition, there is a palpable tension between, on the one hand, the longevity of health and long-term quality of life and, on the other, the more short-term and short-lived performance goals.

The frameworks that guide my work are an eclectic and intentional mix based upon the person and situation and what resonates with us at the time. These include: behavior change and readiness; stress, health, and performance; biopsychosocial models of injury/illness; stress-recovery (im)balance; performance psychology (e.g. characteristics of excellence, expertise/talent development); psychological skills training (e.g. self-regulation of attention and arousal); functional equivalence of motor imagery (physical, environment, task, timing, learning, emotion, perspective: PETTLEP); group/organisational dynamics, social networks, and complex systems; acceptance and commitment therapy (ACT; see Chapter 16), dialectical behavioral therapy (DBT); and mindful-based cognitive behaviour therapy (CBT; see Chapter 15); self-compassion; and neuroscience of (therapeutic) relationships. A detailed review of these is not the aim of this chapter, but readers are encouraged to investigate any that seem useful or perhaps are completely unknown.

In Staging Camp With Tonya

Tonya was an experienced athlete in her mid-twenties and lived in a different city from where I lived and worked as a sport psychologist. I only met her a few times during the previous year but had heard she sustained a major injury two years prior. I had spoken over the phone with her physiotherapist who was concerned Tonya's anxiety was limiting her progress now that they were doing more functional movements. Her physiotherapist had frequently encountered patients with kinesiophobia and was intrigued how anxiety showed up in the body. I suggested a few resources (e.g., Van der Kolk, 2015), and recommended she consult with a psychologist herself, especially as Tonya was not working with anyone.

I knew very little about Tonya's injury or rehabilitation beyond what her physiotherapist had disclosed with her permission. I knew only that she was medically cleared and had been to a few smaller events earlier that year. At the time, she was in the final week of preparation for her first competition since her injury two years prior, and I was the team psychologist. Tonya had not worked with a psychologist during her rehabilitation, or much at all really. However, as a senior member of the team, we had attended the same events that year and enjoyed informal, brief interactions with tones of sarcasm and lighthearted verbal sparring.

One day after training, she asked to meet with me. During our first consultation, Tonya and I chatted about how she was feeling with just over a week until her first major competition back after the injury. She admitted to being fearful that she would get injured again and not be able to compete, as had happened the last time. With an intention to both normalize her fears and reassure her, I validated her feelings but then pointed out that it was highly unlikely for the same thing to happen again. Unaware of this at the time, my well-intentioned reassurance probably only served to invalidate her worries. This realization only came to me when reflecting on our session later. As our conversation continued, we talked about her desire for control, and compared the situation to being a passenger on a plane during turbulence. We joked that the plane was not going to crash, and she was finding it really uncomfortable not to be flying the plane herself. We had a good laugh, and she seemed to relax a little. My sense at the time was that we had connected quite well and that our brief chat was helpful. As the days went on, we had a few more brief contact interventions, again revisiting her fears and desire for control.

One afternoon while I was in the medical staff area chatting to a coach about his athletes, a team member ran over to tell the doctor that Tonya had just injured herself. My stomach dropped immediately. I looked over to see her being carried into the medical tent. Despite feeling horrible, I tried to remain calm and merely observe how she seemed while being assessed by the doctor. She described the same sensations and sounds as the last injury. The doctor informed her she would need to be taken to the hospital for a magnetic resonance imaging (MRI) scan. This scan would later confirm what everyone feared – that it was happening to her, again. As preparations to leave were made, we looked at each other in disbelief. She nervously laughed through tears and said, "The plane is going down, again."

As she left for the hospital, I stayed back in the medical tent in case the other staff wanted to debrief what had just happened, as a few of them had known Tonya for a while and had been on the team with her when she was injured two years ago. I don't recall too much about that evening, other than I felt completely incompetent. I beat myself up a good while for joking with Tonya about how it could not possibly happen again. Why did I try to predict the future, in an attempt to reduce her discomfort about a re-injury? It's as if I was in control, the pilot in the cockpit in charge of the plane.

I remained at the competition venue that day trying to focus on supporting the other athletes who were still preparing and competing shortly. After a few hours, I received a message to chat from the team manager. When we met up, he looked quite worried. He informed me that Tonya was leaving the hospital now, and that I should get back to the hotel to meet her. I was initially surprised, as there were plenty of other athletes requesting support at the venue. However, I reluctantly packed up my stuff and headed back to the hotel. When I arrived, athletes were gathering in the dining hall. I grabbed some food and sat down at a table with a few other senior athletes. Tonya entered on crutches, and as the saying goes, you could hear a pin drop. Complete silence. After grabbing some food, she hobbled over to the table and sat down at the table with her friends and peers right next to me.

I sat at the table for a while, feeling that my support services were not really required there and wished that I had remained at the venue. In the moment, I felt pretty helpless and sad for Tonya and what this meant for her career. I was also frustrated with the team manager telling me what to do (i.e., meet Tonya at the hotel vs. remain at the venue). I felt my presence in the dining room was limiting the support she might have organically received from friends and teammates. I watched how other athletes reacted to seeing her. Many were stunned and most did not talk to her directly, despite being on teams together for years. One athlete was trying to get my attention, and when Tonya turned to speak to someone behind her, he shrugged his shoulders with a thumbs up then a thumbs down, asking what the MRI results had been. I had already been told by the manager that Tonya's competition was over, and she would be out for at least another year. I gave the thumbs down to let him know it wasn't a good outcome. The athlete just sat quiet and stunned. I felt a bitter sadness that this athlete had turned to me rather than asking Tonya directly about the diagnosis and/or prognosis. Fortunately, at this same time, another senior athlete entered the dining room, placed his tray on the table and immediately came over to give her a big long hug – no words exchanged, just physical comfort. I felt such gratitude for witnessing such a simple but authentic gesture, especially as others sat quiet or even avoided her.

Despite my own discomfort, I remained at the table. We all chatted awkwardly about the situation, and various unrelated topics that came up. As athletes continued to enter the dining hall, several wanted to show their support, so she had a steady stream of attention and remained at the table for quite a while. Arrangements had been made for her roommate to sleep in another room, as she was competing the next day. I could see Tonya was tired, and I privately commented to her on what I suspected to be a reluctance to go up to her room alone that night. She smiled slightly, which suggested she was avoiding it but quickly indicated she would be okay. I reminded her to reach out if she needed it, and we made plans to catch up early evening the following day. We both knew that lying in bed that night by herself would be really tough. In fact, I had a lot of trouble falling asleep that night and several subsequent nights, as my brain worked overtime trying to make sense of what had happened, my thoughts rewinding and replaying over and over our prior conversations and future scenarios for how to support her and what to say.

Over the next few days, I met with Tonya when she requested it and did not force myself to hang around otherwise. Outside of this, I focused on the other athletes and looked after my own well-being by exercising and shrinking my sleep deficit. Before bed, I listened to short podcasts (i.e., Pema Chodron) to help quiet and slow down the rumination.

Well after the tour ended, and through a lot of formal and informal supervision, I realized how preoccupied I was at the time with my "foot in mouth" failure. My insecure self and negative inner critic hijacked my attention, leaving little to give others, such as Tonya's coach or other staff who were also struggling (see Chapter 10). I had no empathy for the team manager at the time, and instead became irritated and felt disrespected when he told me how to do my job. In hindsight, his helplessness perhaps meant he tried to exercise what little control he felt he had in the situation by telling me what to do. However, I now know I did the best I could to support Tonya and the other athletes during that time.

Getting Steve Back on the Snow

Steve was a young elite skier admitted to our multidisciplinary rehabilitation center. This was his first severe injury, which would result in missing most of the racing season one year prior to the winter Olympic Games. Steve spent the first few days onsite familiarizing himself with the campus, his support team, and the daily schedule. We spent three sessions during the first two weeks completing the intake and orientation process and agreeing upon psychological aspects of his rehabilitation goals. Two of our objectives were to minimize his future thinking about the next year and Olympic qualifying and integrate healing imagery into his rehabilitation program.

Steve had well-developed imagery skills, which he had refined using mental rehearsal since he first started racing internationally. It was rather straightforward to apply these skills to healing imagery, making use of his scans and the models and illustrations provided by the physiotherapist and doctor. He was eager to be "doing" something and considered imagery during the early phases of rehabilitation very helpful. In terms of future thinking, we identified that staying in the present moment allowed him to be fully absorbed in his skiing while flexibly attending and responding to relevant cues on the hill during a race. Given the role of present-moment awareness in competition, it seemed intuitive to bring this into rehabilitation. Steve wasn't initially sold on the idea but agreed to give it a go during a few specific exercises he found rather difficult in rehabilitation. Over the next several weeks, he maintained a regular and formal practice of noticing his attention, and gently bringing it back to the movements and sensations of the most challenging exercises.

As he continued this practice, he would share situations when his thoughts became distracting, or he found himself stressed out about future "what ifs" playing through in his mind. Often these were happening after a conversation with his coach. Recently, they had been discussing various scenarios of where they could go to train based upon when he got back on the snow and next year's race calendar. I used these opportunities to discuss how he reacted and to identify the reoccurring thoughts and sensations that would arise in these situations. Unfortunately, I began to suspect that the coach's anxiety about the upcoming Olympic year was being transferred onto Steve; they would have these private planning sessions to talk through the calendar and potential plans based on hypothetical timeframes, some of which did not reflect the progression given to both of them by the rehabilitation support team. Steve's own anxiety about the upcoming Olympic Games, along with the disappointing performance he had at the previous Games, made it difficult for him not to react. He began avoiding his coach and changing the topic to deter the conversation from looking too far ahead into the future. I had little contact with Steve's coach, so we continued to focus on the reactions he had to these meetings, and when similar thoughts and sensations came up in rehabilitation.

We continued working with defusion, contact with the present moment, and values clarification, all core principles of acceptance and commitment therapy (ACT; see Chapter 16). We explored situations where unhelpful thoughts (e.g., future planning, what ifs) and unwanted sensations (e.g., fear and worry) came up, and discussed ways to make space for them when they arise so we can consciously and deliberately choose to respond rather than react to them with choices and actions that align to what is important and meaningful. Steve and I continued to work together toward our objectives, meeting once or twice per week over the next few months of his rehabilitation.

As part of the multidisciplinary team, we often have fortnightly roundtable meetings to share observations of how the athlete is progressing and discuss challenges encountered or ones we anticipate in the coming days or weeks in progressing the rehabilitation program. Usually these are formal meetings with everyone in attendance, but when the clinic is busy we aim to find time for informal catch-ups. The last month had been very busy for a lot of the staff who also worked with sports in addition to their roles in the rehabilitation center. As a result, Steve's support team had not met as often as originally planned, but a few of us would catch up when we had a few spare moments. I was seeking to have one of these quick catch-ups and headed into the clinic, where Steve's physiotherapist and strength and conditioning coach were laughing. The physiotherapist proceeded to let me in on the joke. Steve had been given new exercises this week as part of a planned progression, which he was finding very difficult. Every time he completed them, he moaned and yelled out in pain so loudly that everyone in the clinic would stop and stare at him. Both staff members laughed again as the story was retold to me. I smiled but did not say a word, as I felt it strange that Steve had not mentioned these painful exercises to me, despite our frequent conversations about what he found difficult in rehabilitation. Considering the number of times Steve and I had met in the previous weeks, I felt as if I did not know what was actually happening. I stood there in silence, feeling stupid. I pushed down my self-doubt and insecurities and asked them both how they thought Steve was coping with the program. The physiotherapist proceeded to complain that Steve was very anxious and lacked confidence in the movements introduced as rehabilitation was progressed. He described Steve as a high-strung Type-A personality, which was at times difficult to communicate with during appointments. He looked at me almost incredulously and asked, "Has Steve been working with you this whole time?" I nodded yes but did not say anything in response. The physiotherapist quickly stated that once Steve was progressed further and began functional movements, he would get his confidence back and hopefully relax a little bit. The strength and conditioning coach nodded in agreement as he walked out of the clinic to return to the gym. I stood for a moment pondering what they had said, and eventually returned to my office to debrief it with a colleague.

If an athlete continues to have anxiety despite working regularly with a psychologist, it is too easy to assume this is the psychologist's failure. Further reflecting upon what the physiotherapist had said, the prognosis of Steve's confidence being restored when physical movement returned to "normal" was an assumption, commonly made, that emotional recovery follows physical recovery. Was this to let me off the hook in some way, perhaps to make me feel less of a failure or to communicate that psychology (me) was an unnecessary part of Steve's recovery? The focus of ACT is not on symptom reduction but rather to connect with people and engage in activities that are personally meaningful when difficult experiences arise. While this is known by those with ACT training (see Chapter 16), it is largely unknown to non-psychologists, including sport science and medical staff. Further, the idea that psychological support would seek to reduce anxiety contradicts well-established notions of what we do – help people feel better, as evidenced by reduction of symptoms. While Steve and I had an effective working relationship, I realized that we had not considered the broader social context in which he was rehabilitating, namely the attitudes and behaviors of his physiotherapist and his coach.

Educating Eloise

Eloise was a young football player admitted to the multidisciplinary rehabilitation center after her sport's rehabilitation staff had been unable to progress her recent injury and get her back on the pitch. She was well-known as an incredibly dedicated athlete and well-respected by her coaches and peers as a hard worker. Not surprisingly, she did not do "nothing" very well when told to just rest following surgery. In contrast to the surgeon's instruction, but in direct reaction to her own desire to return to the pitch, she had doubled up on exercises and skipped the recovery room following rehabilitation and gym sessions. I met with Eloise when she was first admitted, but it was clear during the intake appointment she was not interested in working with me. I did not immediately see this as a problem and trusted I could build rapport through accepting her perspective and working with what she was willing to give in the session.

I asked Eloise about her prior experiences with injury and returning to sport both at a participation level but also in terms of readiness to return to competition.

I had heard some of this history from my colleagues when she arrived in the center. She had multiple prior injuries over the last eight to ten years that she had returned from, but probably never back to full health and definitely not competition-ready. She described in her own words feeling like she never had enough time to get back, and described situations that to me appeared to suggest she had returned prematurely and/or was not progressed safely. This can occur for a number of reasons, such as when an athlete is not open or honest about pain (see Chapter 5) and recovery following each progression, hiding signs or sensations that might indicate the need to slow down their progression. This can also happen when gaps occur in the continuity of care or communication across providers. For example, an orthopedic specialist might discharge an athlete following a post-surgery follow up and imply readiness to return to sport, which unintentionally makes it difficult for the coach and medical team to agree on what is required to safely transition back to movement, sport training, and, eventually, competition. There can also be a limited handover, or none, between a doctor or physiotherapist and other sport staff or coaches, such as when the athlete spends less time in the clinic and more time in the gym or on the field. Regarding Eloise's situation, she did not have much respect for the physiotherapist on the national team, and it was apparent she did not think the medical and sport coaches communicated frequently enough, or when they did that it was poor at best. My take was she did not feel supported by her medical team and was disappointed in how she re-entered the team's training environment. This perhaps also suggested she expected her experience and transition from rehabilitation back to sport might be better this time because it was being managed by us at the center not by her sport's staff.

When I explained my role and how I work as part of the rehabilitation support team, she smiled while saying quite matter-of-factly she did not think that psychology support would be relevant or important to her recovery and return to sport. I asked about her prior experience with psychology, and she described performance-focused support which she did not find useful when competing and actually did not trust as a safe and supportive outlet for dealing with challenging team dynamics. She had prior interactions with sport psychologists that were limited (only performance-based) and unhelpful – not surprisingly, she did not book in to see me again.

I was not deterred by Eloise's reluctance to work with me, given her prior experiences. She would be on site for a while, and I could provide indirect support to other staff working with her initially. At our first roundtable meeting, I provided a brief summary of my intake evaluation and indicated I did not expect her to meet with me regularly at first. I then offered strategies that would demonstrate explicitly (rather than as an assumption) that we valued honest and regular communication and placed her central to any health-related decisions, and we discussed how the way we worked as a coordinated and integrated team would show her how things would be different under our care.

Although I had not been meeting with Eloise, I was working with a number of other athletes at the center, frequently catching up with staff and staying across what was happening with each of the athletes under our care during roundtable meetings. Eloise was beginning to shift into harder and more intense activities to regain strength in her injured knee while maintaining a high level of fitness. After a few weeks, she was getting frustrated. For example, during the clinic sessions and with one of the sport staff in the gym, she complained we were not progressing her quickly enough to be ready by the team selection deadline.

During our next roundtable meeting, a few of the staff were complaining that she was pushing too hard and trying to take on too much too soon, without adequate rest and recovery. They urged me to meet with her, yet when I asked if anyone had suggested that to Eloise, no one had. I noticed a little resentment, which may have been about me not pulling my weight on the team. Now that Eloise's emotions were getting in the way (or more likely that these were uncomfortable for them to deal with), I needed to step up and take care of it. I am not a fan of mandated psychology sessions, and I suspected they wanted me to "fix" this, hoping that my involvement would magically enable their work with her to be easier or more effective than it was at the moment. They were quick to raise these observations with me and want me to take action but had not mentioned or discussed this with the athlete – who was supposedly central to her own healthcare. Problematic emotions showing up? Psychologist to the rescue!

It is nice to feel needed, but to prevent myself from jumping to the rescue and to avoid falling into a trap I had been caught up in earlier in my career, I instead reminded my colleagues that she did not want psychology support initially but maybe would be willing to give it a go now. If she was not willing, then they would need to give her good reasons to try it now. This was a perfect opportunity for them to demonstrate open and honest feedback as well as involve her in her own care. We discussed how to share their observations of her frustration, and if comfortable, admit to feeling frustrated as well, and agreeing to work together to address it. If they felt my services would be helpful, then suggest that to her, and explain why you are recommending it. I provided them with a few specific examples of things we could work on that reinforced the role of psychology in health and healing (e.g., holistic physical and psychological recovery to enable safe progression of rehabilitation, anxiety about not being ready in time for team selection, prior disappointment and distrust of medical staff in safely and sufficiently preparing her to return at a high level). I also challenged them to consider what they might say if she refused to meet with me, and we role-played a few possible scenarios.

I revisited what I had shared during our first roundtable meeting. Essentially, if we suspect her prior care had likely been mishandled and/or mismanaged in the past, then she may not know what a safe and sufficient rehabilitation program looked like, nor may she have been expected or invited to be actively engaged in her own programming. We needed to be transparent with her about where she was at, what milestones she was achieving, and what was required before progressing, as well as seek her feedback on and engagement in planning each week throughout the process.

After a week or so, Eloise booked in and I considered this a chance to show her where psychology fitted into restoring health and how it was not just about competition performance. I provided an example of how even normal and expected worries can interfere with sleep, pressure us to overlook the boring but basic activities (such as the stretches or recovery sessions she rushed through or skipped) and preference what seems more interesting or relevant at the time (sport-specific activities which she was only to do on a limited basis, and alternating days). She seemed intrigued enough to hear more and admitted to having not always followed the agreed weekly plan as indicated (i.e., regular recovery sessions, limited sport-specific training). I had opened the door, and she was walking in, albeit cautiously I'm sure. I continued psychoeducation on the importance of rest to facilitate healing (the invisible "work" required before the familiar and observed work can begin), and the concepts of active and passive recovery. This was interspersed with opportunities for her to ask questions, or even challenge some of the science, and explore her beliefs about recovery and rest. We talked about her prior injuries, and situations where she may have pushed return to training and competition too quickly, and a few times where she withheld or minimized signs of fatigue that may have indicated rehabilitation was not ready to progress. We also explored her distrust and disappointment in her body and in her rehabilitation team at the time. These experiences probably contributed to her ignoring or underreporting signs of fatigue that may have actually indicated the need to rest or alter activities rather than progress to more training on-field and in the gym – the latter being where she desperately preferred to be.

Over time, and with a lot of careful challenging (with humor), she continued to book in and made space for openness and transparency about what she was doing (or not) day by day, and what she was finding difficult to do (willingness to be supported and participate in the agreed plan). She was also willing to re-familiarize herself with her body and reexamine her reactions, almost learning to respond in a different manner to sensations that were maybe undesirable but very relevant and important to share with the support team so as to effectively adjust and progress the program each week.

Critical Reflections

As I critically reflect on my experience with Tonya, I become increasingly aware that insecurities are normal and how important it is to find ways to acknowledge and accept them. Showing compassion toward oneself frees us up to empathize with others in shared difficult experiences. In addition to self-compassion, we can also show compassion from acknowledging athletes' own personal views and beliefs that may be unhelpful to their health and recovery. For example, the relationship an athlete has with his or her body may be seen through the meaning and response given to physical sensations, such as ignoring or amplifying what is being experienced or what is to be expected (see Eloise's vignette). Athletes may be encouraged to redefine the connection to their physical self and view the body as a valuable partner which communicates relevant information to inform how healing and rebuilding is going (e.g., Hefferon, Grealy, & Mutrie, 2010), particularly when so much is demanded from it in elite sport. Further, athletes' responses to injuries are simply not good or bad, positive or negative, but complex and dynamic (Day & Wadey, 2017). Athletes will also hold unhelpful attitudes, about their bodies and the degree of control they desire over how to move, think, and feel. This is not a desire unique to athletes, it is universal to being human to seek personal control over ourselves and our situations. Athletes' intrapersonal challenges become visible when they express frustration or anxiety with *doing nothing*, what feels like forced or unwanted down time when injured and unable to train or compete, or for those who proudly proclaim that they do not do *recovery* or *mandated rest* very well (Cavallerio & Wadey, 2013).

There are two key lessons that I have identified from reflecting on my experience with Steve. First, restoration of health is not linear, nor is it a simple process. The biological healing process might generally reflect or follow stages, but the process is a complex interplay of factors within and outside of the individual athlete, in terms of their self-care and self-regulating behavior and the supportive or disruptive environment around them. The emotional healing process may not follow the physical or biological healing process, and it is not appropriate to assume problematic emotions or thoughts will disappear once physical strength is restored or when an athlete returns to the sport environment. These assumptions and biases sneak into our own work at times, and this happens with athletes and within their ecosystem, including family and friends, coaches, sport science, and medical staff. Too often I've sat quiet in response to something being said like, "he'll be alright, mate, once he's back on the snow, field, track, in the pool and so on", which can be harmful and misleading, as was case with Steve's coach and physiotherapist.

When our medical and allied healthcare colleagues unintentionally reinforce experiential avoidance, or when a coach and other sport scientists with expectations for a smooth and quick return to sport tell us how to do our jobs, it might suggest they are feeling helpless or are not sure what to do. Medical settings are typically hierarchical, where our healthcare colleagues' perceptions of where, how, and when sport psychology fits in (or doesn't), can be perceived as micromanaging. Over the years, I've gotten better at promoting opportunities to support athletes through a more interdisciplinary or transdisciplinary manner than merely settling for or maintaining a siloed multidisciplinary approach. Medical and health professions can also be patriarchal when it comes to determining what is in an athlete's "best interests". I've often observed decisions about healthcare and related matters decided without asking for or considering the athlete's perspective. This may reflect how healthcare professionals and coaches might view athletes, as people who need protection and/or instruction, which sends the (covert and overt) message they are not capable of understanding or deciding for themselves, such as what happened with Eloise. Most of the time, however, these interactions were not intended to micromanage or belittle my own expertise and experience. Instead, these are well-meaning attempts to be helpful, often with the assumption that as an expert we know what to do and have the answers or solutions to "fix" undesirable and difficult situations.

All in all, the experiences I've shared here were not all terrible, and it has turned out okay for everyone involved. I did not lose my job over any of them, but I may have reinforced a few stereotypes and biases about how sport psychologists work. I admit that during some of these more uncomfortable situations, I was not performing my best. I let insecurities fly the plane, my sleep suffered at the hand of rumination, and I unveil my sword of righteous indignation when I feel invalidated or disrespected by others. Alas, I did not tell tales of my proudest and more enjoyable professional moments in this chapter. Yet in these times too, I have found myself ruminating at night or distracted by self-doubt, wearing an imposter t-shirt that claims I cannot possibly repeat or sustain whatever contribution I had to an athlete's optimal performance or transformative insight.

There are peaks and valleys in the journey to becoming a sport psychologist, as with any profession. Whether you are just starting out, recently graduated and in your first job, or have been practicing for a while now, it is easy to get stuck in the valley, which limits what we see to what's in our immediate view. When we enjoy success, we may start to expect those highs to come again more often and too easily, or to last longer than they do.

My Survival Pack

What helps me navigate the diverse and challenging terrain of professional practice, I refer to as my survival pack – essentials for a long journey. These include: a compass (values), a map (frameworks), fuel/water (recovery strategies), and a first-aid kit (self-care and support network). As frameworks were listed previously in this chapter, following are the other contents in this pack. First, my values guide and redirect me toward what is important to me in life. The perspective and space I give to my work, as well as my role as a sport psychologist, within the context of my life, is critical. I am passionate about sport psychology, and genuinely love the work I get to do most of the time. However, it is a job, it is what I do and not who I am. When things are difficult, I take pause and reflect on the big picture, remember the transient nature of these situations, and make an effort to connect to other meaningful aspects of my life.

One of my core values developed and articulated early in my career is: *do good work with good people*. I have an incredible social network, most notably my husband and best friend. He not only supports me personally, he frequently (and fortunately) calls attention to the organizational and socio-contextual influences at play when I'm fully fused with my intra and interpersonal reactions. I am also grateful for good friends in sport psychology. I chat with a few of them regularly, over coffee and/or a walk, and consult with (and vent to) them when I'm away from home traveling with sport. I also have long-term relationships with two fantastic professionals – one is an executive coach (my very own performance psychologist) and the other my supervisor (clinical and sport psychologist) – both of whom I consider friends. Each of these, in their own unique style, provide a safe space for me to unpack my stories, which often come out with a mix of laughter and, occasionally, self-righteousness as well as reminders to keep it all in perspective.

Packed with the above is self-care. For me, this is an ongoing practice which involves the people, places, and activities that ground me, nourish and comfort me when unstable or uncertain, the things that replenish and restore my energy and attention when exhausted (e.g., connecting with nature, yoga), as well as strategies to stay motivated and challenged (e.g., family holidays, fun adventures). I use different techniques to process and reflect, seek feedback, and learn new things. I work hard at self-awareness, regular recovery strategies, and nurturing support networks so they are there for me in stressful situations, and it helps to have a damn good poker face! I try my best to stay physically active, sleep well, and keep a consistent bedtime routine, regularly engaging in activities to promote rest when needed (quieting the rumination), and restore and/or replenish energy when required. This may seem easy but is quite challenging to keep up in daily life but especially when living 24/7 with a sport team on tour (a.k.a. the bubble!).

My survival pack has developed over time, is periodically re-evaluated and refreshed (as needed), and is personally relevant to me, consisting of what I need to perform optimally while enjoying my life. Everyone's survival pack will look a little different, have more or less of various strategies, and ideally reflect one's individual needs, preferences, and work–life demands.

Future Research Implications

Reflecting on my own experiences and the available literature, the following are a few recommendations for future research. First, while this chapter provides a glimpse into my experience helping athletes with sport injury, we would benefit from more in-depth summaries; for example, qualitative research that includes consultants' experiences alongside the athlete, or ideally perspectives across all parties involved (athlete and key members of the support network, beyond just the psychologist). Research is needed to identify and understand how individual preferences and behaviors, as well as interactions within the eco-system including athletes, medical and healthcare providers, coaches, and sport leaders, may influence health outcomes (cf. Ekstrand, Lundqvist, Davison, D'Hooghe, & Pensgaard, 2018; Ekstrand et al., 2018); further, consideration of the sociocultural factors involved in working within the contexts of health and medicine, as well as with cultural competence as we support various athletes and other health and sport science professionals. New frameworks such as the Multilevel Model of Sport Injury (Wadey, Day, Cavallerio, & Martinelli, 2018) are welcome additions to guide us through the dynamic complex ecosystem of providing psychological support for rehabilitation within an elite sport environment. In addition, increased efforts to establish and nurture partnerships between researchers and consultants are needed to explore what, how, and why things happen as they do in practice. These partnerships would undoubtedly contribute to evidence-based practice, which considers the best available evidence, the client's preferences and values, as well as the practitioner's experience, but also support athletes' involvement in their own healthcare decisions informed by both tacit and explicit knowledge and within the context of available resources (Dawes et al., 2005). Finally, the science of learning would be useful whereby there is more explicit utilization of educational psychology to inform our development not just as psychologists but also as educators in healthcare environments.

Conclusion

My experiences with, and reflection upon, challenges encountered when supporting athletes with injury are unique to me. However, I can almost guarantee everyone will have at least one, if not more, of their own stories. Through reading and self-reflection, peer consultation, or formal supervision, and a decently stocked pack, you will survive, as I have. I hope that by sharing my discomfort, you take pause to reflect and consider the ways in which you work currently. And by doing this, we can re-examine and remodel how we provide psychological services to those in need.

Critical Discussion Questions

1) Identify the reactions you had to the situations described in this chapter and reflect on how you may have reacted and responded.
2) (a) select one of the specific situations and identify how my professional philosophy or preferred frameworks might have guided my response; and (b) reflecting on your own professional philosophy, how might you have applied other frameworks to navigate this situation?
3) What essentials would make up your own survival pack that will help you cope with and develop as a sport psychologist?

References

Brown, C. H., Gould, D., & Foster, S. (2005). A framework for developing contextual intelligence. *The Sport Psychologist, 19*(1), 51–62. doi: 10.1123/tsp.19.1.51

Brown, C. H., Gould, D., & Sandra, F. (2005). A framework for developing contextual intelligence. *The Sport Psychologist, 19*, 51–62. doi: 10.1123/tsp.19.1.51

Cavallerio, F., & Wadey, R. (2013). *Risk culture and overuse injuries in sport: A narrative review.* Paper presented at the British Psychological Society's Division of Sport and Exercise Psychology Annual Conference, Manchester, United Kingdom.

Dawes, M., Summerskill, W., Glasziou, P., Cartabellotta, A., Martin, J., Hopayian, K., … Osborne, J. (2005). Sicily statement on evidence-based practice. *BMC Medical Education, 5*(1), 1. doi: 10.1186/1472-6920-5-1

Day, M. C., & Wadey, R. (2017). Researching growth following adversity in sport and exercise: Methodological implications and future recommendations. *Qualitative Research in Sport, Exercise and Health, 9*(4), 499–513. doi: 10.1080/2159676X.2017.1328460

Ekstrand, J., Lundqvist, D., Davison, M., D'Hooghe, M., & Pensgaard, A. M. (2019). Communication quality between the medical team and the head coach/manager is associated with injury burden and player availability in elite football clubs. *British Journal of Sports Medicine, 53*(5), 304–308. doi: 10.1136/bjsports-2018-099411

Ekstrand, J., Lundqvist, D., Lagerbäck, L., Vouillamoz, M., Papadimitiou, N., & Karlsson, J. (2018). Is there a correlation between coaches' leadership styles and injuries in elite football teams? A study of 36 elite teams in 17 countries. *British Journal of Sports Medicine*, *52*(8), 527–531. doi: 10.1136/bjsports-2017-098001

Hefferon, K., Grealy, M., & Mutrie, N. (2010). Transforming from cocoon to butterfly: The potential role of the body in the process of posttraumatic growth. *Journal of Humanistic Psychology*, *50*(2), 224–247. doi: 10.1177%2F0022167809341996

Van Der Kolk, B. (2015). *The body keeps the score: Mind, brain, and body in the transformation of trauma*. Penguin.

Wadey, R., Day, M., Cavallerio, F., & Martinelli, L. (2018). Multilevel model of sport injury (MMSI): Can coaches impact and be impacted by injury? In R. Thelwell & M. Dicks (Eds.), *Professional advances in sports coaching: Research and practice* (pp. 408–440). London: Routledge.

19 Three Decades Later

Looking Back to Look Forward

Britton W. Brewer

Introduction

It is difficult to pinpoint exactly when sport injury psychology (aka "psychology of sport injury" (Heil, 1993) and "sports medicine psychology" (Wiese-Bjornstal, 2014)) officially became "a thing". Nevertheless, the publication of the first books devoted exclusively to the topic (Heil, 1993; Pargman, 1993) represented a definitive early landmark in the maturity of the field. How the field got to that point and where it has gone in the subsequent decades have important implications for the future of sport injury psychology. Consequently, this chapter involves "looking back" at the history of sport injury psychology as a means of "looking forward" at what may lie ahead for the field. After a brief overview of general trends in sport injury psychology, historical developments and progress in theory, research, and practice are considered.

General Trends

Among the general trends that can be observed about sport injury psychology over the field's existence, two in particular stand out as important. One trend pertains to the multidisciplinarity of the field, and the other involves the tremendous expansion of knowledge on the subject. With respect to the first trend, sport injury psychology has been multidisciplinary (Stember, 1991) from the beginning. The seminal investigations in the field were conducted by psychiatrists (Holmes, 1970; Little, 1969), and sport injury psychology has been populated by scholars and practitioners across many other disciplines, including athletic training, behavioral medicine, coaching, epidemiology, kinesiology, nursing, orthopaedic surgery, physiotherapy, public health, sport psychology, sport sociology, sports medicine, and various subfields of psychology ever since. The field has been multidisciplinary both on aggregate (as the result of the combined independent contributions of professionals across disciplines) and as the product of the joint collaborative efforts of professionals in multiple disciplines. With no single discipline laying claim to sport injury psychology, it would not be surprising to find that many individuals contributing to the field may not even self-identify as doing so. The field has not matured to the point that it can be considered interdisciplinary – with a true synthesis of approaches and integration of knowledge and methods across disciplines (Stember, 1991) – so it is likely to continue in a multidisciplinary vein for the foreseeable future.

The second general trend pertains to the veritable explosion of scientific information on sport injury psychology that has occurred over the past four decades. Long-time veterans of the field will recall the early days when the small array of relevant writings could only be accessed by paging through bound volumes in the library or by sending a postcard to the author(s) to request a reprint. Once discovered, readers pored over articles and book chapters as if they were sacred tomes, not knowing whether or when additional material might be made available. In the subsequent decades, research production in this area has increased exponentially, resulting in a steady stream of pertinent information published in a wide variety of outlets across the academic spectrum. There are numerous book chapters and multiple edited and authored books on the topic. With internet access, free registration on a platform such as ResearchGate, and email subscriptions to journal content updates, scholars and practitioners can download three or four articles per week on topics of relevance to sport injury psychology (broadly defined). Whereas material on sport injury psychology once was sparse and intermittently available, it has become an ongoing challenge to keep up with, manage, and integrate the heavy volume of information that is generated. It is reasonable to expect this trend to continue.

Theory

In response to the accumulation of empirical data and the thirst of coaches and sports health care professionals for information about the psychological aspects of sport injury, theoretical frameworks were developed in the 1980s and early 1990s for the prediction of sport injury occurrence (Andersen & Williams, 1988; van Mechelen, Hlobil, & Kemper, 1992) and psychological responses to sport injury (Gordon, 1986; Weiss & Troxel, 1986). Over the subsequent two decades, the models have been modified, reconceptualized, and expanded in minor and not-so-minor ways (e.g., Bahr & Krosshaug, 2005; Meeuwisse, 1994; Meeuwisse, Tyreman, Hagel, & Emery, 2007; Petrie & Perna, 2004; Wiese-Bjornstal, 2009; Wiese-Bjornstal, Smith, Shaffer, & Morrey, 1998; Williams & Andersen, 1998). Variants of the models focusing on a specific population (e.g., Wiese-Bjornstal, 2004), particular outcomes (e.g., Brewer, 2010; Roy-Davis, Wadey, & Evans, 2017), and different levels of analysis (e.g., Wadey, Day, Cavallerio, & Martinelli, 2018) have also been developed.

On the whole, the models have served the field well, doing what models are supposed to do. Specifically, the models have focused research efforts, facilitated interpretation of research findings, and guided the development of preventive and rehabilitative interventions. The track records of the models suggest that they and their successors will continue to have a favorable impact on sport injury psychology, with revisions occurring on an irregular basis to accommodate advances in knowledge and new ways of conceptualizing the phenomena of interest.

Theoretical integration under a biopsychosocial framework may also occur, as the leading models of sport injury prediction feature different terminology but are wholly compatible (Brewer & Redmond, 2017; Wiese-Bjornstal, 2019a) and the variables in prominent injury prediction models overlap heavily with those in psychological response models (Brewer, 2007). Spiritual perspectives on sport injury (Clement, LaGuerre, & Arvinen-Barrow, 2019; Wiese-Bjornstal, 2019b) may also play a part in theoretical integration.

Lest one gain too rosy an impression of the state of theory in sport injury psychology, it is important to note several limitations and challenges, most of which pertain to the complexity or sophistication of the models (or the lack thereof). Accurately reflecting the sheer complexity of the phenomena under consideration, models of sport injury occurrence and psychological responses to sport injury have tended to feature an abundance of variables that are typically arranged in broad categories (e.g., "coping resources", "emotional responses", "extrinsic risk factors", "sociodemographic factors"). An inevitable consequence of the within-category heterogeneity is that the models lack precision with respect to the nature of associations between categories. Consider, for example, the variable "previous injury", which could increase the likelihood of injury as an intrinsic risk factor (Meeuwisse et al., 2007) or as part of an athlete's history of stressors (Williams & Andersen, 1998). Conversely, if rehabilitation of the prior injury was successful, the previous injury could be associated with a reduced risk of injury due to strengthening a previously weakened region of the body during rehabilitation or increased coping self-efficacy from dealing successfully with the stressor. The circumstances under which previous injuries confer risk and those under which they confer benefit are not explicated in extant models, which make no explicit provisions for such hypothetical situations. Multiplied across the many variables included in the models, the predictive power of the models can be severely compromised.

Another complexity-related issue associated with prominent models in sport injury psychology is that although they may allow for (or at least not rule out) the possibility of interactions between variables both within and across general categories of variables, the nature of the interactions is not specified in the models. Interpretable, theoretically meaningful interactions have been documented (e.g., Brewer, Cornelius, Van Raalte, Tennen, & Armeli, 2013; Petrie, 1992; Rubio, Pujals, de la Vega, Aguado, & Hernández, 2014; Smith, Smoll, & Ptacek, 1990), but the obtained interactions could not have been predicted on the basis of the specifications of relevant models. Similarly, relative weighting of variables is not featured in models, both within and across categories of variables. For example, the relative contributions of intrinsic risk factors and extrinsic risk factors to injury susceptibility in the model of Meeuwisse et al. (2007). It is, of course, recognized that those relative contributions may vary extensively across athletes and situations (e.g., an exceptionally slippery playing surface may outweigh intrinsic risk factors on a given day). These observations about the lack of model specificity with respect to interactions between, and weighting of, variables should not be construed as criticisms of the models so much as a commentary on the complexities of phenomena of interest in sport injury psychology and the current state of knowledge in the field. Put simply, there is plenty of room for theoretical growth in sport injury psychology!

Of the many variables in sport injury psychology models, the one that presents the most vexing challenge for researchers is the temporal aspect. It is difficult, if not impossible, to adequately represent the dynamic nature of many of the variables (and the relations among variables) in the models in a two-dimensional figure. For example, however athletes' vulnerability to injury "looks" at any particular point in time (given their profile of risk factors), their vulnerability is likely to be different at any subsequent point in time due to minor or major alterations in variables prone to change (i.e., most variables!). Even without the specificity required to adequately represent the processes underlying phenomena such as sport injury occurrence and psychological responses to sport injury, the prevailing models are unwieldy and far too complex to be tested fully in any single study. Consequently, it is necessary to piece together findings across many investigations to obtain as complete an understanding as possible of the phenomena of interest, just as the blind men's tactile observations in the famous parable would need to be combined to gain a complete description of the elephant. Again, the challenges of representing and testing the models are not limitations of the models, but are instead reflections of the complexity of the issues being studied. Moreover, the challenges are not insoluble. In particular, advances in representational technology may one day assist in depicting more adequately the dynamic processes under investigation.

Research

Within the general trend of an increasing rate of production of scientific information in sport injury psychology are subtrends characteristic of research endeavours. Specifically, the subtrends are toward topical and methodological diversification in empirical investigations.

Topical Diversification

The range of topics in sport injury psychology has expanded dramatically over the past five decades. Whereas research in the field once focused primarily on psychological predictors of and psychological (especially emotional) responses to sport injury (for an update on this topic, see Chapter 8), sport injury psychology now features a wide array of areas of inquiry (as reflected in the content of the current volume).

Among the areas of inquiry in sport injury psychology that emerged in the 1960s, 1970s, and 1980s and have continued to the present day are pain in sport (for a review, see Chapter 5), psychological factors associated with sport injury rehabilitation outcomes, psychological interventions in sport injury rehabilitation, and adherence to sport injury rehabilitation regimens. Research on pain in sport and psychological predictors of sport injury rehabilitation processes (such as adherence) and outcomes (e.g., recovery) has helped to provide a foundation for the use of psychological interventions in sport injury rehabilitation (Brewer, 2010).

Subareas of sport injury psychology that emerged in the 1990s and have remained topics of interest in the ensuing decades include sports health care professional perceptions and behaviors related to psychology in their work with athletes, psychosocial interventions in sport injury prevention, sociocultural aspects of pain and injury in sport, and perceived benefits of sport injury. Recognizing that the successful application of psychology in association with sport injury required the "buy in" of sports health care professionals, investigators began surveying practitioners such as athletic trainers (Wiese, Weiss, & Yukelson, 1991), sport physiotherapists (Gordon, Milios, & Grove, 1991), and sports medicine physicians (Brewer, Van Raalte, & Linder, 1991) regarding various aspects of psychology in association with sport injury, a research practice that has continued to the current era. Drawing on sport injury prediction theory and research that accumulated over the 1970s, 1980s, and early 1990s, the first experimental study in which a psychosocial intervention was evaluated as means of preventing sport injury appeared in the mid-1990s (Kerr & Goss, 1996), paving the way for additional similar studies in the decades that followed (for a meta-analytic review, see Ivarsson et al., 2016). Spearheaded initially by sport sociologists and sport philosophers, research has addressed ways in which social and cultural factors affect the attitudes and behaviors of athletes with respect to pain and injury (for a review, see Wiese-Bjornstal, 2018). Despite an early preoccupation with the adverse psychological effects of injury on athletes, investigators have increasingly focused on exploring the potential benefits experienced by athletes as a result of incurring injury (as documented in Chapter 7).

In the 2000s, psychological aspects of sport-related concussion and psychological readiness to return to sport after injury became bona fide subareas of sport injury psychology. The emergence and subsequent growth of scholarly interest in sport-related concussion from a psychological perspective parallels the rise of societal awareness of the injury as an important public health issue with potential ramifications for long-term functioning and well-being (for more on this important topic, see Chapter 4). Building on the groundbreaking research of Podlog and Eklund (2005, 2006, 2007), inquiry on psychological readiness to return to sport after injury has exploded over the past 15 years, particularly in the context of anterior cruciate ligament (ACL) reconstructive surgery (for a review, see Ardern, 2015).

Perhaps the most recent new subarea of sport injury psychology to emerge is adherence to sport injury prevention programs. Although adherence to preventive interventions has been assessed in the context of sport injury for decades, it didn't become a topic of focal interest until the 2010s with the publication of articles offering theoretical guidance (Keats, Emery, & Finch, 2012; McKay, Merrett, & Emery, 2016) and meta-analyses documenting positive associations between adherence to prevention programs and sport injury occurrence outcomes (Goode et al., 2015; Sugimoto, Myer, Bush, Klugman, McKeon, & Hewett, 2012). As with the more established subareas of sport injury psychology, adherence to preventive interventions appears to be well on its way to becoming a fruitful avenue of inquiry.

Methodological Diversification

Not only have the topics explored in sport injury psychology expanded markedly, but the methods used to examine those topics have expanded as well. For the most part, the methodological diversification observed in the field has been beneficial in terms of facilitating more sophisticated and productive exploration of questions of interest. Not all potentially useful methodological approaches have been adopted with equal fervour, however. Some approaches have "caught on" more than others. For example, recognizing that many of the outcomes of interest in sport injury psychology are conceptualized as the culmination of processes lasting for days, weeks, months, or even years, prospective, longitudinal research designs have been used with increasing frequency, first in predicting sport injury occurrence and, more recently, in examining postinjury phenomena. Nevertheless, calls for more frequent assessment of predictor variables (e.g., Evans & Hardy, 1999; Johnson, Tranaeus, & Ivarsson, 2014; Petrie & Falkstein, 1998)—an essential aspect of investigating processes—have gone largely unheeded (for a notable exception, see Ivarsson, Johnson, Lindwall, Gustafsson, & Altemyr, 2014).

Similarly, although qualitative methods have been widely adopted in sport injury psychology since the 1990s, experimental designs have been used only sporadically and, relative to other designs, infrequently. Paralleling growth in the use of qualitative methods in both psychology and the sport sciences over the past three decades, investigators have implemented qualitative approaches to obtain richly detailed accounts of the preinjury and postinjury experiences of athletes. Findings from qualitative studies have not only added depth to the knowledge base in sport injury psychology by substantiating, augmenting, and extending those from quantitative studies, but also have offered fresh perspectives in pursuit of new and innovative lines of inquiry (as described, for example, in Chapters 1, 8, 10, and 12). In contrast, although experimental designs are the strongest tool available for examining causal influences on sport injury outcomes of interest and have been advocated for use in sport injury psychology for at least a quarter-century (Brewer, 1994), they have not been used with a frequency proportionate to their value. As discussed in Chapter 13, some of the reasons for low rate of adoption of experimental designs by sport injury psychology researchers pertain to challenges in recruiting samples that are sufficiently large and homogeneous, ensuring the baseline equivalence of experimental and control groups, masking participants and data collectors regarding the group assignment of participants, and delivering standardized treatment protocols.

Other developments in sport injury psychology over the past three decades that reflect the methodological diversification of the field include increased implementation of programmatic research, identification of sources for and methods of data collection, use of samples that are homogeneous with respect to injury-related characteristics, and sophistication of research designs and statistical procedures. Although much of the scientific literature in sport injury psychology is populated with research conducted by scholars making "one-off" forays in the topic area, a large portion of the literature consists of work produced by "lifers" who have devoted many years to the subject. The principal advantage of such programmatic inquiry is that it allows investigators to build directly upon their previous studies and explore questions of interest systematically across samples, methods, and theoretical approaches.

In sport injury psychology, there is a rich tradition of using a variety of sources and methods to collect relevant data. As described in Chapter 2, the mainstream and social media have proven to be fertile sources of data, particularly for research on sociocultural aspects of sport injury. Additional innovative sources and methods of obtaining data in sport injury psychology include injury surveillance systems (Ekegren, Gabbe, & Finch, 2016), photo-elicitation interviews (Curry & Strauss, 1994), and video incident analysis (Caswell, Lincoln, Almquist, Dunn, & Hinton, 2012; Hendricks et al., 2016). An as-yet-untapped source of data for research in sport injury psychology is wearable technology, which can be used to assess a variety of internal and external factors of potential relevance to the occurrence of and responses to sport injury (Halson, Peake, & Sullivan, 2016; Ng & Ryba, 2018). The sheer volume of data generated by wearables and the ease with which such data can be collected leave open the possibility of conducting meaningful intraindividual analyses (Evans & Hardy, 1999) and combining with data collected through other means to gain a more complete and customized description of athletes before and/or after injury.

Given the challenges in enlisting study participants that sport injury psychology researchers sometimes encounter, it is not surprising that empirical investigations often feature athletes with a variety of injuries. It can be difficult, however, to disentangle the potential influences of variations in injury type, severity, course, and prognosis on biological, psychological, and social processes and outcomes. When feasible, researchers can use homogeneous samples to hold injury-related characteristics *relatively* constant and isolate factors of interest. The two injuries for which injury-specific sport injury psychology research arcs have emerged are anterior cruciate ligament tears (Ardern & Kvist, 2016) and sport-related concussions (Kontos, 2017).

Paralleling a rise in the quality of research studies in sports medicine over the past quarter-century (Grant, Tjoumakaris, Maltenfort, & Freedman, 2014), investigations in the psychology of sport injury have gotten increasingly sophisticated, both methodologically and statistically, over the same period of time. In a clear indication of the maturity of the field, Ivarsson et al. (2017) conducted a meta-analysis of studies involving psychosocial factors in sport injury prediction and prevention. Latent growth curve (Ivarsson et al., 2017) and Bayesian latent change score (Clement, Ivarsson, Tranaeus, Johnson, & Stenling, 2018) analyses have been used to examine psychosocial predictors of sport injury. The advantage of such procedures is that they are "well-aligned with the theoretical frameworks developed to understand predictors of sport injury risk, and they provide researchers with statistical tools to test more complex hypotheses related to sport injury risk" (Ivarsson & Stenling, 2018, p. 4). The trend toward ever more complex statistical analyses is expected to continue. Ivarsson and Stenling (2018) proposed the adoption of classification and regression tree (CART), random forest, and neural network analyses "to provide researchers and clinicians with results that are more clinically meaningful and accurate in determining the injury risk for a specific athlete" (p. 5). Similar advances have also been made in postinjury research, in which procedures such multilevel modelling (Cornelius, Brewer, & Van Raalte, 2007) and multiple mediation analysis (Wadey et al., 2014) have been applied to complex longitudinal and cross-sectional sport injury rehabilitation data, respectively.

Practice

Despite the abundance of substantial theoretical and empirical advances in sport injury psychology that have transpired over the past three decades, practical gains have been more modest. Although the importance of psychology in relation to sport injury has long been recognized by sports health care professionals (Brewer et al., 1991; Gordon et al., 1991; Wiese et al., 1991), the question of how the growing knowledge base in sport injury psychology can best be applied and by whom remains largely unanswered. By virtue of their frequent contact with athletes after they have become injured (and, in some cases, prior to the occurrence of injury), sports health care professionals are well-positioned to apply psychology in the context of sport injury. Encouragingly, programming to educate sports health care professionals on the psychological aspects of sport injury rehabilitation has been developed (Gordon, Potter, & Ford, 1998; Heaney, Walker, Green, & Rostron, 2016; Stiller-Ostrowski, Gould, & Covassin, 2009) and athletic trainers have expressed feeling competent and comfortable in addressing issues in the psychosocial domain (Clement & Arvinen-Barrow, 2019). Nevertheless, sports health care professionals tend to have a limited repertoire of psychological interventions (Brewer & Redmond, 2017) and may sometimes wind up "using psychosocial strategies that they are more confident in using, instead of those that are most effective and appropriate" (Clement, Granquist, & Arvinen-Barrow, 2013, p. 518).

In contrast, implementing psychological interventions in association with the prevention and rehabilitation of sport injuries is potentially within the skillset of sport psychology consultants and other professionals with psychological training. Although such individuals tend to view themselves as part of the primary multidisciplinary treatment team for athletes with injury (Arvinen-Barrow & Clement, 2017), they do not customarily act in this capacity and are instead viewed by sports health care professionals as performing a more secondary role (Clement & Arvinen-Barrow, 2013). Barriers to sport psychology consultants implementing empirically validated psychological interventions for use in the prevention (Ivarsson et al., 2017) and rehabilitation (Brewer, 2010) of sport injuries therefore include restricted access to athletes before and after injury, professional territoriality, stigma associated with psychosocial and mental health issues, and lack of provisions for monetary compensation of psychological services.

It is clear that empirical and theoretical support for the application of psychology in sports health care is insufficient to overcome structural and economic barriers to fully addressing the psychological needs of athletes before and after injury. Even in the most elite levels of sport (Gervis, Hau, Pickford, & Fruth, 2019), access to psychological services in association with sport injury is generally limited, and means are not typically in place to furnish compensation for the provision of standard psychological services for athletes with injury. Presumably, some preventive and rehabilitative interventions can be implemented inexpensively through online and multimedia technology (Clark, Bassett, & Siegert, 2019; Maddison, Prapavessis, & Clatworthy, 2006; Vriend, Coehoorn, & Verhagen, 2015), but such an approach may leave out some of the social elements that can increase the potency of psychological intervention. Cost offset research, which has documented the effectiveness of behavioral interventions in reducing health care costs (Blount et al., 2007) and utilization of medical services (Stahl et al., 2015), may prove useful in helping to convince those who make funding decisions about sports health care to offer psychological services on a routine basis in association with sport injury.

Conclusion

Over the past three decades, extensive progress has been made in sport injury psychology. Substantial theoretical, empirical, and practical advances in the field have been documented. With a prolific multidisciplinary corps (and core) of scholars and practitioners, the field stands poised for further advancement in the decades ahead. To be sure, there are formidable theoretical and methodological challenges and considerable applied obstacles to be overcome for sport injury psychology to fulfill its potential.

As the course of the field is plotted, it will be important for proponents to be proactive in identifying explicitly the purpose and objectives of sport injury psychology. As noted by Evans and Hardy (1999), a more cohesive foundation of knowledge can be developed by increasing the consistency of the research questions pursued and the methods and measures used. In the absence of professional organizations, journals, or conferences devoted exclusively to sport injury psychology, it is not abundantly clear from where the impetus for developing a more focused and unified agenda for the field will come. Ultimately, however, the success of the field is likely to be contingent on the ability of parties from disparate backgrounds to come together to best serve the athletes they study and with whom they work.

Critical Discussion Questions

1) How important or desirable is theoretical integration in sport injury psychology? Are there advantages to be gained by attempting to integrate theoretical perspectives in the field or are the phenomena of interest in sport injury psychology too broad to be united under one or a few theoretical banners?
2) What are some potential solutions to bridging the gap between research and practice in sport injury psychology?
3) What are the most vital research questions facing sport injury psychology? What would a "focused and unified" agenda for the field look like?

References

Andersen, M. B., & Williams, J. M. (1988). A model of stress and athletic injury: Prediction and prevention. *Journal of Sport and Exercise Psychology*, *10*(3), 294–306. doi: 10.1123/jsep.10.3.294

Ardern, C. L. (2015). Anterior cruciate ligament reconstruction – Not exactly a one-way ticket back to the preinjury level: A review of contextual factors affecting return to sport after surgery. *Sports Health*, *7*(3), 224–230. doi: 10.1177/1941738115578131

Ardern, C. L., & Kvist, J. (2016). What is the evidence to support a psychological component to rehabilitation programs after anterior cruciate ligament reconstruction? *Current Orthopaedic Practice*, *27*(3), 263–268. doi: 10.1097/BCO.0000000000000371

Arvinen-Barrow, M., & Clement, D. (2017). Preliminary investigation into sport and exercise psychology consultants' views and experiences of an interprofessional care team approach to sport injury rehabilitation. *Journal of Interprofessional Care*, *31*(1), 66–74. doi: 10.1080/13561820.2016.1235019

Bahr, R., & Krosshaug, T. (2005). Understanding injury mechanisms: A key component of preventing injuries in sport. *British Journal of Sports Medicine*, *39*(6), 324–329. doi: 10.1136/bjsm.2005.018341

Blount, A., Schoenbaum, M., Kathol, R., Rollman, B. L., Thomas, M., O'Donohue, W., & Peek, C. J. (2007). The economics of behavioral health services in medical settings: A summary of the evidence. *Professional Psychology: Research and Practice*, *38*(3), 290–297. doi: 10.1037/0735-7028.38.3.290

Brewer, B. W. (1994). Review and critique of models of psychological adjustment to athletic injury. *Journal of Applied Sport Psychology*, *6*(1), 87–100. doi: 10.1080/10413209408406467

Brewer, B. W. (2007). Psychology of sport injury rehabilitation. In G. Tenenbaum & R. C. Eklund (Eds.), *Handbook of sport psychology* (3rd ed., pp. 404–424). New York: Wiley.

Brewer, B. W. (2010). The role of psychological factors in sport injury rehabilitation outcomes. *International Review of Sport and Exercise Psychology*, *3*(1), 40–61. doi: 10.1080/17509840903301207

Brewer, B. W., Cornelius, A. E., Van Raalte, J. L., Tennen, H., & Armeli, S. (2013). Predictors of adherence to home rehabilitation exercises following anterior cruciate ligament reconstruction. *Rehabilitation Psychology*, *58*(1), 64–72. doi: 10.1037/a0031297

Brewer, B. W., & Redmond, C. J. (2017). *Psychology of sport injury*. Champaign, IL: Human Kinetics.

Brewer, B. W., Van Raalte, J. L., & Linder, D. E. (1991). Role of the sport psychologist in treating injured athletes: A survey of sports medicine providers. *Journal of Applied Sport Psychology*, *3*(2), 183–190. doi: 10.1080/10413209108406443

Caswell, S. V., Lincoln, A. E., Almquist, J. L., Dunn, R. E., & Hinton, R. Y. (2012). Video incident analysis of head injuries in high school girls' lacrosse. *American Journal of Sports Medicine*, *40*(4), 756–762. doi: 10.1177/0363546512436647

Clark, H., Bassett, S., & Siegert, R. (2019). The effectiveness of web-based patient education and action and coping plans as an adjunct to patient treatment in physiotherapy: A randomized controlled trial. *Physiotherapy Theory and Practice*, *35*(10), 930–939. doi: 10.1080/09593985.2018.1467521

Clement, D., & Arvinen-Barrow, M. (2013). Sport medicine team influences in psychological rehabilitation: A multidisciplinary approach. In M. Arvinen-Barrow & N. Walker (Eds.), *The psychology of sport injury and rehabilitation* (pp. 156–160). Abingdon, UK: Routledge.

Clement, D., & Arvinen-Barrow, M. (2019). Athletic trainers' views and experiences of discussing psychosocial and mental health issues with athletes: An exploratory study. *Athletic Training and Sports Health Care, 11*(5), 213–223. doi: 10.3928/19425864-20181002-01

Clement, D., Granquist, M., & Arvinen-Barrow, M. (2013). Psychosocial aspects of athletic injuries as perceived by athletic trainers. *Journal of Athletic Training, 48*(4), 512–521. doi: 10.4085/1062-6050-48.3.21

Clement, D., Ivarsson, A., Tranaeus, U., Johnson, U., & Stenling, A. (2018). Investigating the influence of intraindividual changes in perceived stress symptoms on injury risk in soccer. *Scandinavian Journal of Medicine and Science in Sports, 28*(4), 1461–1466. doi: 10.1111/sms.13048

Clement, D., LaGuerre, D., & Arvinen-Barrow, M. (2019). Role of religion and spirituality in sport injury rehabilitation. In B. Hemmings, N. J. Watson & A. Parker (Eds.), *Sport, psychology and Christianity: Welfare, performance and consultancy* (pp. 71–86). New York: Routledge.

Cornelius, A. E., Brewer, B. W., & Van Raalte, J. L. (2007). Applications of multilevel modeling in sport injury rehabilitation research. *International Journal of Sport and Exercise Psychology, 5*(4), 387–405. doi: 10.1080/1612197X.2007.9671843

Curry, T. J., & Strauss, R. H. (1994). A little pain never hurt anybody: A photo-essay on the normalization of sport injuries. *Sociology of Sport Journal, 11*(2), 195–208. doi: 10.1123/ssj.11.2.195

Ekegren, C. L., Gabbe, B. J., & Finch, C. F. (2016). Sports injury surveillance systems: A review of methods and data quality. *Sports Medicine, 46*(1), 49–65. doi: 10.1007/s40279-015-0410-z

Evans, L., & Hardy, L. (1999). Psychological and emotional response to athletic injury: Measurement issues. In D. Pargman (Ed.), *Psychological bases of sport injuries* (2nd ed., pp. 49–64). Morgantown, WV: Fitness Information Technology.

Gervis, M., Hau, T., Pickford, H., & Fruth, M. (2019). A review of the psychological support mechanisms available for long-term injured footballers in the UK throughout their rehabilitation. *Science and Medicine in Football, 4*, 22–29. doi: 10.1080/24733938.2019.1634832

Goode, A. P., Reiman, M. P., Harris, L., DeLisa, L., Kauffman, A., Beltramo, D., … Taylor, B. (2015). Eccentric training for prevention of hamstring injuries may depend on intervention compliance: A systematic review and meta-analysis. *British Journal of Sports Medicine, 49*(6), 349–356. doi: 10.1136/bjsports-2014-093466

Gordon, S. (1986, March). Sport psychology and the injured athlete: A cognitive-behavioral approach to injury response and injury rehabilitation. *Science Periodical on Research and Technology in Sport, 3*, 1–10.

Gordon, S., Milios, D., & Grove, J. R. (1991). Psychological aspects of the recovery process from sport injury: The perspective of sport physiotherapists. *The Australian Journal of Science and Medicine in Sport, 23*, 53–60.

Gordon, S., Potter, M., & Ford, I. (1998). Toward a psychoeducational curriculum for training sport-injury rehabilitation personnel. *Journal of Applied Sport Psychology, 10*(1), 140–156. doi: 10.1080/10413209808406382

Grant, H. M., Tjoumakaris, F. P., Maltenfort, M. G., & Freedman, K. B. (2014). Levels of evidence in the clinical sports medicine literature: Are we getting better over time? *American Journal of Sports Medicine, 42*(7), 1738–1742. doi: 10.1177/0363546514530863

Halson, S. I., Peake, J. M., & Sullivan, J. P. (2016). Wearable technology for athletes: Information overload and pseudoscience? *International Journal of Sports Physiology and Performance, 11*(6), 705–706. doi: 10.1123/IJSPP.2016-0486

Heaney, C. A., Walker, N. C., Green, A. J., & Rostron, C. L. (2016). The impact of a sport psychology education intervention on physiotherapists. *European Journal of Physiotherapy*, *19*(2), 97–103. doi: 10.1080/21679169.2016.1267794

Heil, J. (1993). *Psychology of sport injury*. Champaign, IL: Human Kinetics.

Hendricks, S., O'Connor, S., Lambert, M., Brown, J. C., Burger, N., Mc Fie, S., … & Viljoen, W. (2016). Video analysis of concussion injury mechanism in under-18 rugby. *BMJ Open Sport and Exercise Medicine*, *2*(1), e000053. doi: 10.1136/bmjsem-2015-000053

Holmes, T. H. (1970). Psychological screening. In *Football injuries: Paper presented at a workshop* (pp. 211–214), *Sponsored by Subcommittee on Athletic Injuries, Committee on the Skeletal System, Division of Medical Sciences, National Research Council*, February 1969. Washington, DC: National Academy of Sciences.

Ivarsson, A., Johnson, U., Andersen, M. B., Tranaeus, U., Stenling, A., & Lindwall, M. (2017). Psychosocial factors and sport injuries: Meta-analyses for prediction and prevention. *Sports Medicine*, *47*(2), 353–365. doi: 10.1007/s40279-016-0578-x

Ivarsson, A., Johnson, U., Lindwall, M., Gustafsson, H., & Altemyr, M. (2014). Psychosocial stress as a predictor of injury in elite junior soccer: A latent growth curve analysis. *Journal of Science and Medicine in Sport*, *17*(4), 366–370. doi: 10.1016/j.jsams.2013.10.242

Ivarsson, A., & Stenling, A. (2020). Prediction of injury risk in sports, in N. Balakrishnan, T. Colton, B. Everitt, W. Piegorsch, F. Ruggeri, and J.L. Teugels (eds.), *Wiley StatsRef: Statistics Reference Online* (pp. 1–6).

Johnson, U., Tranaeus, U., & Ivarsson, A. (2014). Current status and future challenges in psychological research of sport injury prediction and prevention: A methodological perspective. *Revista de Psicología del Deporte*, *23*, 401–409.

Keats, M. R., Emery, C. A., & Finch, C. F. (2012). Are we having fun yet? Fostering adherence to injury preventive exercise recommendations in young athletes. *Sports Medicine*, *42*(3), 175–184. doi: 10.2165/11597050-000000000-00000

Kerr, G., & Goss, J. (1996). The effects of a stress management program on injuries and stress levels. *Journal of Applied Sport Psychology*, *8*(1), 109–117. doi: 10.1080/10413209608406312

Kontos, K. P. (2017). Concussion in sport: Psychological perspectives. *Sport, Exercise, and Performance Psychology*, *6*(3), 215–219. doi: 10.1037/spy0000108

Little, J. C. (1969). The athlete's neurosis--A deprivation crisis. *Acta Psychiatrica Scandinavia*, *45*(2), 187–197. doi: 10.1111/j.1600-0447.1969.tb10373.x

Maddison, R., Prapavessis, H., & Clatworthy, M. (2006). Modeling and rehabilitation following anterior cruciate ligament reconstruction. *Annals of Behavior Medicine*, *31*(1), 89–98. doi: 10.1207/s15324796abm3101_13

McKay, C. D., Merrett, C. K., & Emery, C. A. (2016). Predictors of FIFA 11+ Implementation intention in female adolescent soccer: An application of the health action process approach (HAPA) model. *International Journal of Environmental Research and Public Health*, *13*(7), 657. doi: 10.3390/ijerph13070657

Meeuwisse, W. H. (1994). Assessing causation in sport injury: A multifactorial model. *Clinical Journal of Sport Medicine*, *4*(3), 166–170. doi: 10.1097/00042752-199407000-00004

Meeuwisse, W. H., Tyreman, H., Hagel, B., & Emery, C. (2007). A dynamic model of etiology in sport injury: The recursive nature of risk and causation. *Clinical Journal of Sport Medicine*, *17*(3), 215–219. doi: 10.1097/JSM.0b013e3180592a48

Ng, K., & Ryba, T. (2018). The quantified athlete: Associations of wearables for high school athletes. *Advances in Human–Computer Interaction*, 1–8. doi: 10.1155/2018/6317524

Pargman, D. (Ed.). (1993). *Psychological bases of sport injuries*. Morgantown, WV: Fitness Information Technology.

Petrie, T. A. (1992). Psychosocial antecedents of athletic injury: The effects of life stress and social support on female collegiate gymnasts. *Behavioral Medicine, 18*(3), 127–138. doi: 10.1080/08964289.1992.9936963

Petrie, T. A., & Falkstein, D. L. (1998). Methodological, measurement, and statistical issues in research on sport injury prediction. *Journal of Applied Sport Psychology, 10*(1), 26–45. doi: 10.1080/10413209808406376

Petrie, T. A., & Perna, F. (2004). Psychology of injury: Theory, research and practice. In T. Morris & J. Summers (Eds.), *Sport psychology: Theory, applications, and issues* (pp. 547–571). Brisbane: Wiley.

Podlog, L., & Eklund, R. C. (2005). Return to sport after serious injury: A retrospective examination of motivation and psychological outcomes. *Journal of Sport Rehabilitation, 14*(1), 20–34. doi: 10.1123/jsr.14.1.20

Podlog, L., & Eklund, R. C. (2006). A longitudinal investigation of competitive athletes' return to sport following serious injury. *Journal of Applied Sport Psychology, 18*(1), 44–68. doi: 10.1080/10413200500471319

Podlog, L., & Eklund, R. C. (2007). The psychosocial aspects of a return to sport following serious injury: A review of the literature from a self-determination perspective. *Psychology of Sport and Exercise, 8*(4), 535–566. doi: 10.1016/j.psychsport.2009.02.003

Roy-Davis, K., Wadey, R., & Evans, L. (2017). A grounded theory of sport injury-related growth. *Sport, Exercise, and Performance Psychology, 6*(1), 35–52. doi: 10.1037/spy0000080

Rubio, V. J., Pujals, C., Vega, R. de la, Aguado, D., & Hernández, J. M. (2014). Autoeficiacia y lesiones deportivas: ¿Factor protector o de riesgo? *Revista de Psicologia del Deporte, 23*, 439–444.

Smith, R. E., Smoll, F. L., & Ptacek, J. T. (1990). Conjunctive moderator variables in vulnerability and resiliency research: Life stress, social support and coping skills, and adolescent sport injuries. *Journal of Personality and Social Psychology, 58*(2), 360–370. doi: 10.1037/0022-3514.58.2.360

Stahl, J. E., Dossett, M. L., LaJoie, A. S., Denninger, J. W., Mehta, D. H., Goldman, R. & Benson, H. (2015). Relaxation response and resiliency training and its effect on healthcare resource utilization. *PLOS ONE, 10*(10), e0140212. doi: 10.1371/journal.pone.0140212

Stember, M. (1991). Advancing the social sciences through the interdisciplinary enterprise. *The Social Science Journal, 28*(1), 1–14. doi: 10.1016/0362-3319(91)90040-B

Stiller-Ostrowksi, J. L., Gould, D. R., & Covassin, T. (2009). An evaluation of an educational intervention in psychology of injury for athletic training students. *Journal of Athletic Training, 44*(5), 482–489. doi: 10.4085%2F1062-6050-44.5.482

Sugimoto, D., Myer, G. D., Bush, H. M., Klugman, M. F., McKeon, J. M., & Hewett, T. E. (2012). Compliance with neuromuscular training and anterior cruciate ligament injury risk reduction in female athletes: A meta-analysis. *Journal of Athletic Training, 47*(6), 714–723. doi: 10.4085/1062-6050-47.6.10

Van Mechelen, W., Hlobil, H., & Kemper, H. C. G. (1992). Incidence, severity, aetiology and prevention of sports injuries: A review of concepts. *Sports Medicine, 14*(2), 82–99. doi: 10.2165/00007256-199214020-00002

Vriend, I., Coehoorn, I., & Verhagen, E. (2015). Implementation of an App-based neuromuscular training programme to prevent ankle sprains: A process evaluation using the RE-AIM Framework. *British Journal of Sports Medicine, 49*(7), 484–488. doi: 10.1136/bjsports-2013-092896

Wadey, R., Day, M., Cavallerio, F., & Martinelli, L. (2018). The multilevel model of sport injury: Can coaches impact and be impacted by injury? In R. Thelwell & M. Dicks

(Eds.), *Professional advances in sports coaching: Research and practice* (pp. 336–357). New York: Routledge.

Wadey, R., Podlog, L., Hall, M., Hamson-Utley, J., Hicks-Little, C., & Hammer, C. (2014). Reinjury anxiety, coping, and return-to-sport outcomes: A multiple mediation analysis. *Rehabilitation Psychology*, *59*(3), 256–266. doi: 10.1037/a0037032

Weiss, M. R., & Troxel, R. K. (1986). Psychology of the injured athlete. *Athletic Training*, *21*, 104–109.

Wiese, D. M., Weiss, M. R., & Yukelson, D. P. (1991). Sport psychology in the training room: Implications for the treatment team. *The Sport Psychologist*, *5*(1), 15–24.

Wiese-Bjornstal, D. M. (2004). From skinned knees and Pee Wees to menisci and masters: Developmental sport injury psychology. In M. R. Weiss (Ed.), *Developmental sport psychology: A lifespan perspective* (pp. 525–568). Morgantown, WV: Fitness Information Technology.

Wiese-Bjornstal, D. M. (2009). Sport injury and college athlete health across the lifespan. *Journal of Intercollegiate Sports*, *2*(1), 64–80. doi: 10.1123/jis.2.1.64

Wiese-Bjornstal, D. M. (2014). Reflections on a quarter-century of research in sports medicine psychology. *Revista de Psicologia del Deporte*, *23*, 411–421.

Wiese-Bjornstal, D. M. (2018). Sociocultural aspects of sport injury and recovery. In *Oxford research encyclopedia of psychology*. Oxford, UK: Oxford University Press. doi: 10.1093/acrefore/9780190236557.013.174

Wiese-Bjornstal, D. M. (2019a). Psychological predictors and consequences of injuries in sport settings. In M. Anshel (Ed.), *APA handbook of sport and exercise psychology* (Vol. 1, pp. 697–726). Washington, DC: American Psychological Association.

Wiese-Bjornstal, D. M. (2019b). Role of religion and spirituality in sport injury rehabilitation. In B. Hemmings, N. J. Watson, & A. Parker (Eds.), *Sport, psychology and Christianity: Welfare, performance and consultancy* (pp. 54–70). New York: Routledge.

Wiese-Bjornstal, D. M., Smith, A. M., Shaffer, S. M., & Morrey, M. A. (1998). An integrated model of response to sport injury: Psychological and sociological dimensions. *Journal of Applied Sport Psychology*, *10*(1), 46–69. doi: 10.1080/10413209808406377

Williams, J. M., & Andersen, M. B. (1998). Psychosocial antecedents of sport injury: Review and critique of the stress and injury model. *Journal of Applied Sport Psychology*, *10*(1), 5–25. doi: 10.1080/10413209808406375

Index

Page numbers in *italics* mark figures while page numbers in **bold** mark tables.

For Product Safety Concerns and Information please contact our EU
representative GPSR@taylorandfrancis.com
Taylor & Francis Verlag GmbH, Kaufingerstraße 24, 80331 München, Germany

www.ingramcontent.com/pod-product-compliance
Lightning Source LLC
Chambersburg PA
CBHW060240220326
41598CB00027B/3990